Perinatal Nutrition

Optimizing Infant Health and Development

NUTRITION AND DISEASE PREVENTION

1. Genomics and Proteomics in Nutrition, *edited by Carolyn D. Berdanier and Naima Moustaid-Moussa*

2. Perinatal Nutrition: Optimizing Infant Health and Development, *edited by Jatinder Bhatia*

Related Volumes

Introduction to Clinical Nutrition: Second Edition, Revised and Expanded, *by V. Sardesai*

Pediatric Gastroenterology and Nutrition in Clinical Practice, *edited by Carlos Lifschitz*

Nutrients and Cell Signaling, *edited by Janos Zempleni and K. Dakshinamurti*

Mitochondria in Health and Disease, *edited by Carolyn D. Berdanier*

Thiamine, *edited by Frank Jordan and Mulchand Patel*

Phytochemicals in Health and Disease, *edited by Yongping Bao and Roger Fenwick*

Handbook of Obesity: Etiology and Pathophysiology, Second Edition, *edited by George Bray and Claude Bouchard*

Handbook of Obesity: Clinical Applications, Second Edition, *edited by George Bray and Claude Bouchard*

Perinatal Nutrition

Optimizing Infant Health and Development

Edited by

JATINDER BHATIA, M.D.

Vice Chairperson for Clinical Research
Section Chief of Neonatology
and
Professor of Pediatrics and Neonatology
Medical College of Georgia
Augusta, Georgia, U.S.A.

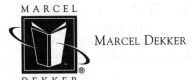

MARCEL DEKKER   NEW YORK

Library of Congress Cataloging-in-Publication Data
A catalog record for this book is available from the Library of Congress.

ISBN: 0-8247-5474-3

This book is printed on acid-free paper.

Headquarters
Marcel Dekker, 270 Madison Avenue, New York, NY 10016, U.S.A.
tel: 212-696-9000; fax: 212-685-4540

Distribution and Customer Service
Marcel Dekker, Cimarron Road, Monticello, New York 12701, U.S.A.
tel: 800-228-1160; fax: 845-796-1772

World Wide Web
http://www.dekker.com

The publisher offers discounts on this book when ordered in bulk quantities. For more information, write to Special Sales/Professional Marketing at the headquarters address above.

Foreword

Our future is determined by our past. This statement truly describes the health of today's adults, for many diseases have their origins during early embryonic, fetal, and perinatal development.

Nutrition is so important to this process that one must look to the nourishment of the very young to see the effects of that nourishment on the development of that individual. Now, more than ever before, we have come to realize that the nutrient intake of the mother profoundly affects her child and that this effect extends even to the period before conception. The periconceptional nutrition effect on pregnancy outcome is shown in the occurrence of spina bifida in infants of mothers whose needs for folacin were not met even before pregnancy commenced. There may be other instances of nutrient effects on fetal development as well, and the reader will find these examples in the text.

Pregnancy places unusual demands on the mother. Endocrine changes affect nutrient need and use for the lactating mother. Likewise, the endocrine system affects the growth of the infant. All of these demands are nutritionally sensitive. If these needs are not met, fetal development will be negatively affected. *Perinatal Nutrition* provides the latest information about the nutrient needs of pregnancy and the early stages of infant growth. It provides the scientific documentation of the role of nutrition in perinatal development. As such, it should be an essential component of every physician's library as well as that of the clinical nutritionist's library. Scientists studying perinatal growth and development will find this book to be a superb summation of the information to date all of the many aspects of pregnancy, lactation, and infant nutrient needs.

Caroly D. Berdanier, Ph.D.
Professor Emerita, Nutrition and Cell Biology
University of Georgia

Preface

Improving the outcome of pregnancy continues to be a global objective among health scientists, and more scientists today recognize that nutrition can prevent certain congenital anomalies. Nutrition also plays an important role in improving survival of low birth weight and extremely premature infants. In addition, proper nutritional care before and after conception can reduce health risks and may improve the outcome of pregnancy. And appropriate nutritional care during the neonatal period and beyond may reduce morbidity and mortality.

Although there are numerous texts and monographs dedicated to nutrition in infancy, a comprehensive treatise on the role of nutrition during the perinatal period, including preconception, is not readily available. This book focuses on the importance of the placenta as an organ in nutrition, aberrations in utero-placental function, the role of macro- and micronutrients in the prevention of congenital anomalies, and the role of nutrition in preventing morbidity in the neonatal period and in infancy.

This book has three main objectives: [1] to examine the mechanisms and actions of nutrients in fetal development and its aberrations; [2] to examine the role of nutrients in the prevention of adverse pregnancy outcome; and [3] to outline current practices in infant nutrition along with evidence that exists for the formulation of these recommendations. This book was written for nutritional scientists and health care professionals who work with the perinatal patient.

The challenge that faces us in future decades is to reduce fetal, neonatal, and infant mortality and morbidity. We will meet this challenge only with better understanding and attention to the whole cycle of reproduction and the critical role nutrition plays in outcomes.

Jatinder Bhatia, M.D.

Contents

Contributors

David H. Adamkin University of Louisville and Kosair Children's Hospital, Louisville, Kentucky, U.S.A.

Suzanne Domel Baxter University of South Carolina, Columbia, South Carolina, U.S.A.

Carol Lynn Berseth Mead Johnson Nutritionals, Evansville, Indiana, U.S.A.

Jatinder Bhatia Medical College of Georgia, Augusta, Georgia, U.S.A.

Jane Blackwell Medical College of Georgia, Augusta, Georgia, U.S.A.

Brian S. Carter Vanderbilt Children's Hospital and Vanderbilt University Medical Center, Nashville, Tennessee, U.S.A.

Laura E. Caulfield The Johns Hopkins University, Baltimore, Maryland, U.S.A.

Lawrence D. Devoe Medical College of Georgia, Augusta, Georgia, U.S.A.

Vadivel Ganapathy Medical College of Georgia, Augusta, Georgia, U.S.A.

William W. Hay, Jr. University of Colorado School of Medicine, Denver, Colorado, U.S.A.

William C. Heird   Baylor College of Medicine, Houston, Texas, U.S.A.

Chandra R. Jones   Medical College of Georgia, Augusta, Georgia, U.S.A.

Steven R. Leuthner   Medical College of Wisconsin, Milwaukee, Wisconsin, U.S.A.

Sharon S. McDonald   Raleigh, North Carolina, U.S.A.

Andrew Muir   Medical College of Georgia, Augusta, Georgia, U.S.A.

Anjali P. Parish   Medical College of Georgia, Augusta, Georgia, U.S.A.

Mary Frances Picciano   National Institutes of Health, Bethesda, Maryland, U.S.A.

Puttur D. Prasad   Medical College of Georgia, Augusta, Georgia, U.S.A.

David K. Rassin   The University of Texas Medical Branch, Galveston, Texas, U.S.A.

Krystal Revai   The University of Texas Medical Branch, Galveston, Texas, U.S.A.

Jin-Xiong She   Medical College of Georgia, Augusta, Georgia, U.S.A.

Jon A. Vanderhoof   University of Nebraska Medical Center, Omaha, Nebraska, U.S.A.

Robert G. Voigt   Mayo Clinic, Rochester, Minnesota, U.S.A.

1

Periconceptional Nutrition and Infant Outcomes

Laura E. Caulfield
The Johns Hopkins University, Baltimore, Maryland, U.S.A.

I. INTRODUCTION

The problems of low birth weight (LBW < 2500 g), intrauterine growth retardation (IUGR) or being small for gestational age (SGA), and preterm delivery (<37 completed weeks' gestation) are well known, and a vast amount of research has been undertaken to understand the etiology of these poor pregnancy outcomes and to identify effective strategies for their prevention. Although much progress has been made in improving the survival of these babies, effective preventive strategies are still lacking. Research suggests that maternal nutritional factors before and during pregnancy affect her risk of poor pregnancy outcomes, from spontaneous abortion, congenital malformations, and birth defects to IUGR and preterm delivery and reduced likelihood of her baby's survival during infancy. Yet there appear to be few examples of effective programs for improving maternal nutrition during pregnancy.

Nutritional recommendations during pregnancy are often predicated upon maternal preconceptional nutritional status; thus, attention to preconceptional risk factors may reduce the burden of "catching up" during pregnancy. However, improving nutritional status before pregnancy is problematic because a large proportion of pregnancies in the United States are not planned, and, even among women planning pregnancy, few seek medical or nutritional advice before attempting pregnancy. Further, most women do not have their first prenatal care visit until well into the first trimester.

1

There is a plethora of books available to the general public detailing nutritional recommendations for optimizing pregnancy outcome that are outside the domain of public health and medical professionals. Therefore, it is helpful to consider what is known about the importance of preconceptional nutritional factors in affecting pregnancy outcomes, with the goal of informing clinicians on the scientific basis for making nutritional recommendations as part of preconceptional care wherever and whenever possible.

II. PERICONCEPTIONAL NUTRITION AND ADVERSE OUTCOMES OF PREGNANCY

In the late 1980s, Kramer (1,2) conducted an exhaustive review of the literature on the etiologies of IUGR and preterm delivery and estimated the fraction of IUGR and preterm delivery attributable to identified risk factors, including maternal malnutrition. The etiologic fraction, or population attributable risk (PAR), is a function of the magnitude of the risk carried by that factor as well as the prevalence of exposure to that risk factor in the population setting. These analyses confirmed that nutritional factors, including low prepregnancy weight or body mass index (BMI = weight in kilograms/height in meters squared) and gestational weight gain were important in the etiology of poor fetal growth and preterm delivery, not only because of the conferred risks for adverse outcomes but also due to the universal nature of the exposure variable.

Not included in that review were several other known nutritional risk factors related to micronutrient malnutrition, either because there was insufficient information available at the time of publication or because the focus of the report was on LBW and preterm delivery and did not include other outcomes, such as birth defects. In 1991, the Institute of Medicine published "Nutrition During Pregnancy" (3), which provides an extensive evaluation of scientific knowledge on maternal nutrition and pregnancy outcomes, as well as several companion documents outlining how to implement recommendations during pregnancy (4,5).

The strongest inference regarding a causal relation between any risk factor and health outcome comes from randomized controlled trials (RCT). The Cochrane Database of Systematic Reviews (CDSR) summarizes results of RCT in order to improve clinical care. In the following sections, evidence is provided regarding the role of maternal preconceptional nutritional factors in influencing pregnancy outcomes. Results from observational studies are considered, and summary evidence from RCT and the CDSR are incorporated where available.

A. Prepregnant Body Mass Index

Nutritional recommendations during pregnancy are in part based on maternal nutritional status prior to pregnancy. The need for increased energy intakes during pregnancy and higher gestational weight gains is inversely related to maternal nutritional status at entry into pregnancy; that is, women with lower BMI need to increase their dietary intake more and have higher weight gain to ensure adequate fetal growth than women entering pregnancy with higher prepregnancy BMI. In 1991, the IOM (3) provided recommended ranges of total gestational weight gain based on maternal BMI: weight gains of 12.5–18 kg for women with BMI $<$ 19.8 kg/m^2 (thin); 11.5–16.0 kg for women with average BMI between 19.8 and 26.0 kg/m^2; 7.0–11.5 kg for women with BMI 26.1–29.0 kg/m^2 (overweight); at least 6.8 kg for women with BMI $>$ 29.0 kg/m^2 (very overweight).

These recommendations provide guidelines for clinicians advising pregnant women on weight gain during pregnancy, but they do not address the unique role of maternal prepregnant nutritional status in influencing risk of adverse outcomes or whether there is evidence of an "optimal" BMI for entering pregnancy. As already stated, there is a large body of evidence from observational studies to suggest that maternal preconceptional body habitus, whether characterized in terms of prepregnancy weight or in terms of BMI, confers unique risk for adverse pregnancy outcomes. Regardless of energy intake during pregnancy or gestational weight gain, women with low prepregnancy BMI are 1.8 times more likely to have a baby with IUGR than women with higher BMI, and their risk of preterm delivery is also elevated (6). It is also true that maternal overweight confers risks for complications of pregnancy (e.g., pre-eclampsia, gestational diabetes, cesarean delivery) as well as infant macrosomia and increased risk of shoulder dystocia (7). Thus, it may seem reasonable to recommend that women gain or lose weight to achieve average BMI prior to pregnancy, but there are no studies to demonstrate the feasibility or effectiveness of such recommendations for improving pregnancy outcomes.

That said, there are potential risks to the pregnancy when it occurs during caloric restriction and weight loss. A poignant example of the influence of periconceptional nutritional status on pregnancy outcomes comes from the pregnancy experiences of women during the Dutch famine of 1944–46, when energy rations were reduced from 1700 kcal/d to 700 kcal/d (Table 1). The effects of acute reductions in energy intake on pregnancy outcomes depended on the timing of the energy restrictions (8). Of interest here are the effects when restrictions occurred periconceptionally and during the first trimester. As shown, energy restriction contributed to reductions in fertility and increased incidences of neural-tube defects when it occurred periconcep-

Table 1 Effects on Pregnancy Outcomes by Time of Severe Energy Restriction: Dutch Famine 1944–46

Periconceptional	First trimester	Third trimester
↓ Fertility	↑ Stillbirths (nearly twofold)	↓ Birth weight
↑ Neural tube defects	↑ Preterm birth	↑ Preterm birth
	↑ Early neonatal mortality (0–7 days)	↑ 0–3 month mortality (threefold)

Note: Energy intakes were reduced from 1700 kcal/d to 700 kcal/d.
Source: Ref. 8.

tionally, and to increased stillbirths, preterm births, and early neonatal mortality when it occurred during the first trimester of pregnancy.

There is ample evidence from RCT to support the relevance of energy intakes during pregnancy for ensuring healthy pregnancy outcomes (9), and there is some evidence to suggest that dietary intakes during pregnancy can be improved through the provision of nutritional advice during prenatal care or as part of broader community-based mass media strategies (see recent reviews, Refs. 10–12). Unfortunately, there is no evidence from RCT to document whether changes in maternal BMI prior to pregnancy would improve pregnancy outcomes ceteris paribus. Thus there is no answer to the question as to whether an optimal range of weight or BMI for entering pregnancy exists.

It should be noted that interventions to change maternal BMI before pregnancy may be impractical in most settings because they require targeting a very large segment of women—women of childbearing age–rather than the *much* smaller percentage of those who actually become pregnant. Worldwide, there are examples of programs targeting newly married women and adolescent girls as a means of improving nutritional status (including BMI) before the first pregnancy, but the impact of such programs on birth outcomes has not been evaluated. Further, although it is clear that reductions in adverse pregnancy outcomes are likely with increases in BMI among thin women (BMI < 19.8 kg/m^2), it is not clear whether an optimal BMI can be defined. It may be more practical for focus on interconceptional care, and analyses of data from a nutritional supplementation trial in Guatemala suggests that when nutritional supplementation of undernourished women continues through one pregnancy and the subsequent interbirth interval, greater gains in birth weight are seen with the second pregnancy (13). Presumably, this is in part due to improvements in maternal BMI prior to the subsequent pregnancy. More work is needed in this area to (1) establish a causal relation between prepregnancy BMI and adverse pregnancy outcomes, (2) establish whether an "optimal" range of BMI for entering pregnancy exists, (3) identify and evaluate strategies to optimize maternal BMI before pregnancy as a means of improving birth outcomes.

B. Maternal Stature

Short maternal stature, reflecting genetic contributions as well as nutritional stunting in early childhood, also contributes significantly to small size at birth, particularly in developing countries (1,2,6). Preventing adverse pregnancy outcomes due to short maternal stature (if the relation is causal) cannot be addressed without sustained nutritional and health interventions during pregnancy and early childhood that would allow the next generation of women to be taller as adults.

C. Iron-Deficiency Anemia

After considering maternal BMI and gestational weight gain, concerns regarding maternal iron status and anemia are of primary concern because of the pervasive nature of iron deficiency and anemia as public health problems. Recommendations for iron supplements during pregnancy are also based on whether women are anemic or not at entry into prenatal care (14), and international guidelines for prenatal iron supplementation differ depending on the prevalence of iron-deficiency anemia in the population (15). Thus, as with gestational weight gain recommendations, care with respect to anemia status prior to pregnancy reduces the need for heightened care during pregnancy. This is important in populations where severe anemia (hemoglobin < 90 g/L) is a concern. Iron supplements during pregnancy are known to be efficacious for preventing low hemoglobin at delivery (16), but clearly the preventive ability of iron supplements is dependent on maternal periconceptional anemia status.

Our concern here is whether maternal iron-deficiency anemia during the periconceptional period also adversely affects pregnancy outcomes. Many observational studies report associations between maternal iron-deficiency anemia during pregnancy and increased risk of LBW and preterm delivery; in some of those studies, a unique role of first trimester anemia has been identified (17). For example, Scanlon et al. (18), in a study of about 170,000 low-income U.S. women, found that women with very low hemoglobin concentrations in the first trimester were 1.68 times more likely, and those with first-trimester hemoglobin concentrations in the low-to-low-normal range were 1.29 times more likely, to deliver preterm. Interestingly, those with high and very high hemoglobin concentrations in the first trimester were at increased risk of delivery an SGA baby. Because this association persisted throughout pregnancy, the finding may reflect an association between high hemoglobin concentrations and reduced plasma volume expansion, and there is some indication of a negative association between maternal hemoglobin concentration in the first trimester and human chorionic gonadotropin concentrations and placental size (19,20). Allen (20) describes other potential mechanisms for the relation between iron status and anemia and pregnancy outcomes, including hypoxia, stress responses, and maternal infection, but more work in this area is needed to delineate the biological mechanism involved. Further, data from RCT to establish whether iron-deficiency anemia causes LBW or preterm delivery (17) are lacking, regardless of when during pregnancy the anemia occurs.

D. Folic Acid

Periconceptional folate status affects risk of neural-tube defects (NTD), such as spina bifida, encephalocele, and anencephaly, which result in severe motor disability and in intellectual impairment among surviving infants (21). This association is due, at least in part, to a gene–environment interaction; mutations of the methylene tetrahydrofolate reductase gene in the absence of a folate-rich diet are associated with elevated maternal plasma homocysteine and the occurrence of neural-tube defects in offspring (22,23). Supplementation of 400 µg/d of synthetic folic acid increases the activity of the variant methylene tetrahydrofolate reductase, corrects maternal hyperhomocysteinemia, and, when initiated prior to conception or very early in pregnancy, prevents the occurrence of a substantial portion of neural-tube defects (24,25).

It has been estimated that 70% of neural-tube defects can be prevented in the United States by ensuring a periconceptional intake of 0.4 mg/d of synthetic folic acid (24,26). Public health efforts have translated this scientific knowledge into public policy, principally the fortification of the U.S. food supply with synthetic folic acid (27). This is logical because, in general, women do not know whether they are at risk for having NTD-affected pregnancy, and attention to folate status after recognition of pregnancy is too late. Women who are at higher risk include those: (1) with an NTD themselves, (2) with a previously affected pregnancy, (3) with a family history of NTD, (4) with a family history of hyperhomocysteinemia. Women with NTD or a history of NTD pregnancies are recommended to receive 4 mg/d folic acid prior to pregnancy and continuing throughout the first trimester (28).

E. Iodine Deficiency

Maternal iodine deficiency during pregnancy is associated with a range of birth defects (29). Severe maternal iodine deficiency can result in cretinism, a severe congenital disability involving cognitive and motor deficits, and often hearing loss and speech impairment; milder forms of maternal iodine deficiency result in a range of intellectual, motor, and hearing deficits (30). The principal means to prevent iodine deficiency is through iodation of salt in the United States and elsewhere, although in some regions iodation of water in has been implemented. Such efforts are known to have reduced the incidence of cretinism. More recently, the results of an iodated water project in an area of China with severe iodine deficiency found approximately 50% reductions in infant and neonatal mortality rates in treated areas (31). Although not known, the authors speculate that the prevention of neonatal hypothyroidism due to iodine deficiency resulted in the observed reductions in mortality.

F. Zinc

Severe maternal zinc deficiency is associated with infertility, spontaneous abortion, and congenital malformations, including neural-tube defects (32). A high incidence of birth defects, including nervous system malformations, has been observed in the fetuses of women suffering from *acrodermatitis enteropathica*, an inborn error of zinc absorption (33); treatment with zinc can lead to normal pregnancy outcomes. Recently, a study among women with marginal zinc intakes indicated that maternal zinc status may affect neuro-behavioral development, as measured by indices of fetal heart rate variability and motor activity, although additional research is needed to replicate the findings (34).

It is important to note that zinc deficiency can be secondary to maternal morbidity, because plasma zinc concentrations are lowered as zinc is seques-tered in the liver as part of the acute-phase response of the body's immune system to disease, injury, or stress (35). Thus, maternal morbidity or maternal stress may increase the risk of poor neurological development in the fetus by making less zinc available for uptake by the fetus. Studies in animal models support the hypothesis, but its relevance for human pregnancy has not been evaluated.

G. Vitamin A

The role of vitamin A in the occurrence of birth defects is well established. Severe maternal vitamin A deficiency is associated across species with a variety of defects, including ocular, cardiac, genitourinary, and skeletal defects, hydrocephaly, and increased risk of mortality (36–40). High maternal vitamin A intakes (leading to the formation of retinoic acid and retinyl esters) are associated with defects in many of these same organ systems, as well as craniofacial defects, such as cleft palate (41,42), suggesting that periconceptional intakes of vitamin A in women should be evaluated. The clinical or public health importance of either hypovitaminosis A or hypervitaminosis A to adverse pregnancy outcomes in the United States is not known, but it is likely that hypervitaminosis A may be the greater concern, particularly among women who consume liver on a regular basis. Women who regularly consume diets containing vitamin A–containing fruits and vegetables should have adequate vitamin A status for entering pregnancy; for those women requiring supplements, it is recommended that total daily intake not exceed 10,000 IU of vitamin A (43).

H. Multiple Micronutrients

Recently, a number of studies have reported reductions in the frequency of congenital heart defects in the offspring of women taking multivitamin supplements periconceptionally (44–47). Interestingly, Botto et al. (47) found that the increased risk of congenital heart defects associated with febrile illness was diminished for the offspring of women taking supplements. The micronutrient(s) responsible for these effects are not identified, but the body of the research to date suggests that—barring constraints—a recommendation to women planning a pregnancy to regularly consume an over-the-counter (OTC) multivitamin/mineral supplement would be prudent. Botto et al. (46) estimate that if their results are causal, then one-fourth of major cardiac defects could be prevented by regular consumption of multivitamin supplements during the periconceptional period.

III. HIGH-RISK NUTRITIONAL CONDITIONS

A. Diabetes

Women with pre-existing diabetes are at risk for having a variety of adverse outcomes of pregnancy. Evidence suggests that the direct cause of these problems is poor glycemic control resulting in intermittent hypo- and hyperglycemic states, but impaired magnesium status secondary to poor control has also been proposed (48,49). Poor glycemic control at the time of conception can increase the likelihood of spontaneous abortion as well as malformations (heart, neural-tube, and limb defects) and decreased bone mineral content in the infant at birth (48,50). Recently, a program of focused periconceptional care for women with type 1 diabetes, emphasizing strict glucose control and fetal surveillance, demonstrated a reduction in malformations and perinatal mortality rates (51).

Because glycemic states are defined based on cut points of a continuous distribution of glucose concentration, it has been suggested that poorer glycemic control (particularly hyperglycemia) among nondiabetic women may also result in adverse outcomes of pregnancy, particularly malformations in the offspring. To our knowledge this has not been specifically tested and warrants further research.

B. Phenylketonuria

Phenylketonuria (PKU) represents another high-risk condition that should be identified and managed perinconceptionally. PKU is an inherited metabolic disorder in which the individual is unable to metabolize phenylalanine. The condition leads to abnormal brain development unless a low-phenylalanine diet is maintained from birth through childhood. Adults with PKU are not generally maintained on special diets and, thus, are likely to have elevated serum phenylalanine concentrations. This is of concern if pregnancy occurs for two reasons: (1) the fetus may have PKU; (2) studies report a high incidence of mental retardation, microcephaly, LBW, and congenital heart defects in such pregnancies, even when the fetus does not have PKU (52–54). It is recommended that women with PKU modify their dietary intakes well in advance of pregnancy in order to reduce these risks (55,56).

C. Eating Disorders

Women with eating disorders such as anorexia nervosa, bulimia, and bulimia nervosa are likely to have poor nutritional status entering pregnancy. Without proper management, they are likely to be at high risk for nutritional deficiencies and poor weight gain. Because they require long-term therapy, they should be identified and referred for care preconceptionally.

IV. NUTRITIONAL EVALUATIONS IN PRECONCEPTIONAL CARE

As described earlier, there are ample reasons to incorporate nutritional evaluation and intervention as part of preconceptional care, and there are demonstrable examples of effective preconceptional interventions to prevent adverse outcomes of pregnancy (57). In recent years, several reports have provided recommendations for nutrition services as part of preconceptional or interconceptional care (5,58–60). Provided in Table 2 is a framework for nutrition assessment and guidance as part of such care services based on the 1992 IOM report (5).

Few health care professionals actively provide preconceptional or interconceptional nutritional advice to women, and thus training in the implementation of such services is needed. It may be most effective to form

Table 2 Nutritional Evaluation in Preconceptional and Interconceptional Care Adapted from Ref. 5

Assessment	Components	Guidance
Health history and lifestyle factors	Plan for pregnancy Prior pregnancy outcomes Prior anemia Chronic or other health conditions Alcohol use Tobacco use Use of other harmful substances Use of nutritional supplements or dietary supplements Eating disorders Physical activity level or exercise	Discourage use of harmful substances, including alcohol Recommend regular consumption of multivitamin/mineral supplement, with folic acid Refer for appropriate care of eating disorder or other health conditions requiring nutritional management
Physical exam	General physical exam Measurement of height and weight and determination of BMI	Consider plans for gaining or losing weight prior to pregnancy, including benefits and potential risks
Dietary practices	Dietary pattern Consumption of organ meats Special diets (vegetarianism, lactose intolerance, others)	Provide dietary guidance following the Dietary Guidelines for Americans, and the Food Guide Pyramid Limit consumption of vitamin A–containing organ meats Refer to nutrition professional regarding special dietary concerns
Laboratory evaluation	Hemoglobin or hematocrit assessment Other tests (glucose, lipids screen, urinalysis) as appropriate	Provision of specialized iron supplements to treat anemia Manage as indicated

interdisciplinary health care teams, including nutritionists for the provision of timely nutritional assessment of the preconceptional women, general nutritional guidance during this important period, as well as the appropriate management of nutrition concerns and high-risk conditions.

REFERENCES

1. Kramer MS. Determinants of low birth weight: methodological assessment and meta-analysis. Bull WHO 1987; 65(5):663–737
2. Kramer MS. Intrauterine growth retardation and gestational duration determinants. Pediatrics 1987; 80(4):502–511.
3. Institute of Medicine (IOM). Subcommittee on nutritional status and weight gain during pregnancy. Nutrition During Pregnancy. Washington, DC: National Academy Press, 1991.
4. Institute of Medicine (IOM). Committee on nutritional status during pregnancy and lactation. Nutrition Services in Perinatal Care. 2nd ed. Washington, DC: National Academy Press, 1992.
5. Institute of Medicine (IOM). Subcommittee for a clinical application guide, Committee on nutritional status during pregnancy and lactation. Nutrition During Pregnancy and Lactation: An Implementation Guide. Washington, DC: National Academy Press, 1992.
6. Kramer M, Victora C. Low birth weight and perinatal mortality. In: Semba RD, Bloem MW, eds. Nutrition and Health in Developing Countries. Totowa, New Jersey: Humana Press, 2001. Chap 3.
7. Abrams B, Parker J. Overweight and pregnancy complications. Int J Obes 1988; 12:293–303.
8. Susser M, Stein Z. Timing in prenatal nutrition: a reprise of the Dutch Famine Study. Nutr Rev 1994; 52:84–94.
9. Kramer MS. Balanced protein/energy supplementation in pregnancy. Cochrane Database Syst Rev 2000; (2):CD000032.
10. Boyd NR Jr, Windsor RA. A meta-evaluation of nutrition education intervention research among pregnant women. Health Education Q 1993; 20:327–345.
11. Rush D. Maternal nutrition and perinatal survival. J Health Pop Nutr Sep 2001; 19(3):S217–S264.
12. Kramer MS. Nutritional advice in pregnancy. Cochrane Database Syst Rev 2000, (2):CD000149.
13. Villar J, Rivera J. Nutritional supplementation during two consecutive pregnancies and the interim lactation period: effect on birth weight. Pediatries 1988; 81:51–57.
14. Centers for Disease Control and Prevention (CDC). Recommendations to prevent and control iron deficiency in the United States. MMWR 1998; 47(No. RR-3):1–29.

15. Stoltzfus RJ, Dreyfuss ML. Guidelines for the Use of Irons Supplements to Prevent and Treat Iron Deficiency Anemia. Washington, DC: International Life Sciences Institute (ILSI) Press, 1998.

16. Kulier R, de Onis M, Gulmezoglu AM, Villar J. Nutritional interventions to reduce maternal morbidity. Int J Gynaecol Obstet 1998; 63:231–246.

17. Rasmussen KM. Is there a causal relationship between iron deficiency or iron-deficiency anemia and weight at birth, length of gestation and perinatal morality? J Nutr 2001; 131:590S–603S.

18. Scanlon KS, Yip R, Schieve LA, Cogswell ME. High and low hemoglobin levels during pregnancy: differential risks for preterm birth and small for gestational age. Obstet Gynecol 2000; 96:741–748.

19. Godfrey Km, Redman EW, Barker DJ, Osmond C. The effect of maternal anaemia and iron deficiency on the ratio or fetal weight to placental weight. Br J Obstet Gynaecol 1991; 98:886–891.

20. Allen LH. Biological mechanisms that might underlie iron's effects on fetal growth and preterm birth. J Nutr 2001; 131:581S–589S.

21. Locksmith GJ, Duff P. Preventing neural tube defects: the importance of peri-conceptional folic acid supplements. Obstet Gynecol 1998; 91:1027–1034.

22. van der Put NM, Gabreels F, Stevens EM, Smeitink JA, Trijbels FJ, Eskes TK, van den Heuvel LP, Blom HJ. A second common mutation in the methylene-tetrahydrofolate reductase gene: an additional risk factor for neural-tube defects? Am J Hum Genet 1998; 62(5):1044–1051.

23. Wilcken DE. MTHFR 677C– – > T mutation, folate intake, neural-tube defect, and risk of cardiovascular disease. Lancet 1997; 350(9078):603–604.

24. MRC Vitamin Study Research Group. Prevention of neural-tube defects: results of the Medical Research Council Vitamin Study. Lancet 1991; 338(8760):131–137.

25. Czeizel AE, Dudas I. Prevention of the first occurrence of neural-tube defects by periconceptional vitamin supplementation. N Engl J Med 1992; 327:1832–1835.

26. Centers for Disease Control and Prevention (CDC). Recommendations for the use of folic acid to reduce the number of cases of spina bifida and other neural-tube defects. MMWR Morb Mortal Wkly Rep 1992; 41(Rr–14):1–7.

27. US Department of Health and Human Services, Food and Drug Administration. Food standards: amendment of the standards of identity for enriched grain products to require addition of folic acid. Federal Register 1993; 58:53306–53312.

28. American College of Obstetricians and Gynecologists. Folic acid for the prevention of neural-tube defects. ACOG committee opinion no. 120. Washington, DC: American College of Obstetricians and Gynecologists, 1993.

29. Hetzel BS. Iodine deficiency disorders (IDD) and their eradication. Lancet 1983; 2(8359):1126–1129.

30. Stanbury JB, ed. The Damaged Brain of Iodine Deficiency: Cognitive, Behavioral, Neuromotor, Educative Aspects. New York: Cognizant Communication Corporation, 1994.

31. DeLong GR, Leslie PW, Wang SH, Jiang Xm, Zhang ML, Rakeman M, Jiang JY, Ma T, Cao XY. Effect on infant mortality of iodination of irrigation water in a severely iodine-deficient area of China. Lancet 1997; 350:771–773.

32. Caulfield LE, Zavaleta N, Shankar A, Merialdi M. Potential contribution of maternal zinc supplementation during pregnancy for maternal and child survival. Am J Clin Nutr 1998; 68(suppl):499S–508S.

33. Hambidge KM, Nelder KH, Walravens PA. Zinc acrodermatitis enteropathica, and congenital malformations. Lancet 1975; 1(7906):577–578.

34. Merialdi M, Caulfield LE, Zavaleta N, Figueroa A, DiPietro J. Adding zinc to prenatal iron and folate supplements improves fetal neurobehavioral development. Am J Obstet Gynecol 1999; 180:483–490.

35. Keen CL, Taubeneck MW, Daston GP, Rogers JM, Gershwin ME. Primary and secondary zinc deficiency as factors underlying abnormal CNS development. Ann NY Acad Sci 1993; 678:37–47.

36. Millen JW, Woollam DHM, Lamming GE. Hydrocephalus in young rabbits associated with maternal vitamin A deficiency. Br J Nutr 1953; 8:363.

37. Warkany J, Nelson RC. Appearance of skeletal abnormalities in offspring of rats reared on deficient diet. Science 1940; 92:383.

38. Warkany J, Schaaffenberger E. Congenital malformations induced by rats by maternal vitamin A deficiency. I. Defects of the eye. Arch Ophthalmol 1946; 35:150.

39. Wilson JG, Warkany J. Malformations of the genito-urinary tract induced by maternal vitamin A deficiency in the rat. Am J Anat 1948; 83:357.

40. Wilson JG, Warkany J. Aortic arch and cardiac anomalies in offspring of vitamin A–deficient rats. Am J Anat 1949; 83:113.

41. Rosa FW. Retinoid embryopathy in humans. In: Koren G, ed. Retinoids in Clinical Practice. New York: Marcel Dekker, 1993:77–109.

42. Olson JA. Biochemistry of vitamin A and carotenoids. In: Sommer A, West KP Jr, eds. Vitamin A Deficiency: Health, Survival and Vision. New York: Oxford University Press, 1996. Chap 6.

43. Underwood BA. The Safe Use of Vitamin A by Women During the Reproductive Years. Washington, DC: International Vitamin A Consultative Group (IVACG), International Life Sciences Institute (ILSI) Foundation, 1986.

44. Czeitzel AE. Periconceptional folic acid–containing multivitamin supplementation. Eur J Obstet Gynecol Reprod Biol 1998; 78:151–161.

45. Shaw GM, O'Malley CD, Wasserman CR, Tolarova MM, Lammer EJ. Maternal periconceptional use of multivitamins and reduced risk for conotruncal heart defects and limb deficiencies among offspring. Am J Med Genet 1995; 59:536–545.

46. Botto LD, Mulinare J, Erickson JD. Occurrence of congenital heart defects in relation to maternal multivitamin use. Am J Epidemiol 2000; 151:878–884.

47. Botto LD, Lynberg MC, Erickson JD. Congenital heart defects, maternal febrile illness, and multivitamin use: a population-based study. Epidemiol 2001; 12:485–490.

48. Mimouni F, Tsang RC. Pregnancy outcome in insulin-dependent diabetes:

temporal relationships with metabolic control during specific pregnancy periods. Am J Perinatol 1988; 5:334–338.

49. Miodovnik M, Mimouni F, Siddiqi TA, Tsang RC. Periconceptional metabolic status and risk of spontaneous abortion in insulin-dependent diabetic pregnancies. Am J Perinatol 1988; 5:368–373.
50. American Diabetes Association. Preconception care of women with diabetes. Diabetes Care 2000; 23(suppl 1).
51. McElvy SS, Miodovnik M, Rosenn B, Khoury JC, Siddiqi T, Dignan PS, Tsang RC. A focused preconceptional and early pregnancy program in women with type 1 diabetes reduces perinatal mortality and malformation rates to general population levels. J Matern Fetal Med 2000; 9:14–20.
52. Dimperio D. Preconceptional nutrition. J Pediatr Perinatal Nutr 1990; 2:65–78.
53. Drogari E, Smith I, Beasley M, Lloyd JK. Timing of strict diet in relation to fetal damage in maternal phenylketonuria. Lancet 1987; 2:927–930.
54. Trahms CM. Maternal hyperphenylalanimemia. In: Worthington-Roberts BS, Williams SR, eds. Nutrition in Pregnancy and Lactation. 4th ed. St. Louis, MO: Times Mirror/Mosby, 1989:193–199.
55. Lenke RR, Levy HL. Maternal phenylketonuria and hyperphenylalaninemia. An international survey of the outcome of untreated and treated pregnancies. N Engl J Med 1980; 303:1202–1208.
56. Lynch BC, Pitt DB, Maddison TG, Wraith JE, Danks DM. Maternal phenyl-ketonuria: successful outcome in four pregnancies treated prior to conception. Eur J Pediatr 1988; 148:72–75.
57. Korenbrot CC, Steinberg A, Bender C, Newberry S. Preconception care: a systematic review. Matern Child Health J 2002; 6:75–88.
58. Brundage SC. Preconception health care. Am Fam Physician 2002; 65:2507–2514.
59. Bendich A. Micronutrients in women's health and immune function. Nutrition 2001; 17:858–867.
60. Czeizel AE. Ten years of experience in periconceptional care. Eur J Obstet Gynecol 1999; 84:43–49.

2

Nutritional Requirements During Pregnancy and Lactation

Mary Frances Picciano
National Institutes of Health, Bethesda, Maryland, U.S.A.

Sharon S. McDonald
Raleigh, North Carolina, U.S.A.

I. INTRODUCTION

The success of a pregnancy may be measured by the degree of maternal health and well-being during and after pregnancy, the delivery of a healthy newborn, and the ability of the lactating mother to provide for her newborn's nutritional needs (1). Improving maternal and infant health is both a national priority in the United States and an international priority throughout the world. In the United States, measurable health promotion and disease prevention objectives for the year 2010 are aimed at enhancing reproductive outcome. Certain of these objectives, such as appropriate weight gain during pregnancy and achievement of optimum prepregnancy folic acid levels, are based on cumulative evidence from public health programs and intervention trials that support the health benefits of maternal nutritional modifications (2). Globally, achieving adequate nutrition of women before and during pregnancy and lactation is a vitally important goal, particularly in developing countries, where average estimated maternal mortality rates are 50 times greater, and for some regions of Africa 100 times greater, than in developed countries (3). Anemia, vitamin A deficiency, iodine deficiency, and protein-energy malnutrition (PEM) are prevalent in female children and adults in developing countries, with consequences for both maternal and infant health (3,4). For example, malnourished women have a higher probability of delivering babies with intrauterine growth retardation (IUGR) or low birth weight (LBW), which increases risk of infant morbidity and mortality as well as adverse effects on long-term physical growth and cognitive development (3). In addition, the "fetal origins" hypothesis of Barker and colleagues, based primarily on epidemiologic data, proposes that impaired fetal growth and development resulting from alterations in fetal nutrition and endocrine status may predispose individuals to certain diseases in adulthood, including coronary heart disease (CHD), hypertension, and type 2 diabetes (5). Evidence supporting this hypothesis, however, is equivocal, with unreported gestational age being a major confounding factor (6,7).

Determining the total nutrient intake required to achieve optimal maternal nutritional status for fetal and infant growth as well as associated changes in maternal structure and metabolism is not as simple as adding the amounts needed for maintainance of nonreproducing women to the amounts accumulated in the products of pregnancy and lactation and in maternal tissues. During pregnancy and lactation, hormones act as mediators to adjust maternal metabolism, redirecting nutrients to the placenta and mammary gland, highly specialized maternal tissues specific to reproduction, and transferring nutrients to the developing fetus or infant. Also, increased nutrient requirements may vary among individuals, depending on maternal prepregnancy nutrition status and genetic individuality. This chapter summarizes current knowledge on the physiological adjustments and nutritional requirements of pregnant and lactating women.

II. PHYSIOLOGICAL AND METABOLIC ADJUSTMENTS OF HUMAN PREGNANCY

During pregnancy, changes in the physiology and anatomy of the mother, as well as complex adjustments in nutrient metabolism brought about by hormones secreted by the placenta, support fetal growth and development while maintaining maternal homeostasis and preparing for lactation (8). Physiological adjustments of pregnancy include significant changes in the maternal hormonal profile, blood volume and composition, renal function, and body weight. Adjustments in nutrient metabolism evolve throughout pregnancy and, depending on the nutrient, include incorporation into new tissue or deposition in maternal stores, redistribution among tissues, and/or increased turnover rate or rate of metabolism (8).

A. Hormonal Profile of Pregnancy

Changes in levels of certain key reproductive hormones in maternal plasma occur throughout pregnancy. Human chorionic gonadotropin (hCG) begins to increase as soon as implantation occurs, and it can be detected in urine and plasma within days. The serum level of hCG peaks at about 8 weeks after conception and then declines to a stable level that is maintained until birth. hCG maintains the corpeus luteum function in early pregnancy (8–10 wk). Secretion of human placental lactogen (also called human chorionic soma-tomammotropin [hCS]), which is structurally similar to growth hormone, parallels placental growth and can be used as a measure of placental function. This hormone affects carbohydrate and lipid metabolism and may be important in maintaining a flow of substrates to the fetus. Cortisol, a maternally derived hormone, is antagonistic to insulin and stimulates glucose synthesis from amino acids. Plasma levels of cortisol increase during preg-nancy because of increased production of free hormone as well as an estrogen-stimulated increase in levels of cortisol-binding protein.

During early pregnancy, progesterone and estrogens are synthesized in the maternal corpeus luteum; these steroid hormones are essential for maintaining the early uterine environment and development of the placenta. At 8–10 weeks' gestation, however, the placenta becomes the main source of progesterone and estrogens, and production increases throughout pregnancy. Progesterone, often called the hormone of pregnancy, stimulates maternal respiration; relaxes smooth muscle, particularly in the uterus and gastroin-testinal tract; is responsible for the inhibition of milk secretion during pregnancy; may promote lobular development in the breast; and may act as an immunosuppressant in the placenta. The high estrogen levels in pregnancy stimulate uterine growth and enhance uterine blood flow. In addition, they stimulate somatotrophs (a population of cells) in the maternal pituitary to become mammotrophs, that is, prolactin-secreting cells; the increased pro-lactin secretion probably helps promote mammary development and also is necessary at the end of pregnancy to initiate and maintain lactation. Secretion of estrogens from the placenta is complex. Estrone (E_1) and estradiol (E_2) are synthesized from dehydroepiandrosterone sulfate (DHEA-S), a precursor derived from both fetal and maternal blood, whereas estriol (E_3) is synthe-sized from fetal 16-α-hydroxy-dehydroepiandrosterone sulfate (16-OH-DHEA-S). The fetus must obtain pregnenolone, required for synthesis of both DHEA-S and 16-OH-DHEA-S, from the placenta.

B. Blood Volume and Composition

Blood volume, plasma volume, and red cell mass increase and hematocrit decreases in pregnant women. The increase in blood volume, 35–40% of the nonpregnant volume, results primarily from expansion of plasma volume by 45–50% and of red cell mass by 15–20%, as measured in the third trimester. Because red cell mass expands less than plasma, the hemoglobin and hematocrit concentrations decrease through the first and second trimesters and then gradually rise in the third trimester (9). For hemoglobin, the mean level of 135 g/L for nonpregnant women decreases to 116 g/L in the second trimester and gradually rises to 125 g/L at 36 weeks of gestation (10). Plasma levels of total lipids and of most lipid fractions, including triacylglycerol, cholesterol, fatty acids, phospholipids, and lipoproteins, increase during pregnancy, possibly a result of hormonal changes. The plasma level of total proteins decreases near the end of pregnancy, primarily because of a drop in albumin. In addition, levels of α-globulins and β-globulins increase and the level of γ-globulin decreases, changes likely mediated by estrogens.

C. Renal Function

Renal function is altered dramatically during pregnancy, likely to help clear nitrogenous and other waste products of maternal and fetal metabolism. In fact, one of the earliest adjustments in pregnancy is an increase (~75%) in effective renal plasma flow (ERPF). Because the glomerular filtration rate (GFR) also increases in early pregnancy, but less substantially (~50%), the filtration fraction (GFR/ERPF) decreases in early pregnancy; it returns to nonpregnant values in the third trimester, however. Changes in renal function are associated with increased urinary excretion of glucose, amino acids, and water-soluble vitamins (10).

D. Weight Gain and Its Components

Weight gain during pregnancy comprises the products of conception—fetus, amniotic fluid, and placenta; and the maternal accretion of tissues—expansion of blood and extracellular fluid, enlargement of uterus and mammary glands, and an increase in stores of adipose tissue. More than 30 years ago, Hytten and Leitch (11) reported that the average weight gain during pregnancy for healthy primigravadas who ate without restriction was 12.5 kg, a value still accepted as the norm. They estimated that the 12.5-kg weight gain included: fetus (3400 g); amniotic fluid (800 g); placenta (650 g); expansion of blood volume (1450 g); increased extracellular and extravascular water (1480 g); uterus (970 g); mammary tissue (405 g); and maternal fat (3345 g) (11,12).

Low gestational weight gain is associated with increased risk of IUGR, LBW, and perinatal mortality. High gestational weight gain is associated with high birth weight, but also with increased risk of complications during labor related to fetopelvic disproportion. Although such complications pose minimal risks in developed countries, where surgical delivery is an option, obstructed labor is still a source of considerable risk in developing countries, particularly in very short women (4). The current Institute of Medicine (IOM) recommendations for weight gain during pregnancy (Table 1) were formulated after a review of available evidence and consider the need to balance the benefits of fetal growth against the risks of labor and delivery complications and of postpartum maternal weight retention (10). The desirable weight gain in each prepregnancy weight-for-height category is that associated with delivery of a full-term infant weighing 3–4 kg. Higher weight gains are recommended for thin women because, at the same gestational weight gain, thin women give birth to infants smaller than those born to heavier women. Also, higher weight gain will help to build maternal fat stores in thin women prior to lactation. Lower weight gains are recommended for overweight and obese women to help minimize maternal fat gain. A cohort study that determined fat deposition in pregnant women who gained weight according to the IOM recommendations reported that women who were underweight, normal weight, or overweight before pregnancy showed mean fat gains of 6.0 kg, 3.8 kg, and 3.5 kg, respectively, whereas obese women had a mean fat loss of 0.6 kg (13). Interestingly, only 35% of women in this study gained weight according to the IOM recommendations; 39% gained more than recommended and 26% gained less. In adolescent pregnancies in which the mother herself is still growing, gestational weight gain and fat stores are greater but birthweights of infants are less than in nongrowing pregnant adolescents and mature women (14). Data suggest that, in the latter part of pregnancy in growing pregnant adolescents, some of the maternal fat stores are reserved for continued maternal growth, resulting in greater glucose use by the mother and, consequently, less glucose availability—and diminished growth—for the fetus (14).

Table 1 Recommended Total Weight Gain Ranges for Pregnant Women, by Prepregnancy Body Mass Index (BMI)

Weight-for-height category	Recommended total weight gain, kg (lb)
Low (BMI < 19.8)	12.5–18 (28–40)
Normal (BMI 19.8–26.0)	11.5–16 (25–35)
High (BMI > 26.0–29.0)	7–11.5 (15–25)
Obese (BMI > 29.0)	≥6 (15)

Young adolescent and African American women should strive for gains at the upper end of the range. Short women (<157 cm, or 62 in.) should strive for gains at the lower end of the range. BMI is defined as (weight in kilograms)/(height in meters)^2.
Source: Ref. 10.

E. Adjustments in Nutrient Metabolism

Hormonal changes, fetal demands, and maternal nutrient supply drive the adjustments in nutrient metabolism that take place during pregnancy (8). Because the nutritional status of women varies at the time of conception, the metabolic adjustments required throughout individual pregnancies also will vary. However, certain generalizations can be made with regard to the pregnancy-related adjustments of carbohydrate, lipid, and protein as well as some micronutrients (e.g., calcium). Data indicate that, as pregnancy progresses in normal women, insulin secretion increases to counteract a progressive decrease in insulin sensitivity, basal endogenous hepatic glucose production increases to meet the needs of the fetus and the placenta, and the contribution of carbohydrate to oxidative metabolism increases (15,16). As noted earlier, changes in lipid metabolism result in increasing plasma levels of most lipid fractions. In addition, in early pregnancy increased levels of estrogen, progesterone, and insulin inhibit lipolysis and favor lipid deposition, whereas in late pregnancy human placental lactogen promotes lipolysis and fat mobilization; this metabolic shift results in the use of lipids as a maternal energy source and helps to preserve maternal glucose and amino acids for the fetus (16). Regulation of protein and nitrogen metabolism evolves gradually during pregnancy and is aimed at conservation of nitrogen and increased protein synthesis by the mother early in pregnancy and by both mother and fetus later in pregnancy (8,17). Metabolic adjustments in the regulatory process include a decrease in urea production; a decrease in plasma α-amino nitrogen; a decreased rate of branched-chain amino acid transamination; and an unchanged rate of weight-specific protein turnover per kilogram of body weight (17). In a recent study that imposed a constant dietary intake of nitrogen, urinary nitrogen excretion decreased toward the end of pregnancy and thus nitrogen balance improved, suggesting that dietary protein is used more efficiently in late pregnancy (18). Calcium metabolism also undergoes changes during pregnancy. Evidence indicates that the fetal calcium demand (25–30 g during pregnancy) is met primarily by high intestinal calcium absorption, which increases approximately twofold in pregnant women by early to mid-pregnancy and may be mediated in part by the increased serum levels of 1,25-dihydroxyvitamin D (1,25-D) found in pregnancy (19,20).

III. NUTRITIONAL NEEDS DURING PREGNANCY

Assessment of a woman's nutritional status during pregnancy is more complicated than assessment for a nonpregnant woman. The physiological changes of pregnancy, including hormone-induced changes in metabolism, shifts in plasma volume, and modifications in renal function and patterns of urinary excretion result in alterations of nutrient levels in the tissues and fluids available for evaluation and interpretation (10). Plasma concentrations of some nutrients show a steady decrease as pregnancy progresses, possibly a result of hemodilution. Concentrations of other nutrients, however, may be either unaffected or increased because of pregnancy-induced changes in the availability of carrier molecules. And relative nutrient concentrations may vary over the course of pregnancy, with different patterns for various nutrient (10). Simply stated, our understanding of the biochemical changes associated with maternal nutrient metabolism and requirements during human pregnancy is far from complete. Consequently, a general lack of pregnancy-specific laboratory indices of nutritional evaluation exists. Thus, when increased maternal intake of a nutrient results in altered nutrient concentration patterns, interpretation may be difficult, unless the change can be related to a functional consequence. Much of the existing knowledge related to associations between either low or high maternal intakes and adverse or favorable pregnancy outcomes is based on observational studies and intervention trials. The current recommended dietary reference intakes (DRIs) for pregnant, lactating, and nonpregnant adult women (ages 19–50 years) are presented in Table 2 (21–25). The DRIs listed are either the adequate intake (AI), which refers to the recommended daily average intake level, assumed to be adequate, that is based on either observed or experimentally determined estimates of nutrient intake by apparently healthy individuals; or the recommended dietary allowance (RDA), which refers to the average daily dietary nutrient intake level sufficient to meet the nutrient requirement of nearly all (97–98%) healthy individuals. The RDA is calculated from the estimated average requirement (EAR), which refers to the average nutrient intake level estimated to meet the requirement of 50% of healthy individuals; the RDA is equal to the EAR plus twice the coefficient of variation (CV). The AI is used as the DRI instead of an RDA if not enough scientific evidence is available to calculate an EAR (21). The following discussion briefly summarizes the rationales used to determine recommended nutrient intakes during pregnancy and highlights those nutrients that are likely to be either limited or excessive in maternal diets as well as the consequences for pregnancy outcome.

A. Energy

Compared with a nonpregnant woman, the estimated average additional energy requirement during a full-term pregnancy is approximately 335 MJ (80,000 calories). This includes energy deposited in the products of conception (0.16%), energy deposited as maternal fat stores (0.39%), and extra energy

Table 2 Comparison of Recommended Daily Energy and Nutrient Intakes of Adult, Pregnant, and Lactating Women

Nutrient	Dietary reference intakes			Increase over nonreproducing adult women (%)	
	Adult (19–50 y) women	Pregnant women	Lactating women	Pregnant women	Lactating women
Energy (kcal)	No value	↑340 kcal/d 2nd trimester ↑452 kcal/d 3rd trimester	↑500 kcal/d 0–6 mo ↑400 kcal/d 7–12 mo	↑ —	↑ ↑
Protein (g)[b]	46	71	71	54.4	54.4
Vitamin C (mg)[b]	75	85	120	13.3	60.0
Thiamin (mg)[b]	1.1	1.4	1.4	27.3	27.3
Riboflavin (mg)[b]	1.1	1.4	1.6	27.3	45.5
Niacin (mg NE)[a,b]	14	18	17	28.6	2.1.4
Vitamin B_6 (mg)c	1.3	1.9	2	46.2	53.9
Folate (μ/g DFE)[a,b]	400	600	500	50.0	25.0
Vitamin B_{12} (μg)[b]	2.4	2.6	2.8	8.3	16.7
Pantothenic acid (mg)[c]	5	6	7	20.0	40.0
Biotin (μg)[c]	30	30	35	0.0	16.7
Choline (mg)[c]	425	450	550	5.9	29.4
Vitamin A (μg RE)[a,b]	700	770	1300	10.0	85.7
Vitamin D (μg)[d]	5	5	5	0.0	0.0
Vitamin E (mg α-TE)[a,b]	15	15	19	0.0	26.7
Vitamin K (μg)[c]	90	90	90	0.0	0.0
Calcium (mg)[c]	1000	1000	1000	0.0	0.0
Phosphorus (mg)[b]	700	700	700	0.0	0.0
Magnesium (mg)[b]	310	350	310	12.9	0.0
Iron (mg)[b]	18	27	9	50.0	−50.0
Zinc (mg)[b]	8	11	12	37.5	50.0
Iodine (mg)[b]	150	220	290	46.7	93.3
Selenium (μg)[b]	55	60	70	9.1	27.3
Fluoride (mg)[c]	3	3	3	0.0	0.0

[a] NE, niacin equivalents; DFE, dietary folate equivalents; RE, retinol equivalents; TE, tocopherol equivalents.

[b] recommended dietary allowance (RDA), the average daily dietary intake level that is sufficient to meet the nutrient requirements of nearly all (97–98%) individuals in a life stage and gender group and is based on the estimated average requirement (EAR).

[c] adequate intake (AI), the value used instead of RDA if sufficient evidence is not available to calculate an EAR.

Source: Refs. 21–25.

needed for basal metabolism to maintain new tissues (0.45%) (11,26). Changes that may help meet the energy demands of pregnancy include increased food intake, decreased physical activity, decreased diet-induced thermogenesis (DIT), and decreased maternal fat storage (8,11,26). The relative contributions of these changes may vary significantly among women. To illustrate, an assessment of energy balance during late pregnancy in 10 well-nourished pregnant women reported wide variations among individuals in resting (basal) metabolic rate (456–3389 kJ/d), energy intake (−259–1176 kJ/d), activity energy expenditure (−2301–2929 kJ/d), diet-induced thermogenesis (−266–110 kJ/meal), and altered body fat mass (−0.6 to 10.6 kg) (27). Thus, the current recommended dietary reference intakes of an additional 340 kcal/d (1420 kJ/d) and 452 kcal/d (1888 kJ/d) during the second and third trimesters, respectively, may be greater than required for some women but less than required for others. Interestingly, although the maternal basal metabolic rate rises throughout pregnancy in well-nourished women, it has been found to decrease in poorly nourished women until late in pregnancy, suggesting an energy-sparing metabolic plasticity that benefits the developing fetus (12).

B. Macronutrients

1. Carbohydrates

The glucose fuel requirement for the fetal brain, a carbohydrate-dependent organ, at the end of gestation is estimated to be approximately 33 g/day. To ensure that the fetal brain is provided with this amount of glucose, as well as to supply the glucose fuel requirement for the maternal brain (the same as for nonpregnant women), the calculated RDA for metabolically available dietary carbohydrate (consumed as either starch or sugar) for pregnant women is 175 g/day(25).

2. Protein

During pregnancy, the mother accretes an estimated 925 g of protein, which is deposited in fetal, placental, and maternal tissues primarily during the second and third trimesters (10). Thus, protein requirements during the first trimester do not increase significantly. During the last two trimesters, the calculated protein RDA for a pregnant woman is 1.1 g/kg/day, equivalent to 25 g/day of additional protein for a pregnant 57-kg reference woman. This results in a recommended protein intake of 71 g/day for a pregnant woman, compared with 46 g/d for a nonpregnant woman (25). Survey data show that women of reproductive age in the United States select diets that provide mean protein intakes of about 70 g/d, well in line with the estimated pregnancy requirement (28).

3. Lipids

Fat intake as a percentage of total energy intake can vary widely without affecting health. Although insufficient data are available to define a specific recommended intake level of total fat during pregnancy, the acceptable macronutrient distribution range (AMDR) is 20–35% of total energy, the same as for nonpregnant women (25). However, DRIs during pregnancy have been formulated for certain essential polyunsaturated fatty acids (PUFAs). AIs for n-6 PUFAs (13 g linoleic acid/day) and n-3 PUFAs (1.4 g α-linolenic acid/day) were set based on the median intakes of these PUFAs by pregnant women in the United States, where deficiency is basically nonexistent (25). Linoleic acid and α-linolenic acid are precursors for arachidonic acid (AA; 20:4n-6) and docosahexaenoic acid (DHA; 22:6n-3), respectively; AA and DHA are vitally important for the accelerated development of the central nervous system (CNS), which occurs in the fetus during the last trimester and in the newborn infant during the first postnatal months (29). Both the fetus and the newborn (through lactation) depend on a maternal supply of AA and DHA; thus adequate dietary intake of AA and DHA by both pregnant and lactating women is highly desirable (30). Good dietary sources of AA and DHA include fish (especially fatty fish), poultry, red meat, and eggs. A recent small survey of pregnant Canadian women, however, found that approximately 17% of the women consumed less than 67 mg DHA/d during the latter part of pregnancy, the estimated daily amount accumulated by the fetus during the last trimester (30). In addition, some data indicate that trans fatty acids, present in hydrogenated vegetable oils (e.g., margarines, short-enings) and in foods containing these fats, compete with long-chain PUFA binding sites in placental membranes, thus inhibiting transport of long-chain PUFAs to the fetus (30,31). A review of the essential fatty acid requirements of pregnant women who are vegetarians concluded that, although further research is required, a prudent vegetarian diet should contain a ratio of linoleic acid to α-linolenic acid of between 4:1 nd 10:1, as suggested by the Food and Agriculture Organization/World Health Organization (32). Although some advocate supplementation of pregnant women with long-chain PUFAs (e.g., cod liver oil), this is not currently recommended, because the potential interactive metabolic effects of high intakes of long-chain PUFAs during pregnancy are still unclear (29).

C. Minerals

Sixteen mineral elements are considered to be essential; that is, they must perform at least one function vital for life, growth, or reproduction. Of these, calcium, phosphorus, magnesium, potassium, sulfur, sodium, and chlorine, are macronutrient minerals (concentration in body > 0.005% of body weight), whereas iron, zinc, selenium, iodine, manganese, copper, molybdenum, chromium, and cobalt are micronutrient, or "trace," minerals (concentration in body < 0.005% of body weight). DRIs have been established for intakes of these essential minerals by pregnant women, except for sodium, chlorine, potassium, sulfur, and cobalt, which are widely available in commonly consumed foods and for which deficiencies are unlikely.

1. Macronutrient Minerals

Calcium. Calcium metabolism, as noted earlier, is greatly altered during pregnancy, such that the high fetal demand is met primarily through enhanced efficiency of intestinal calcium absorption, which more than doubles during pregnancy and is mediated through elevated serum concentrations of 1,25-D (21). In addition, parathyroid-hormone-related protein (PTHrP) as well as other hormones and growth factors are elevated during pregnancy and could potentially stimulate alterations in both calcium and bone metabolism (19). Studies on changes in maternal skeletal calcium content during pregnancy have yielded inconsistent results; thus, the extent to which the maternal skeletal calcium is resorbed is not entirely clear (20). Available data, however, generally support the premise that the maternal skeleton is not a major source of fetal calcium. For example, a long-term, comprehensive longitudinal analysis of calcium homeostasis during pregnancy and lactation found no significant changes in either maternal trabecular bone mineral density (BMD) of the lumbar spine or integral (trabecular and cortical bone combined) BMD of the arms, legs, trunk, or total body between prepregnancy and 1–2 weeks postdelivery (33). Surprisingly, evidence indicates that calcium-related metabolic changes during pregnancy are independent of maternal calcium intake and that calcium supplements have a minimal effect on these changes in well-nourished women (20,33). Thus, the AI for calcium for pregnant (and nonpregnant) women has been set at 1000 mg/day, the intake sufficient for optimal bone accretion rates in nonpregnant women (21).

Phosphorus. Phosphorus is so ubiquitous in the food supply that dietary phosphorus deficiency rarely occurs. Because available evidence does not support a need for additional phosphorus by pregnant women, the RDA is 700 mg/day, as for nonpregnant women (21).

Magnesium. Magnesium requirements during pregnancy are based simply on increased needs that may result from maternal weight gain caused by lean tissue accretion (estimated at 7.5 kg); evidence is inconsistent as to whether magnesium intakes greater than those of nonpregnant women are beneficial during pregnancy. The RDA for pregnant women has been calculated to be 350 mg/day (21).

2. Micronutrient Minerals

Iron. Iron requirements during pregnancy vary during each trimester. Because menstruation stops during pregnancy, the need for absorbed iron during the first trimester (1.2 mg/d) is actually lower than in prepregnancy. However, absorbed iron requirements begin to increase in the second trimester (4.7 mg/d) and continue to increase through the third trimester (5.6 mg/d) (24). Enhanced intestinal iron absorption during the last two trimesters (25% absorption) of pregnancy is an important physiological adjustment that helps pregnant women to meet the increased requirements (24). The mean total iron cost of pregnancy is estimated to be 1190 mg; component requirements include the fetus (270 mg), placenta (90 mg), expansion of red blood cell mass (450 mg), and obligatory basal losses (230 mg). In addition, about 150 mg is lost in blood at delivery (34). Assessing the iron status of a pregnant woman is extremely difficult because the expansion of plasma volume that occurs influences indices of iron status. For example, plasma hemoglobin concentration declines during pregnancy, as do concentrations of serum iron, percentage saturation of transferrin, and serum ferritin. Transferrin levels, however, increase from mean values of 3 mg/L (in nonpregnant women) to 5 mg/L in the last trimester of pregnancy, perhaps to facilitate iron transfer to the fetus. Serum transferrin carries iron from the maternal circulation to placental transferrin receptors; after the iron is released, apotransferrin is returned to the maternal circulation. Most iron transfer to the fetus takes place after week 30 of gestation (35). Factorial modeling that considered basal losses, the iron deposited in the fetus and related tissues, and the iron necessary for hemoglobin expansion estimated the mean iron requirements for pregnant women to be 6.4 mg/d, 18.8 mg/d, and 22.4 mg/d for the first, second, and third trimesters, respectively. An RDA of 27 mg/d was established by using third trimester estimates at the 97.5 percentile and assuming 25% absorption; this RDA helps to build iron stores during the first two trimesters and to prevent the development of iron deficiency (24). It is difficult to obtain this level of iron from foods. This is particularly true for vegetarian pregnant women, because bioavailability of iron from a vegetarian diet is estimated to be only 10%, compared with 18% from a mixed Western diet. Data from U.S. surveys found that the median intake of iron by pregnant women is approximately only 15 mg/d, indicating a need for iron supplementation (24). Considerable data have demonstrated that iron supplementation improves maternal iron status during pregnancy and also postpartum, an important benefit when interpregnancy intervals are short (35). Adequate maternal iron intake is important for both the mother and the fetus. Severe iron deficiency anemia (hemoglobin < 70–80g/L) during pregnancy is associated with increased maternal mortality (4) and reduced birthweight resulting from growth restriction and preterm labor (36). More moderate iron deficiency (80–110 g/L), especially in the first trimester, also is associated with low birth weight and preterm delivery (24,35). Considerable disagreement exists, however, regarding routine use of iron supplements, because high maternal hemoglobin levels (> 120–130 g/L) also have been linked to adverse birth outcomes as well as increased risk of preeclampsia (36,37). High hemoglobin levels, however, likely indicate inadequate plasma volume expansion rather than iron status. Evidence is lacking to support the supposition that iron supplementation can result in abnormally high hemoglobin concentrations (37).

Iodine. Iodine deficiency during pregnancy has implications for the developing brain of the fetus, because iodine is required for synthesis of thyroid hormones, which are critical for maturation of the central nervous system, particularly for myelination. Severe iodine deficiency leads to cretinism, the most extreme adverse outcome, which is characterized by severe mental retardation, deaf-mutism, stunted growth, and impaired gait and motor function. Even mild maternal iodine deficiency, however, may affect fetal brain development and result in decreased intelligence (38,39). Evidence indicates that maternal thyroid status during the first trimester is vitally important to pregnancy outcome (40); thus, maternal iodine deficiency should be corrected either before or during the first trimester. The iodine RDA during pregnancy has been set at 220 µg/d; this amount is based on the requirement for nonpregnant women and the needs of the developing fetus (24). A U.S. survey found that the median intake of iodine from foods (not including iodized salt) was 290 µg/d for both pregnant and lactating women. However, approximately 25% of pregnant women had an iodine intake from foods below 220 µg/d (24).

Zinc. Severe maternal zinc deficiency can cause infertility, prolonged labor, congenital anomalies, IUGR, and death of the embryo or fetus (41). Even moderate deficiency may adversely affect fetal growth, infant birth weight, and labor and delivery. Nevertheless, findings in human studies of maternal zinc status and pregnancy outcome, including randomized, controlled trials in both developed and developing countries, have not been consistent (41,42). The general lack of agreement among studies may stem from methodological differences, particularly use of various techniques to assess zinc status (43). For example, circulating zinc in plasma provides only an insensitive measure of zinc status; thus, clinical features of zinc deficiency can occur while plasma zinc levels appear to be normal (24). In addition, plasma zinc declines during pregnancy and, at term, is approximately 35% lower than in nonpregnant women, contributing to difficulty of data interpretation. In a study of 3448 pregnant women, plasma zinc concentrations between the late first trimester and the early third trimester were not associated with any measure of pregnancy outcome or neonatal condition (43). It is estimated that an additional 100 mg of zinc is needed during pregnancy, which is deposited primarily in the fetus and in the uterine muscle. Potential metabolic adjustments in maternal zinc utilization that could help meet the increased demand include increased intestinal absorption, reduced endogenous gastrointestinal zinc excretion, renal conservation, and release of maternal tissue zinc (41). The zinc RDA for pregnant women has been set at 11 mg/d, based on the requirement for nonpregnant women plus the additional amount calculated to be accumulated in maternal and fetal tissues. Approximately half of pregnant women in the United States meet this requirement, with a median intake slightly less than 11 mg/d (24). Zinc bioavailability may be reduced in pregnant women who consume a vegetarian diet containing high amounts of phytate, fiber, calcium, and other inhibitors of zinc absorption; in these women, the requirement for dietary zinc may be as much as 50% greater than for nonvegetarians. (24). Currently, zinc supplementation (15 mg/d) is recommended for pregnant women who ordinarily consume an inadequate diet or who are at increased risk for poor reproductive outcomes (e.g., smokers, alcohol and drug abusers, and women carrying multiple fetuses). In addition, zinc supplementation (15 mg/d) is recommended for women taking iron supplements (>30 mg/d), because some evidence suggests that iron may interfere with zinc absorption. In one study, iron supplements (60 mg/d) decreased zinc absorption in fasting pregnant women by more than 50% (44). Data from a study in nonpregnant women, however, indicated that although iron supplements did not affect zinc status, zinc supplements reduced iron status, underscoring the need for more research to gain a clearer understanding of the interactive effects of these minerals (45).

Trace Minerals. Just as for other minerals, DRIs for pregnant women for the trace minerals selenium, manganese, copper, molybdenum, and chromium, included in Table 2, have been calculated based on requirements for nonpregnant women and analysis of available evidence regarding pregnancy-related needs. Data from national U.S. surveys indicate that mean dietary intakes of manganese and copper by pregnant women are at recommended levels and intakes of selenium and molybdenum are approximately 200% and 150%, respectively, of recommended levels; no national survey data are available for chromium intakes (24).

C. Vitamins

1. Fat-Soluble Vitamins

Vitamin A. Vitamin A, transported between mother and fetus through the placenta, is essential for vertebrate embryonic and fetal development. In animal models, vitamin A deficiency can result in abnormalities in the heart, the CNS, the circulatory, respiratory, and urogenital systems, and in the development of skull, skeleton, and limbs (46). In addition, animal studies have reported a teratogenic association between maternal intake of excess vitamin A and a pattern of birth defects (retinoic acid syndrome) that includes cardiovascular, CNS, craniofacial, and thymus malformations (47,48). Although abnormalities associated with vitamin A deficiency in animals are not commonly found in humans, epidemiologic data support the possible human teratogenicity of high vitamin A intake (24). The vitamin A requirement for human pregnancy has been estimated to be 770 μg retinol activity equivalents (RAE)/d, based on the amount that accumulates in the fetal liver (0.3600 μg) plus maternal needs and maternal storage for use during lactation (24). Overt vitamin A deficiency during pregnancy, associated with night blindness and other ocular symptoms as well as increased risk of infectious morbidity and mortality (24), is a widespread problem in developing countries. In such areas, the World Health Organization (WHO) recommends either a daily supplement no greater than 3,000 retinol equivalents (RE) or a weekly supplement no greater than 7,500 RE (47). In contrast, deficiency of vitamin A during pregnancy is not often observed in the United States or other developed countries, where concern focuses more on excess intake from either supplements or medications such as isotretinoin, a vitamin A analogue used to treat severe cystic acne. Vegetarians, however, who consume few or no animal-derived foods, the only source or preformed vitamin A, are at risk for low vitamin A intake, and should include significant quantities of dark green and yellow/orange vegetables and fruits (high in β-carotene, i.e., provitamin A) in their diets.

Vitamin D. During pregnancy, maternal serum concentrations of 25-hydroxyvitamin D, the major circulating form of vitamin D in plasma, are either similar to or lower than those in nonpregnant women; concentrations vary according to vitamin D intake and sun exposure, which is the source of ultraviolet (UV) light required for synthesis of vitamin D in the skin, and depend to some extent on season and geographic location. However, serum concentrations of both free and bound 1,25-dihydroxyvitamin D, the biologically active form of the vitamin, are elevated during pregnancy (49,50). Maternal vitamin D, which is transported across the placenta, is the sole source of vitamin D for the fetus. Adverse fetal effects of maternal vitamin D deficiency include possible delayed growth, delayed bone ossification, abnormal enamel formation, and disturbances in neonatal calcium homeostasis (hypocalcemia, tetany) (50). In the pregnant woman, vitamin D deficiency can cause a decrease in serum calcium, leading to mobilization of calcium form the skeleton and osteomalacia (21,49). The prevalence of vitamin D deficiency in women can be high in northern latitudes, where the amount of exposure to UV light is limited in the winter months (51), and among certain ethnic groups (52). For example, data from the third National Health and Nutrition Examination Survey (NHANES III) found that 42.4% of African American women aged 15–49 years had a serum 25-hydroxyvitamin D concentration ≤37.5 nmol/L, the value used to define hypovitaminosis D in this study, compared with 4.2% of white women (52). Surprisingly, prevalences of hypovitaminosis D were 28.2% and 10.6% even among African American women who consumed either 5 µg or 10 µg vitamin D/d, respectively, from supplements. In the United States, the AI for dietary vitamin D for pregnant women has been set at 5 µg/d when sunlight exposure is inadequate, the same as for nonpregnant women, based on evidence suggesting that the small amounts of vitamin D transferred to the fetus do not appear to affect overall maternal vitamin D status (21). Except for fatty fish, very few natural foods contain vitamin D; vitamin D–fortified milk is the most significant food source. Women who either are vegetarians or restrict their milk intake should consider vitamin D supplementation. A supplement of 10 µ/d, the amount supplied by prenatal vitamin supplements, is viewed as a safe amount.

Vitamin E. The RDA for vitamin E (15 mg α-tocopherol/d) and the AI for vitamin K (90 µg/d) for pregnant women are the same as those for nonpregnant women; no clinical deficiencies of these vitamins have been reported in pregnant women, and additional fetal needs are not yet known (23,24). Placental transfer of vitamin E appears to be relatively constant throughout pregnancy (IOM, 2000) (23). However, transfer of vitamin K through the placenta is minor, and newborns have low vitamin K tissue stores (53).

2. Water-Soluble Vitamins

Folate. "Folate," a B-complex vitamin, includes the naturally occurring form found in foods as well as the synthetic form (folic acid) found in fortified foods and supplements. Folate acts as a cofactor for essential cellular reactions that involve transfer of single-carbon units, including those necessary for synthesis of nucleic acids required for DNA and, thus, cell division. The accelerated cell division that occurs in both fetal and maternal tissues during pregnancy results in a considerable increase in maternal folate requirements (54,55). Maternal folate inadequacy is associated with increased risks of neural-tube defects (NTDs), preterm delivery, low birth weight, and fetal growth retardation (22). NTDs originate during the first 4 weeks of pregnancy, before a woman may even realize that she is pregnant. Between 1990 and 1996, almost 9500 infants in the United States were born with NTDs (56). Maternal folate absorption does not change during pregnancy, and folate levels in blood plasma and erythrocytes normally fall as pregnancy progresses, likely because of expanded blood volume and increased urinary excretion. Folate is provided to the fetus through placental transport, likely with the aid of folate-binding proteins (FBP) located in the placental membranes. Folate blood levels in the fetus are characteristically high, frequently at maternal expense. Because humans cannot synthesize folate, a sufficient intake from dietary sources and supplements is essential during pregnancy. In some women, folate requirements may be increased as a result of polymorphisms in genes that govern folate metabolism (e.g., 5,10-methylenetetrahydrofolate reductase (MTHFR)) (55). Based on evidence from population-based studies and a controlled metabolic study, the RDA for folate has been set at 600 µg/d of dietary folate equivalents (DFEs), an amount adequate to maintain normal folate status in pregnant women (22,54). Naturally occurring dietary folate is only 50% bioavailable, whereas folic acid from supplements is 100% bioavailable (when taken on an empty stomach); thus 300 µg of folic acid are equivalent to 600 DFEs (22,54). NHANES III (1988–1994) found a median dietary folate intake for U.S. women of reproductive age of approximately 225 µg/d (22). Periconceptional folic acid intake of 400 µg/d, however, is believed to be the amount required to reduce risk of NTDs. In 1992, as a preventive measure, the Centers for Disease Control and Prevention (CDC) recommended that all women capable of becoming pregnant should take a daily 400 µg folic acid supplement, a recommendation also made by the Institute of Medicine (IOM) in 1998 (22). In addition, the FDA mandated the addition of folic acid to enriched grain products (effective January 1998), an action expected to add approximately 100 µg folic acid/d to the average diet of Americans (56). Some have voiced concern that high intakes of folate can mask signs of vitamin B_{12} deficiency and delay treatment while irreversible neurological damage progresses.

Other B-Complex Vitamins. In addition to folate, the B-complex vitamins include B_6, B_{12}, thiamine (B_1), riboflavin (B_2), niacin, pantothenic acid, and biotin. RDAs/AIs for these vitamins are based on evidence of sufficiency and are set higher than the amount needed to prevent signs and symptoms of deficiency disease, to include a safety margin. The RDAs/AIs for pregnant women are based on those for nonpregnant women plus an amount expected to accommodate fetal needs and increased maternal needs (22). In the United States, except for vitamin B_6, these B vitamins are generally considered to be consumed in adequate amounts from dietary sources by women who are omnivorous (10). Functional measures of vitamin B_6 status, including plasma levels of the vitamin and pyridoxal phosphate (PLP), its active metabolite, decrease throughout pregnancy. Because as much as 10 mg vitamin B_6/d (an amount too great to be provided by food intake) is required to maintain status indicators at nonpregnant levels, and because decreases during pregnancy are not associated with signs of deficiency, the changes in measurable vitamin B_6 status likely represent normal physiological changes. Fetal concentrations of PLP are significantly higher than maternal concentrations, especially during the last two trimesters (22). The RDA for vitamin B_6 for pregnancy has been set at 1.9 mg/d, based on the RDA of 1.3 mg/d for nonpregnant women plus fetal requirements and increased maternal needs. U.S. surveys, however, have reported median dietary intakes of 1.56 and 1.76 for pregnant women, indicating that more than 50% do not meet the current RDA (22). In addition, a recent assessment of vitamin B status in nonpregnant women in a controlled feeding study, combined with data from previous studies, indicated that a higher RDA of 1.5–1.7 mg/d may be more appropriate for nonpregnant women (57). If so, the RDA for pregnant women also would increase and relatively few women would meet the requirement. Pregnant women who are strict vegetarians (vegans) may be deficient in vitamin B_{12}, which is found only in animal products or fortified foods, and both they and their infants may benefit from supplementation. Deficiency symptoms have frequently been reported in infants born to vegan mother (58). Much remains to be learned about requirements for the B-complex vitamins during pregnancy. For example, clinical data suggest that mild biotin deficiency, not severe enough to produce symptoms, develops in many women during normal pregnancy. Because mild biotin deficiency is teratogenic in several animal species, the possibility of mild biotin deficiency as a contributing factor to human birth defects should be considered (59,60).

Choline. Although not normally called a vitamin, choline is a nutrient obtained from foods that plays a role in numerous biochemical processes and is essential for liver function. Fetal choline needs are met through placental transfer of maternal choline. The choline AI for pregnant women (450 mg/d) was estimated based on the amount required by nonpregnant women to prevent liver damage plus the amount that accumulates in fetal and placental tissues (22). Although choline is widely distributed in foods, it is not included in major nutrient databases, and U.S. intakes have not been quantitated.

Vitamin C. Maternal plasma concentrations of vitamin C decrease during pregnancy, likely a result of both hemodilution and vitamin C transfer to the fetus. The amount of vitamin C required by the fetus is not known. Thus, the RDA for vitamin C for pregnant women has been set at 85 mg/d, by considering the amount required for nonpregnant women plus the amount known to prevent scurvy in young infants (23).

IV. NUTRITION-RELATED PROBLEMS DURING PREGNANCY

A. Diabetes

Women who suffer from either diabetes mellitus or gestational diabetes mellitus (GDM) require close monitoring during pregnancy. GDM affects 3–4% of pregnant women and likely results from metabolic maladaptation to the insulin resistance caused by pregnancy-related hormonal changes (61). For both groups of women, regulation of maternal plasma glucose is essential for successful pregnancy outcome. High maternal glucose correlates with high fetal plasma glucose, which stimulates fetal insulin secretion and increases the need for oxygen to metabolize the glucose. Elevated maternal plasma glucose in the first 2 months of pregnancy is associated with a greatly increased risk of congenital abnormalities, and increased maternal plasma glucose later in pregnancy is linked to macrosomia (birth weight > 4000g), infant hypoglycemia, perinatal mortality, and prematurity. These adverse effects can be prevented if maternal plasma glucose is controlled aggressively throughout pregnancy with diet and insulin therapy; oral hypoglycemia drugs, however, are contraindicated. All pregnant women should be screened for gestational diabetes between 24 and 28 weeks of pregnancy (62).

B. Phenylketonuria

Women with phenylketonuria (PKU) must make dietary choices that help to maintain low blood phenylalanine concentrations both before and during pregnancy to reduce the risk of adverse outcomes for their infants, including mental retardation and microcephaly (63). Consumption of high protein, phenylalanine free medical foods can help to achieve this objective. Data from the international Maternal Phenylketonuria Study, however, indicate that overall diet, not just protein intake, is important to reproductive outcome in women with PKU (64). Findings showed that maternal intakes of both protein and fat throughout pregnancy and energy intake during the second and third trimesters were inversely correlated with maternal plasma phenylalanine concentrations, suggesting that inadequate protein, fat, and energy intakes in women with PKU may contribute to high plasma phenylalanine concentrations and poor reproductive outcomes.

C. Pregnancy-Induced Hypertension

Hypertensive disorders induced during pregnancy include gestational hypertension, preeclampsia (gestational hypertension with proteinuria, edema, or both in a previously normotensive woman), and eclampsia (development of grand mal seizure in preeclampsia). The etiology of these disorders is not yet clear. Many nutrients have been investigated as possible contributing factors for gestational hypertension and preeclampsia, including energy/protein, salt, calcium, fish oil, and vitamins E and C; in addition, possible effects of iron, folate, and zinc (on gestational hypertension) and magnesium (on preeclampsia) have been evaluated. A recent review of the outcomes of nutritional interventions during pregnancy concluded that calcium supplementation reduced the incidence of hypertension (only in women with initially low calcium intake) and preeclampsia (primarily in women at high risk of hypertension) and that fish oil and vitamins E and C showed promise for reducing the risk of preeclampsia (65). Salt restriction, as well as iron, folate, magnesium, and zinc supplements, showed no beneficial affects on these hypertensive disorders. In addition, even though maternal obesity increases the risk of gestational hypertension and preeclampsia, available evidence suggested that energy/protein restriction is unlikely to reduce their risk in overweight pregnant women (65).

D. Alcohol

Fetal alcohol syndrome (FAS) refers to a pattern of mental and physical defects that include prenatal and postnatal growth retardation, distinct facial anomalies, multiple organ dysfunction, and CNS abnormalities that result in learning disabilities and reduced intelligence quotient (66). The prevalence of FAS in the United States is not known with certainty. In various studies, U.S. prevalence rates have ranged from 0.3 to 2.2 cases per 1000 live births; this means that each year between 1200 and 8800 babies in the United States are born with FAS (67). The extent of damage varies with the volume of alcohol ingested, the timing during pregnancy, genetics, and environmental factors. One drink a day (e.g., a 5-oz glass of wine) or more than 5 drinks on one occasion is considered to be "risk drinking" by the CDC (67). Birth defects associated with alcohol exposure can occur in the early weeks of pregnancy, before a woman may even know she is pregnant. Although the adverse effects of alcohol may be related to decreased dietary intake, impaired metabolism and absorption of nutrients, and interactions between alcohol and certain nutrient deficiencies, specific mechanisms by which alcohol influences fetal growth and development have not yet been established (10). Some individuals might be more sensitive to alcohol than others; however, it is not possible to determine which fetuses might be at greatest risk from exposure to alcohol. Thus, although some professional groups view occasional small doses of alcohol during pregnancy as not being harmful, the safest approach is complete abstinence. The U.S. Surgeon General recommends that pregnant women abstain completely from alcohol.

E. Caffeine

Commonly consumed beverages that are caffeine sources and their typical caffeine levels include brewed coffee (135 mg/8 oz), instant coffee (95 mg/8 oz), expresso (320 mg/8 oz), tea (50 mg/8 oz), and cola drinks (25 mg/8 oz) (63). Although substantial evidence exists that caffeine is a teratogen in animals, no similar effects have been observed in humans (68). Data from some studies indicate that caffeine consumption during pregnancy, especially at levels greater than 300 mg/d, may reduce fetal birth weight; the overall evidence, however, is not consistent (69). The U.S. Food and Drug Administration (FDA) recommends that the most prudent action for pregnant women is to either avoid caffeine-containing products or use them sparingly (10).

V. ENDOCRINE REGULATION OF HUMAN LACTATION

Lactogenesis and lactation are regulated through complex endocrine system control mechanisms that coordinate the actions of various hormones, including the reproductive hormones prolactin, progesterone, placental lactogen, oxytocin, and estrogen (70,71). Although hormonal regulation of the first stage of lactogenesis (lactogenesis 1), which begins in midpregnancy, is not well understood, it is known that progesterone suppresses active milk secretion during this stage (71). After parturition, progesterone withdrawal combined with high levels of prolactin results in the onset of secretion of colostrum ("early milk") and then milk; this process is termed *lactogenesis 2*, or secretory activation. The initiation of lactogenesis 2 does not require infant suckling, but the infant must begin to suckle by 3–4 days postpartum to maintain milk secretion. Prolactin, required to maintain milk production after lactation is established, is released into the circulation from mammotrophs in the anterior pituitary in response to suckling. During lactation, release of prolactin is mediated by a transient decline in the secretion of

Table 3 Representative Values for Constituents of Human Milk

Constituent (per liter)[a]	Early milk	Mature milk
Energy (kcal)		653–704
Carbohydrate		
Lactose (g)	20–30	67
Glucose (g)	0.2–1.0	0.2–0.3
Oligosaccharides (g)	22–24	12–14
Total nitrogen (g)	3.0	1.9
Nonprotein nitrogen (g)	0.5	0.45
Protein nitrogen (g)	2.5	1.45
Total Protein (g)	16	9
Casein (g)	3.8	5.7
β-Casein (g)	2.6	4.4
κ-Casein (g)	1.2	1.3
α-Lactalbumin (g)	3.62	3.26
Lactoferrin (g)	3.53	1.94
Serum albumin (g)	0.39	0.41
sIgA (g)	2.0	1.0
IgM (g)	0.12	0.2
IgG (g)	0.34	0.05
Total lipids (%)	2	3.5
Triglyceride (% total lipids)	97–98	97–98
Cholesterol[b] (% total lipids)	0.7–1.3	0.4–0.5
Phospholipids (% total lipids)	1.1	0.6–0.8
Fatty acids (weight %)	88	88
Total saturated	43–44	44–45
C12:0		5
C14:0		6
C16:0		20
C18:0		8
Monounsaturated		40
C18:ω-9	32	31
Polyunsaturated	13	14–15
Total ω-3	1.5	1.5
C18:3ω-3	0.7	0.9
C22:5ω-3	0.2	0.1
C22:6ω-3	0.5	0.2
Total ω-6	11.6	13.06
C18:2ω-6	8.9	11.3
C20:4ω-6	0.7	0.5
C22:4ω-6	0.2	0.1
Water-soluble vitamins		
Vitamin C		100
Thiamin (μg)	20	200

Table 3 Continued

Constituent (per liter)[a]	Early milk	Mature milk
Riboflavin (µg)		400–600
Niacin (mg)	0.5	1.8–6.0
Vitamin B6 (mg)		0.09–0.31
Folate (µg)		80–140
Vitamin B_{12} (µg)		0.5–1.0
Pantothenic acid (mg)		2.0–2.5
Biotin (µg)		5–9
Fat-soluble vitamins		
Vitamin A (mg)	2	0.3–0.6
Carotenoids (mg)	2	0.2–0.6
Vitamin K (µg)	2–5	2–3
Vitamin D (µg)		0.33
Vitamin E (mg)	8–12	3–8
Minerals		
Macronutrient minerals		
Calcium (mg)	250	200–250
Magnesium (mg)	30–35	30–35
Phosphorus (mg)	120–160	120–140
Sodium (mg)	300–400	120–250
Potassium (mg)	600–700	400–550
Chloride (mg)	600–800	400–450
Micronutrient minerals		
Iron (mg)	0.5–1.0	0.3–0.9
Zinc (ng)	8–12	1–3
Copper (mg)	0.5–0.8	0.2–0.4
Manganese (µg)	5–6	3
Selenium (µg)	40	7–33
Iodine (µg)		150
Fluoride (µg)		4–15

[a] All values are expressed as per liter of milk, with the exception of lipids, which are expressed as a percentage on the basis of either milk volume or weight of total lipids.
[b] The cholesterol content of human milk ranges from 100 to 200 mg/L in most samples of human milk after day 21 of lactation.
Source: MF Picciano. Appendix, Representative Values for Constituents of Human Milk. Pediatr Clin North Am 48:263–264, 2001.

dopamine, an inhibiting factor, from the hypothalamus. Because plasma prolactin levels do not correlate with rate of milk secretion, it has been suggested that prolactin may be a permissive factor for milk secretion, rather than a regulatory factor (71).

Milk volume increases significantly between 36 and 96 hours postpartum (<100 mL/d to 500 mL/d). Milk composition changes substantially as early milk develops the characteristics of mature milk, which are evident by day 10 of lactation (see Table 3) (53). For example, lactose increases, sodium and chloride decrease, the immune factors lactoferrin and secretory immunoglobulin A decrease (in part, a dilution effect as milk volume increases), and oligosaccharides, considered to be protective against infections, decrease (70). During lactation, the typical daily volume of milk transferred to the infant increases from 0.50 mL on day 1, to 500 mL by day 5, to 650 mL by 1 month, and to 750 mL by 3 months. Most women are capable of secreting considerably more milk than needed by a single infant.

Although milk secretion is a continuous process, the amount produced is regulated primarily by infant demand. Suckling causes neural impulses to be sent to the hypothalamus; this triggers oxytocin release from the posterior pituitary. Oxytocin brings about contraction of the myoepithelial cells that surround mammary alveoli and ducts, forcing milk into the ducts of the nipple so that it is available for the infant. This response (milk ejection; let-down) also can be triggered simply by seeing the infant or hearing the infant cry. When milk is not removed by either infant suckling or other means, involution of the mammary epithelium occurs, and milk secretion stops within 1–2 days.

Lactation and the associated high levels of prolactin suppress the release of luteinizing hormone and interfere with the secretion of gonadotropin; thus, ovarian activity is inhibited. This provides 98% protection from pregnancy during the first 6 months of lactation if the nursing mother remains amenorrheic (72).

VI. NUTRITIONAL NEEDS DURING LACTATION

Reference standards to determine the nutritional status of lactating women using chemical or anthropometric criteria have not yet been developed (73). Thus, the current recommended DRIs for lactating adult women, summarized in Table 2, were calculated based on the amount of milk produced during lactation, its energy and nutrient contents, and the amount of maternal energy and nutrient reserves stored during pregnancy that are available to support milk production. Generally, the birth weight of an infant doubles in the first 4–6 months after birth; during this period, human milk is adequate as the sole source of nutrition, provided that the maternal diet and reserves are adequate. Lactation is deemed successful when a completely breast-fed infant grows well and maintains appropriate nutritional status, as judged by specific biochemical indicators. Under these circumstances, the nutrient composition of the milk and the quantity of milk consumed by the infant frequently are used as proxies to assess maternal nutritional adequacy during lactation.

Maternal nutritional needs to support lactation are exceedingly high. In fact, the estimated energy cost of 6 months of lactation exceeds that of pregnancy by 42% (53), and DRIs for many minerals and vitamins are higher in lactation than in pregnancy. During lactation, if maternal nutrient intake is lower than the total needed for maternal maintenance plus milk production, required nutrients will be mobilized from maternal tissues (73). Thus, maintaining a maternal diet characterized by high nutrient density (nutrient intake per 1000 kcal) is important during lactation to prevent nutritional deficiencies for both the lactating mother and the breast-fed infant. It should be noted that constituents of human milk generally exhibit a range of values, as indicated in Table 3, and may show considerable variation not only among women but also within women at different times. Such variation, however, is compatible with successful lactation. Nutrients in milk that can be influenced by maternal nutrition as well as nutrients associated with recognizable deficiencies in breast-fed infants, based on available evidence, are identified in Table 4 (74).

A. Energy

The energy requirements of lactating women appear to be met primarily through diet, with a small (but not mandatory) contribution from mobilization of tissue stores. The estimated energy requirement for an average active adult woman is 2400 kcal/d. The additional energy required by a lactating woman is proportional to the amount of milk produced. Average milk production for American women is about 780 mL/d during the first 6 months of lactation and 600 mL/d in the second 6 months (25). Based on a measured mean energy density for human milk of approximately 67 kcal/100 g, the milk energy output (after rounding) is approximately 500 kcal/d and 400 kcal/d in the first and second 6 months of lactation, respectively. In the first 6 months postpartum, the average weight loss of well-nourished lactating women is 0.8 kg/mo, equivalent to 170 kcal/d, after which weight appears to stabilize. Consequently, the estimated maternal energy requirement for lactation is 330 kcal/d (500–170 kcal/d) during the first 6 months and 400 kcal/d during the second 6 months, and the total estimated daily energy requirements during these two periods are 2730 kcal/d and 2800 kcal/d, respectively (25). At energy

Table 4 Possible Influences of Maternal Intake on the Nutrient Composition of
Human Milk and Nutrients for Which Clinical Deficiency Is Recognizable in
Breast-Fed Infants

Nutrient or nutrient class	Effects of maternal intake on milk composition[a]	Recognizable nutritional deficiency in breast-fed infants
Macronutrients		
Proteins	+	Unknown
Lipids	+[b]	Unknown
Lactose	o	Unknown
Minerals		
Calcium	o	Unknown
Phosphorus	o	Unknown
Magnesium	o	Unknown
Sodium	o	Unknown
Potassium	o	Unknown
Chlorine	o	Unknown
Iron	o	Yes[c]
Copper	o	Unknown
Zinc	o	Unknown
Manganese	+	Unknown
Selenium	+	Unknown
Iodine	+	Yes
Fluoride	+	Unknown
Vitamins		
Vitamin C	+	Yes
Thiamin	+	Unknown
Riboflavin	+	Unknown
Niacin	+	Yes
Pantothenic Acid	+	Yes
Vitamin B_6	+	Yes
Biotin	+	Yes
Folate	+	Yes
Vitamin B_{12}	+	Yes
Vitamin A	+	Yes
Vitamin D	+	Yes
Vitamin E	+	Yes
Vitamin K	+	Yes[d]

[a] " + " denotes a positive effect of intake on nutrient content of milk; the magnitude of the effect
varies widely among nutrients. "o" denotes no known effect of intake on nutrient content of
milk.
[b] Intake appears to affect the type of fatty acids present in milk but not the total milk content of
triacylglycerol or cholesterol.
[c] Deficiency is not related to maternal intake.
[d] Maternal intake is not the primary determinant of infant vitamin K status.
Source: Adapted from Ref. 74.

intakes lower than 2700 kcal/d, maternal intakes of calcium, magnesium, zinc, vitamin B-6, and folate may be lower than required (73).

It should be noted that changes in weight resulting from the demands of lactation are highly variable among individual women within a population as well as among diverse populations. For example, in some under-privileged populations, mean weight loss in the first 6 months postpartum is only 0.1–0.2 kg/mo, compared with the 0.8 kg/mo in well-nourished populations. Gestational weight gain is the most consistent predictor of postpartum weight loss across all studies, suggesting that biological mechanisms strive to restore prepregnancy body weight (75).

B. Macronutrients

1. Carbohydrates

The requirement for carbohydrates increases during lactation. Human milk contains approximately 74 g lactose/L, which is synthesized from glucose obtained from precursors consumed by the mother. Calculation of the RDA during lactation is based on the glucose fuel requirement for a nonlactating, nonpregnant woman plus the additional amount (0.60 g/day) required to replace the carbohydrate secreted in human milk. The RDA for carbohydrate for lactating women is 210 g/d (25).

2. Protein

The additional protein requirement for lactation, defined as the output of total protein and nonprotein nitrogen in milk, has been calculated to be 0.39 g protein/kg/d for a reference 57-kg woman. This is equivalent to an RDA of 25 g/d of additional protein for a lactating woman. Thus, the recommended protein intake is 71 g/d for a lactating woman, compared with 46 g/d for a nonlactating, nonpregnant woman (25).

3. Lipids

The discussion regarding lipid requirements during pregnancy also is generally valid for lactation. The acceptable macronutrient distribution range (AMDR) is 20–35% of total energy, the same as for pregnant and non-lactating women (25). For lactating women, AIs for n-6 PUFAs (13g linoleic acid/d) and n-3 PUFAs (1.3g α-linolenic acid/d) were set based on the median intakes of these PUFAs by lactating women in the United States, where deficiency is basically nonexistent (25). Evidence from isotope studies indicates that a large part of milk PUFAs is derived from endogenous body stores, rather than maternal diet, suggesting that long-term dietary intake influences milk fat composition (76).

C. Minerals

1. Macronutrient Minerals

Calcium.   Calcium transfer between the lactating mother and nursing infant averages about 200 mg/d during full breast-feeding (19); over 6 months, this is equivalent to approximately 4% of the maternal skeletal reserve of calcium (77). Calcium resorbed from the maternal skeleton is the primary source for this mineral in human milk (19,20). Evidence indicates that increasing dietary calcium does not prevent loss of calcium from the skeleton of lactating women (21). For example, studies in well-nourished lactating Caucasian adult women with calcium intakes between 750 and 700 mg/d (77) and in lactating Gambian women consuming either their usual low calcium intake (mean, 288 mg/d) or a supplemented intake (mean, 992 mg/d) (78) found that supplementation had little effect on calcium homeostasis and did not decrease bone turnover in these populations. Considering the lack of supporting evidence for a benefit of supplementation, the AI for calcium for lactating women has been set at 1000 mg/d and is based on the intake sufficient for optimal bone accretion rates in nonlactating women. Importantly, studies consistently show that the skeletal calcium lost during lactation is regained after the infant is weaned (19–21).

Phosphorus.   Phosphorus requirements have not been observed to increase during lactation. Thus, the RDA for phosphorus is 700 mg/d, the same as for pregnant women and nonpregnant women (21). In lactating women, increased bone resorption and decreased urinary excretion of phosphorus appear to provide the necessary phosphorous for milk production, independent of dietary phosphorous intake (21).

Magnesium.   Magnesium requirements during lactation are estimated to be the same as those for nonlactating women of similar age and body weight, because evidence does not consistently support an increased requirement for dietary magnesium for lactating women. As for phosphorus, the magnesium necessary for milk production may be independent of dietary intake, being provided through increased bone resorption during lactation and decreased urinary excretion. The RDA for magnesium for lactating women has been calculated to be 310 mg/d (21). A recent review reported that concentrations of magnesium in human milk do not appear to be influenced by either maternal constitutional factors (e.g., undernutrition, diabetes, race, stage of lactation) or environmental factors (e.g., dietary

supplementation, smoking habits, vegetarianism, use of hormonal contra-
ceptives) (79).

2. Micronutrient Minerals

Iron. Iron needs during lactation are estimated based on the iron
secreted in human milk, the basal iron losses for nonpregnant, nonlactating
women, and the assumption that menstruation does not resume until after
6 months of breast-feeding. The RDA for iron for lactating women has been
set at 9 mg/d, based on basal losses, the amount secreted in milk, and the
assumption that menstruation does not resume until 6 months postpartum
(24). This is less than the 18 mg/d, estimated to cover both basal and
menstrual losses, recommended for nonreproducing women. However,
considering that NHANES III data indicate only approximately 10% of
women of childbearing age meet the recommended intake of 18 mg/d (mean
intake, 13 mg/d) and that 16% of women who enter pregnancy appear to be
iron deficient (ferritin < 15 μg/L) (24), it is difficult to reconcile recommending
an RDA of only 9 mg/d for lactating women, many of whom may have
inadequate iron status and would benefit from higher iron intake. A more
judicious approach to the formulation of recommended iron intake for
women during lactation might include recovery of iron stores and
mitigation of iron deficiency after pregnancy as contributing factors. This
becomes particularly important if the lactating mother likely will have only a
short interval before her next pregnancy.

Iodine. The iodine requirement for a lactating woman is estimated
based on the average needs of a nonlactating woman and the average daily
loss of iodine in human milk. The iodine RDA during lactation has been set at
290 μg/d. A U.S. survey found that approximately 50% of lactating women
had an iodine intake from foods below 290 μg/d, indicating that supplementation might be beneficial for some women (24).

Zinc. The RDA for zinc during lactation has been set at 12 mg/d. This
value was determined by considering the average needs of a nonlactating
woman, the loss of zinc in human milk, the release of maternal zinc that results
from postpartum involution of the uterus and decreased maternal blood
volume, and the increase in zinc absorption that occurs during lactation (24).
For example, a small study in lactating Chinese women with a mean low zinc
intake (7.6 mg/d) found a much higher fractional zinc absorption in these
women (0.53) than in never-pregnant women (0.31). Endogenous fecal zinc
loses also decreased in the lactating women, relative to the amount of zinc
absorbed (80). In the United States, about 75% of women meet the RDA for
zinc (24). As in pregnancy, lactating women who are vegetarians may require

as much as 50% more zinc than nonvegetarians. In addition, supplemental iron may interfere with zinc absorption in lactating women. In one study, fractional zinc absorption was significantly lower in women given a single 60-mg iron supplement at 7–9 weeks of lactation (21.7%) than in unsupplemented women (26.9%) (81).

Trace Minerals. DRIs for lactating women for the trace minerals selenium, manganese, copper, molybdenum, and chromium, included in Table 2, have been estimated based on requirements for nonlactating women and the amount of these minerals secreted in milk. As for pregnant women, data from national U.S. surveys indicate that mean dietary intakes of manganese, copper, selenium, and molybdenum by lactating women are either at or above recommended levels; national data for dietary chromium intake are not available (24).

D. Vitamins

1. Fat-Soluble Vitamins

Vitamin A. An infant needs sufficient vitamin A intake for several months after birth to attain adequate stores. Because the vitamin A content of human milk is influenced by maternal vitamin A status during the last trimester of pregnancy and lactation, adequate maternal vitamin A intake is essential to prevent vitamin A deficiency in both the lactating woman and her breast-fed infant (47). Maternal vitamin A requirements during lactation have been estimated to be 1300 µg RAE/d, based on the needs of nonpregnant women and an average vitamin A loss in breast milk of 400 µg/d (24). National survey data indicate that the majority of lactating women in the United States, with a mean intake of about 1100 µg RAE/d, do not meet this requirement (24). As during pregnancy, lactating vegetarian women are at greater risk for low dietary vitamin A intake and should consume considerable quantities of foods rich in β-carotene. Because of the potential adverse effects of excess vitamin A during pregnancy, supplementation is recommended only for lactating women (and their infants) in developing countries, where overt deficiency is endemic (47).

Vitamin D. Human milk contains only low amounts of vitamin D (25 IU/L or less) and data are lacking to estimate a woman's need for this vitamin during lactation (21,50). Thus, the AI for vitamin D has been set at 5 µg/d when sunlight exposure is inadequate, the same as for nonlactating women (21). Infant vitamin D is affected by both diet and sunlight exposure. Breast-fed infants who do not receive either supplemental vitamin D or adequate sunlight exposure are at increased risk of developing vitamin

D deficiency; in fact, rickets in infants continues to be reported in the United States. The American Academy of Pediatrics recommends that all breast-fed infants receive a daily supplement of 200 IU vitamin D/d, beginning within the first two months of life, unless they are weaned to at least 500 mL per day of vitamin D–fortified formula (infants < 1 year old) or milk (infants > 1 year old) (82).

Vitamins E and K. The RDA for vitamin E for lactating women (19 mg α-tocopherol/d) is based on the needs of nonpregnant women plus the amount secreted in breast milk (0.4 mg/d) (23). The vitamin K AI during lactation (90 μg/d) is the same as for nonpregnant women, because little correlation exists between maternal dietary vitamin K intake and milk vitamin K content (24). Maternal supplementation with pharmacologic doses of vitamin K (5 or 20 mg/d), however, has been reported to significantly increase milk concentrations and improve vitamin K status of breast-fed infants (53). Because newborn infants are functionally vitamin K deficient and thus susceptible to hemorrhagic disease, they routinely receive a prophylactic dose of vitamin K at birth (10).

2. Water-Soluble Vitamins

Folate. If maternal intake is inadequate during lactation, milk folate concentrations are maintained by drawing from maternal folate reserves, highlighting the importance of assessing maternal status in addition to infant status during lactation (83). Preserving adequate maternal folate stores is critical when pregnancies are closely spaced, to reduce risk of NTDs. Based on the folate needs of nonlactating women plus the average amount of folate secreted in human milk (85 μg/L), the RDA for folate for lactating women has been set at 500 μg/d of DFEs (22).

Other B-Complex Vitamins. As in pregnancy, RDAs/AIs for B_6, B_{12}, thiamine (B_1), riboflavin (B_2), niacin, pantothenic acid, and biotin in lactating women are set higher than the amount needed to prevent signs and symptoms of deficiency disease; the values are based on the requirements for nonpregnant women plus the amount secreted in human milk (22). The human milk content of these vitamins are related directly to maternal dietary intake (73).

Choline. The mean choline content of human milk is relatively high (.150 mg/L). Because mechanisms for conserving maternal choline status have not been identified, the need for choline likely increases during lactation, and the AI has been set at 550 mg/d, an amount adequate to cover the requirement for a nonpregnant woman plus the daily amount secreted in breast milk (22).

Vitamin C.   The RDA for vitamin C for lactating women of 120 mg/d was estimated based on the needs for nonlactating women plus the average daily vitamin C secreted in human milk (40 mg). Maternal intake of vitamin C greater than 100 mg/d does not alter the milk content, possibly due to a regulatory mechanism in the mammary gland. However, vitamin C content of milk decreases when maternal intake is below 100 mg/d (23).

VII. KNOWLEDGE GAPS, RESEARCH RECOMMENDATIONS, AND FUTURE DIRECTIONS

Without doubt, pregnancy and lactations are life stages that require generally increased intakes of energy and nutrients. Nevertheless, many questions remain to be answered regarding how maternal nutrient status influences maternal health as well as fetal and infant growth and development. Research is needed in numerous areas, including physiological adjustments in nutrient absorption and excretion during pregnancy, definitive quantitation of maternal and fetal needs for specific nutrients, nutrient–nutrient interactions that can influence nutrient availability, metabolic differences among women stemming from genetic polymorphisms that might affect nutrient requirements during pregnancy and lactation, and long-term effects of the intrauterine environment on adult disease risk.

Much remains to be learned about the biomolecular mechanisms that regulate maternal nutrient status as well as potential postpartum implications of such regulation. For example, the physiological adaptations in maternal calcium and bone metabolism during pregnancy and lactation occur independent of maternal calcium intakes; thus, even if maternal intakes are low, adequate calcium is available for fetal growth and milk production. But the possibility that low calcium intakes before and during pregnancy might have adverse longer-term effects on the growth and bone mineral development of infants, as well as osteoporosis in later life, has not been investigated. In addition, some studies have suggested that maternal calcium intake may influence childhood hypertension development (19). Gaining a clearer understanding of the underlying cellular and molecular changes of pregnancy and lactation could provide important insights into future disease risk.

Many studies of nutrient requirements during pregnancy have focused on the second two trimesters, when increased maternal and fetal needs often become more readily apparent. It is important, however, to understand how maternal nutritional status in early pregnancy and even before conception may affect outcome, as was illustrated clearly by the finding that folic acid supplementation before and during early pregnancy reduces the risk of NTDs. Before it will be possible to gain a better understanding of how maternal nutrition influences pregnancy outcome, reliable and valid laboratory methods must be developed to assess nutrient status for both mothers and infants. For instance, even women in developed countries may suffer from borderline vitamin A deficiencies that are unrecognized, because an acceptable biomarker to assess vitamin A status is not available, except in cases of extreme hypovitaminosis (47). In animal studies, inadequate vitamin A nutrition during early pregnancy results in heart abnormalities that resemble common heart-related birth defects in humans, underscoring the potential clinical importance of this vitamin (46).

Although conducting investigations that attempt to unravel the interactions of nutrients poses certain challenges, research on the effects of single nutrients may tell only part of the story. For example, in a study of the effects of supplementation on night blindness in pregnant women, zinc alone and vitamin A alone restored vision in 12.5% and 36.4% of women, respectively; zinc combined with vitamin A, however, restored vision in 46.2% of women, suggesting that zinc potentiated the effect of vitamin A (84). The area of potential nutrient interactions during pregnancy and lactation holds countless research opportunities.

The possibility that nutrient requirements during pregnancy and lactation may differ somewhat for individual women because of genetic polymorphisms related to metabolism also is a research area that should be emphasized. As noted earlier, genetic heterogenicity in folate metabolism resulting from a polymorphism in MTHFR can increase folate requirements, with implications for pregnancy outcome. Numerous other genetic variations likely play a role in maternal and thus fetal nutrient status and must be explored.

While research continues to more completely define nutritional requirements during pregnancy and lactation as well as the factors contributing to those requirements, clinicians who care for and advise women should base their patient management on the most recent dietary recommendations along with any existing special circumstances relevant to individual patients.

ACKNOWLEDGMENT

We are grateful to Mrs. Suzette Smikle-Williams for her very able assistance in the review and compilation of literature for use in this manuscript.

REFERENCES

1. Jackson AA, Robinson SM. Dietary guidelines: a review of current evidence. Public Health Nutr 2001; 4:625–630.
2. U.S. Department of Health and Human Services. Healthy People 2010: With

Understanding and Improving Health and Objectives for Improving Health. U.S. Government Printing Office, Washington, DC, 2000.

3. Mora JO, Nestel PS. Improving prenatal nutrition in developing countries: strategies, prospects, and challenges. Am J Clin Nutr 2000; 71:1353S–1363S.
4. Rush D. Nutrition and maternal mortality in the developing world. Am J Clin Nutr 2000; 72:212S–240S.
5. Godfrey KM, Barker DJ. Fetal nutrition and adult disease. Am J Clin Nutr 2000; 71:1344S–1352S.
6. Jones SE, Nyengaard JR. Low birth weight and cardiovascular disease: myth or reality? Curr Opin Lipidol 1998; 9:309–312.
7. Wilson J. The Barker hypothesis: an analysis. Australian N Z J Obstet Gynecol 1999; 39:1–7.
8. King JC. Physiology of pregnancy and nutrient metabolism. Am J Clin Nutr 2000; 71:1218S–1225S.
9. Whittaker PG, MacPhail S, Lind T. Serial hematologic changes and pregnancy outcome. Obstet Gynecol 1996; 88:33–39.
10. Institute of Medicine. Nutrition During Pregnancy. Washington, DC: National Academy Press, 1990.
11. Hytten FE, Leitch I. The Physiology of Human Pregnancy. Oxford, UK: Blackwell Scientific Publications, 1971.
12. Prentice AM, Goldberg GR. Energy adaptations in human pregnancy: limits and long-term consequences. Am J Clin Nutr 2000; 71:1226S–1232S.
13. Lederman SA, Paxton A, Heymsfield SB, Wang J, Thornton J, Pierson RN Jr. Body fat and water changes during pregnancy in women with different body weight and weight gain. Obstet Gynecol 1997; 90:483–488.
14. Scholl TO, Stein TP, Smith WK. Leptin and maternal growth during adolescent pregnancy. Am J Clin Nutr 2000; 72:1542–1547.
15. Butte NF, Hopkinson JM, Mehta N, Moon JK, Smith EOB. Adjustments in energy on. Am J Clin Nutr expenditure and substrate utilization during late pregnancy and lactation. Am J Clin Nutr 1999; 69:299–307.
16. Butte NF. Carbohydrate and lipid metabolism in pregnancy: normal compared with gestational diabetes mellitus. Am J Clin Nutr 2000; 71:1256S–1261S.
17. Kalhan SC. Protein metabolism in pregnancy. Am J Clin Nutr 2000; 71:1249S–1255S.
18. Mojtahedi M, de Groot LCPGM, Boekholt HA, van Raadj JMA. Nitrogen balance of healthy Dutch women before and during pregnancy. Am J Clin Nutr 2002; 75:1078–1083.
19. Prentice A. Calcium in pregnancy and lactation. Annu Rev Nutr 2000; 20:249–272.
20. Kovacs CS. Calcium and bone metabolism in pregnancy and lactation. J Clin Endocrinol Metab 2001; 86:2344–2348.
21. Institute of Medicine. Dietary Reference Intakes for Calcium, Phosphorus, Magnesium, Vitamin D, and Fluoride. Washington, DC: National Academy Press, 1997.
22. Institute of Medicine. Dietary Reference Intakes for Thiamin, Riboflavin, Niacin, Vitamin B_6, Folate, Vitamin B_{12}, Pantothenic Acid, Biotin, and Choline. Washington, DC: National Academy Press, 1998.

23. Institute of Medicine. Dietary Reference Intakes for Vitamin C, Vitamin E, Selenium, and Carotenoids. Washington, DC: National Academy Press, 2000.

24. Institute of Medicine. Dietary Reference Intakes for Vitamin A, Vitamin K, Arsenic, Boron, Chromium, Copper, Iodine, Iron, Manganese, Molybdenum, Nickel, Silicon, Vanadium, and Zinc. Washington, DC: National Academy Press, 2001.

25. Institute of Medicine. Dietary Reference Intakes for Energy, Carbohydrate, Fiber, Fat, Fatty Acids, Cholesterol, Protein, and Amino Acids. Washington, DC: The National Academies Press, 2002.

26. Kopp-Hoolihan LE, van Loan MD, Wong WW, King JC. Longitudinal assessment of energy balance in well-nourished, pregnant women. Am J Clin Nutr 1999; 69:697–704.

27. Kopp-Hoolihan LE, Van Loan MD, Wong WW, King JC. Fat mass deposition during pregnancy using a four-component model. J Appl Physiol 1999; 87:196–202.

28. McDowell MA, Briefel RR, Alaimo K. Energy and macronutrient intakes of persons ages 2 months and over in the United States: NHANES III, Phase 1, 1988–91. Advance Data from Vitae and Health Statistics, No. 255. Hyattsville, MD: National Center for Health Statistics, 1994.

29. Herrara E. Implications of dietary fatty acids during pregnancy on placental, fetal and postnatal development. Placenta 2000; 23(suppl A):9–19.

30. Innes SM, Elias SL. Intakes of essential n-6 and n-3 polyunsaturated fatty acids among pregnant Canadian women. Am J Clin Nutr 2003; 77:473–478.

31. Dutta-Roy AK. Transport mechanisms for long-chain polyunsaturated fatty acids in the human placenta. Am J Clin Nutr 2000; 71:315S–322S.

32. Sanders TAB. Essential fatty acid requirements of vegetarians in pregnancy, lactation, and infancy. Am J Clin Nutr 1999; 70:555S–559S.

33. Ritchie LD, Fung EB, Halloran BB, Turnlund JR, Van Loan MD, Cann CE, King JC. A longitudinal study of calcium homeostasis during human pregnancy and lactation and after resumption of menses. Am J Clin Nutr 1998; 67:693–701.

34. Bothwell TH. Iron requirements in pregnancy and strategies to meet them. Am J Clin Nutr 2000; 72:257S–264S.

35. Allen LH. Anemia and iron deficiency: effects on pregnancy outcome. Am J Clin Nutr 2000; 71:1280S–1284S.

36. Steer PJ. Maternal hemoglobin concentration and birth weight. Am J Clin Nutr 2000; 71:1285S–1287S.

37. Yip R. Significance of an abnormally low or high hemoglobin concentration during pregnancy: special consideration of iron nutrition. Am J Clin Nutr 2000; 72:272S–279S.

38. Smallridge RC, Ladenson PW. Hypothyroidism in pregnancy: consequences to neonatal health. J Clin Endocrinol Metab 2001; 86:2349–2353.

39. Dunn JT, Delange F. Damaged reproduction: the most important consequence of iodine deficiency. J Clin Endocrinol Metab 2001; 86:2360–2363.

40. Calvo RA, Jauniaux E, Gulbis B, Asunción M, Gervy C, Contempré B, de Escobar GM. Fetal tissues are exposed to biologically relevant free thyroxine

concentrations during early phases of development. J Clin Endocrinol Metab 2002; 87:1768–1777.

41. King JC. Determinants of maternal zinc status during pregnancy. Am J Clin Nutr 2000; 71:1334S–1343S.
42. Osendarp SJM, West CE, Black RE. The need for maternal zinc supplementation in developing countries: an unresolved issue. J Nutr 2003; 133:817S–827S.
43. Tamura T, Goldenberg RL, Johnston KK, DuBard M. Maternal plasma zinc concentrations and pregnancy outcome. Am J Clin Nutr 2000; 71:109–113.
44. O'Brien KO, Zavaleta N, Caulfield LE, Wen J, Abrams SA. Prenatal iron supplements impair zinc absorption in pregnant Peruvian women. J Nutr 2000; 130:2251–2255.
45. Donangelo CM, Woodhouse LR, King SM, Viteri FE, King JC. Supplemental zinc lowers measures of iron status in young women with low iron reserves. J Nutr 2002; 132:1860–1864.
46. Zile MH. Function of vitamin A in vertebrate embryonic development. J Nutr 2001; 131:705–708.
47. Azaïs-Braesco V, Pascal G. Vitamin A in pregnancy: requirements and safety limits. Am J Clin Nutr 2000; 71:1325S–1333S.
48. Dolk HM, Nau H, Hummler H, Barlow SM. Dietary vitamin A and teratogenic risk. Eur J Obstet Gynecol Reprod Biol 1999; 83:31–36.
49. Salle B, Delvin EE, Lapillone A, Bishop NJ, Glorieux FH. Perinatal metabolism of vitamin D. Am J Clin Nutr 2000; 71:1317S–1324S.
50. Specker BL. Do North American women need supplemental vitamin D during pregnancy or lactation? Am J Clin Nutr 1994; 59:484S–491S.
51. Waiters B, Godel JC, Basu TK. Perinatal vitamin D and calcium status of northern Canadian mothers and their newborn infants. JAm Coll Nutr 1998; 18:122–126.
52. Nesby-O'Dell S, Scanlon KS, Cogswell ME, Gillespie C, Hollis BW, Looker AC, Allen C, Dougherty C, Gunter EW, Bowman BA. Hypovitaminosis D prevalence and determinants among African American and white women of reproductive age: third National Health and Nutrition Examination Survey, 1988–1994. Am J Clin Nutr 2002; 76:187–192.
53. Picciano MF. Nutrient composition of human milk. Pediatr Clin North Am 2001; 48:53–67.
54. Bailey LB. New standard for dietary folate intake in pregnant women. Am J Clin Nutr 2000; 71:1304S–1307S.
55. Scholl TO, Johnson WG. Folic acid: influence on the outcome of pregnancy. Am J Clin Nutr 2000; 71:1295S–1303S.
56. Honein MA, Paulozzi LJ, Mathews TJ, Erickson JD, Wong L-YC. Impact of folic acid fortification of the U.S. food supply on the occurrence of neural tube defects. J Am Med Assoc 2001; 285:2981–2986.
57. Hansen CM, Schultz TD, Kwak H-K, Memon HS, Leklem JE. Assessment of vitamin B-6 status in young women consuming a controlled diet containing four levels of vitamin B-6 provides an estimated average requirement and recommended dietary allowance. J Nutr 2001; 131:1777–1786.
58. Allen LH. Nutrient Regulation During Pregnancy, Lactation, and Infant

Growth. In: Allen L, King J, Lönnerdal B, eds. New York: Plenum Press, 1994:173–186.

59. Mock DM, Quirk JG, Mock NI. Marginal biotin deficiency during normal pregnancy. Am J Clin Nutr 2002; 75:295–299.

60. Zempleni J, Mock DM. Marginal biotin deficiency is teratogenic. Proc Soc Exp Biol Med 2000; 223:14–21.

61. Weijers RNM, Bekedam DJ, Smulders YM. Determinants of mild gestational hyperglycemia and gestational diabetes mellitus in a large Dutch multiethnic cohort. Diabetes Care 2002; 25:72–77.

62. American Diabetes Association. Position statement: gestational diabetes mellitus. Diabetes Care 1991; 14:5–6.

63. Kaiser LL, Allen L. Position of the American Dietetic Association: nutrition and lifestyle for a healthy pregnancy outcome. J Am Diet Assoc 2002; 102:1479–1490.

64. Acosta PB, Matalon K, Castiglioni L, Rohr FJ, Wenz E, Austin V, Azen C. Intake of major nutrients by women in the Maternal Phenylketonuria (MPKU) Study and effects on plasma phenylalanine concentrations. Am J Clin Nutr 2001; 73:792–796.

65. Villar J, Merialdi M, Gulmezoglu AM, Abalos E, Guillermo C, Kulier R, de Oni M. Nutritional interventions during pregnancy for the prevention or treatment of maternal morbidity and preterm delivery: an overview of randomized controlled trials. J Nutr 2003; 133:1606S–1625S.

66. Eustace LW, Kang D-H, Coombs D. Fetal alcohol syndrome: a growing concern for health care professionals. J Obstet Gynecol Neonatal Nurs 2003; 32:215–221.

67. Centers for Disease Control and Prevention, National Center on Birth Defects and Developmental Disabilities. Fetal Alcohol Syndrome.http://www.cdc.gov/ncbddd/fas. Accessed May 19, 2003.

68. Christian MS, Brent RL. Teratogen update: evaluation of the reproductive and developmental risks of caffeine. Teratology 2001; 64:51–78.

69. Leviton A, Cowan L. A review of the literature relating caffeine consumption by women to their risk of reproductive hazards. Food Chem Toxicol 2002; 40:1271–1310.

70. Neville MC, Morton J. Physiology and endocrine changes underlying human lactogenesis II. J Nutr 2001; 131:3005S–3008S.

71. Neville MC, McFadden TB, Forsyth I. Hormonal regulation of mammary differentiation and milk secretion. J Mammary Gland Biol Neoplasia 2002; 7:49–66.

72. Vekemans M. Postpartum conception: the lactational amenorrhea method. Eur J Contracept Reprod Health Care 1997; 2:105–111.

73. Institute of Medicine. Nutrition During Lactation. Washington, DC: National Academy Press, 1991.

74. Picciano MF. Pregnancy and lactation. In: Ziegler EE, Filer LJ, eds. Present Knowledge in Nutrition. 7th ed. Washington, DC: ILSI Press, 1996:384–395.

75. Butte NF, Hopkinson JM. Body composition changes during lactation are highly variable among women. J Nutr 1998; 128:381S–385S.

76. Koletzko B, Rodriguez-Palmero M, Demmelmair H, Fidler N, Jensen R,

Sauerwald T. Physiological aspects of human milk lipids. Early Hum Dev 2001; 65:S3–S18.

77. Kalkwarf HJ, Specker BL, Ho M. Effects of calcium supplementation on calcium homeostasis and bone turnover in lactating women. J Clin Endocrinol Metab 1999; 84:464–470.

78. Prentice A, Jarjou LMA, Stirling DM, Buffenstein R, Fairweather-Tait S. Biochemical markers of calcium and bone metabolism during 18 months of lactation in Gambian women accustomed to a low calcium intake and in those consuming a calcium supplement. J Clin Endocrinol Metab 1998; 83:1059–1066.

79. Dórea JG. Magnesium in human milk. J Am Coll Nutr 2000; 19:210–219.

80. Sian L, Krebs NF, Westcott JE, Fengliang L, Tong L, Miller LV, Sonko B, Hambidge M. Zinc homeostasis during lactation in a population with a low zinc intake. Am J Clin Nutr 2002; 75:99–103.

81. Chung CS, Nagey DA, Veillon C, Patterson CY, Jackson RT, Moser-Veillon PB. A single 60-mg iron dose decreases zinc absorption in lactating women. J Nutr 2002; 132:1903–1905.

82. Gartner M, Greer FR. Section on Breastfeeding and Committee on Nutrition. Prevention of rickets and vitamin D deficiency: new guidelines for vitamin D intake. Pediatrics 2003; 111:908–910.

83. Mackey AD, Picciano MF. Maternal folate status during extended lactation and the effect of supplemental folic acid. Am J Clin Nutr 1999; 69:285–292.

84. Christian P, Khatry SK, Yamini S, Stallings R, Le Clerq SC, Shrestha SR, Pradhan EK, West KP Jr. Zinc supplementation might potentiate the effect of vitamin A in restoring night vision in pregnant Nepalese women. Am J Clin Nutr 2001; 73:1045–1051.

3
Maternal Nutrition for Normal Intrauterine Growth

Chandra R. Jones and Lawrence D. Devoe
Medical College of Georgia, Augusta, Georgia, U.S.A.

I. INTRODUCTION

Maternal–fetal nutrition is a complex and interactive process. It is limited by the preconceptual status of the mother and continuously modified by many factors during pregnancy. Consequently, optimal conditions for maternal nutrition should be established prior to pregnancy. To maintain optimal nutrition for the normal fetus, the mother is expected to provide energy-supplying and nonenergetic nutrients in sufficient quantities.

The efficiency of this nutritional supply system depends on two factors: (1) the maternal adaptive physiological changes that occur during pregnancy, and (2) the effectiveness of the placental nutrient transfer. Placental transport and transfer functions maintain maximum efficiency until the 36th week of gestation, following which they gradually decline.

While the maternal fetal nutrition system can be impaired by many problems, the common end result of its premature compromise is restricted fetal growth. Deficient or insufficient amounts of certain key nutrients may produce developmental effects on the immune, hematologic, and central nervous systems.

This chapter reviews the following:

1. Normal maternal physiological changes in pregnancy
2. Normal intake and distribution of nutrients in the healthy fetus
3. Consequences of maternal–fetal nutrition disturbances and their impact on adult disease.

II. MATERNAL PHYSIOLOGICAL CHANGES IN PREGNANCY

A. Cardiovascular System

Extensive anatomic and physiologic changes occur in the cardiovascular system during pregnancy. These include slight cardiac dilation and an increase in maternal blood volume. Maternal blood volume increases as a result of a rise in plasma volume and erythrocyte mass. Cardiac output increases from 30% to 50% by 32 weeks of gestation. Between 14 and 20 weeks, the resting maternal pulse increases by 10–15 beats per minute (1). Central hemodynamic changes that occur during pregnancy have been measured and are shown in Table 1.

B. Hematological System

Plasma volume begins to rise at 6 weeks and increases to 1200–1300 mL (40% over nonpregnant values) by 30 week's gestation. Erythrocyte mass begins to rise at 10 weeks and increases more gradually than plasma volume. Red blood cell (RBC) count (normal 4.0–$5.2 \times 10^{6}/L$) increases by 18% in women without iron supplementation and by 30% by women receiving iron supplementation. The so-called transfusion of pregnancy accommodates the increased blood requirements of the placental bed and protects the mother from the consequences of blood loss during delivery. The disproportionate increase of plasma volume over red cell mass results in a paradoxical dilutional

Table 1 Central Hemodynamic Changes

	36–38 weeks' gestation	% change nonpregnant
Cardiac output (L/min)	6.2 ± 1.0	$+43^{a}$
Heart rate (beats/min)	83 ± 10.0	$+17^{a}$
Systemic vascular resistance (dyne $\cdot$ cm $\cdot$ sec^{-5})	1210 ± 266	-21^{a}
Pulmonary vascular resistance (dyne $\cdot$ cm $\cdot$ sec^{-5})	78 ± 22	-34^{a}
Colloid oncotic pressure (mm Hg)	18 ± 1.5	-14^{a}
Mean arterial pressure (mm Hg)	90.3 ± 5.8	NS
Pulmonary capillary wedge pressure (mm Hg)	7.5 ± 1.8	NS
Central venous pressure (mm Hg)	3.6 ± 2.5	NS
Left ventricle stroke work index (g $\cdot$ m $\cdot$ m^{-2})	48 ± 6	NS

Data are presented as mean ± standard deviation.
[a] $p < 0.05$. NS, not significant.
Source: Ref. 21.

"anemia" in which maternal oxygen-carrying capacity is increased in the face of reduced red cell volume indices. This laboratory picture is corrected within the first few postpartum days.

C. Gastrointestinal System

Most women experience an increase in appetite during pregnancy. Maternal dietary intake increases by 200 kcal/d to 300 kcal/d from the first to the third trimester, respectively. During pregnancy, gastric tone and motility are decreased due to the relaxing effects of progesterone. Nausea and vomiting complicate up to 70% of pregnancies, with a typical onset at 4-8 weeks postconception and gradual improvement through the end of the first trimester. Rarely, these symptoms may progress to hyperemesis gravidarum, leading to dehydration, electrolyte imbalance, and malnutrition if not treated appropriately with fluid/electrolyte support and antiemetics.

Pregnant women have greater risk of developing gastroesophageal reflux disease due to the physiologic changes involving the stomach and lower esophagus. Constipation is a common complaint, resulting from decreased motility of the small and large intestines. Gallbladder emptying time is also decreased during pregnancy, with an increased predisposition for the development of cholelithiasis. Total body protein and albumin concentrations are also decreased in pregnancy as a result of hemodilution, as noted in the hematologic system section. In the last trimester of pregnancy, maternal serum albumin levels may decrease by as much as 25% from prepregnancy levels.

D. Urinary System

Urinary tract changes in pregnancy include anatomic ureterocalyceal dilation and a functional increase in renal plasma flow and glomerular filtration rate. Creatinine clearance increases from nonpregnant levels of 120 mL/min to 150–200 mL/min during pregnancy. Changes in tubular function include an increase in the excretion of amino acids, bicarbonate, and calcium. Calcium absorption is doubled by 12 weeks of gestation, thus enabling the fetus to meet its calcium requirements. The early increase in calcium absorption allows the maternal skeleton to store calcium for the peak third-trimester fetal demand. Total maternal calcium levels decline throughout pregnancy as a result of the decrease in serum albumin; however, the serum ionized calcium level is unchanged.

E. Endocrine System

Pregnancy is associated with increased maternal levels of more than 30 different hormones (1). Table 2 illustrates the hormonal effects on nutrient

Table 2 Hormonal Effects on Nutrient Metabolism in Pregnancy

Hormone	Source of secretion	Effects
Progesterone	Placenta	Reduces gastric motility; favors maternal fat deposition; increases sodium excretion; reduces alveolar and arterial P_{CO_2}; interferes with folic acid metabolism
Estrogen	Placenta	Reduces serum proteins; increases hydroscopic properties of connective tissue; affects thyroid function; interferes with folic acid metabolism
Human placental lactogen (HPL)	Placenta	Elevates blood glucose from breakdown of glycogen
Human chorionic thyrotropin (HCT)	Placenta	Stimulates production of thyroid hormones
Human growth hormone (HGH)	Anterior pituitary	Elevates blood glucose; stimulates growth of long bones; promotes nitrogen retention
Thyroid-stimulating hormone (TSH)	Anterior pituitary	Stimulates secretion of thyroxine; increases uptake of iodine by thyroid gland
Thyroxine	Thyroid	Regulates rate of cellular oxidation (basal metabolism)
Parathyroid hormone (PTH)	Parathyroid	Promotes calcium resorption from bone; increases calcium absorption; promotes urinary excretion of phosphate
Calcitonin (CT)	Thyroid	Inhibits calcium resorption from bone
Insulin	Beta cells, pancreas	Reduces blood glucose levels to promote energy production and synthesis of fat
Glucagon	Alpha cells, pancreas	Elevates blood glucose levels from glycogen breakdown
Aldosterone	Adrenal cortex	Promotes sodium retention and potassium excretion
Cortisone	Adrenal cortex	Elevates blood glucose from protein breakdown
Renin-angiotensin	Kidneys	Stimulates aldosterone secretion; promotes sodium and water retention; increases thirst

Source: Ref. 1, p. 70.

metabolism during pregnancy. Among those most relevant to maternal nutrition are those involving insulin secretion, which increases significantly with each trimester. This is needed to counterbalance the growing anti-insulinic influence of the placenta, which is maximal in the third trimester. As a consequence, the rapid increase in insulin secretion may lead some pregnant women to develop hypoglycemia and/or ketosis in the first trimester, if meals are missed or are separated by excessive intervals. With the increasing insulin resistance produced by the placenta, there is an approximate 3% risk for pregnant women to develop carbohydrate intolerance in the third trimester. This state of gestational diabetes can be successfully managed with a combination of diet and lifestyle modifications for most patients and rarely requires the use of exogenous insulin. If inadequately treated, fetal over-growth (macrosomia) may occur, which increases the risk for birth trauma.

III. PLACENTAL TRANSFER OF NUTRIENTS

The human placenta is of the hemochorial type, which brings maternal and fetal circulations into close relationship. The membranes that separate the maternal and fetal compartments consist of the syncytiotrophoblast, a thin layer of connective tissue, and the fetal endothelium (2). The fetus receives nutrition during the embryonic period by a histiotrophic phase. Following the embryonic period, the fetus receives nutrition by a hemotrophic phase (3). The histiotrophic phase occurs during the first two months of gestation. During this time the conceptus absorbs nutrients by phagocytosis and pinocytosis from ductal and uterine secretions. The hemotrophic phase occurs during the third month of gestation, at which time the placenta

Table 3 Exchange of Physiological Constituents and Other Substances Across the Placenta

Maternal-to-fetal transport	Fetal-to-maternal transport
Oxygen	Carbon dioxide
Water + electrolytes	Water + urea
Hormones	Hormones
Carbohydrates	
Lipids	
Vitamins	
Drugs	
Viruses	

Source: Ref. 2.

Table 4 Transport Mechanism and Substance Transported

Passive diffusion	Oxygen
	Carbon dioxide
	Fatty acids
	Steroids
	Nucleosides
	Electrolytes
	Fat-soluble vitamins
Facilitated diffusion	Sugars
Active transport	Amino acids
	Cations (calcium, iron, iodine, phosphate)
	Water-soluble vitamins
Solvent drag	Electrolytes

Source: Ref. 1, p. 79.

assumes the nutritive role and develops transport systems for the fetus. If the placenta does not function properly, it can limit maternal–fetal exchange and lead to pathologic risks to the fetus (2).

The estimated blood flow of the term placenta is 500 mL/min. The placenta demonstrates a low-pressure system, with pressure in the uterine artery of 70 mmHg and that pressure in the intervillous space of 10 mmHg. This high-flow-rate and low-pressure system favors maternal fetal exchange (2).

The exchange from the maternal to fetal circulation in the placenta occurs by passive diffusion and active transport systems. The exchange from fetal to maternal circulation occurs mostly by passive diffusion. Table 3 depicts the exchanges of vital substrates and nutrients that occur across the placenta. In considering these mechanisms and the nutrients that are involved, it should be remembered that the relative energy requirements of the transport modes can be rate limiting for a specific nutrient. Maternal conditions or disease states that produce increased stress for the fetus, such as chronic hypertension and complex insulin-dependent diabetes, can lead to reduced placental function and effective transport, in spite of adequate maternal nutrient and caloric intake (Table 4).

IV. NUTRITIONAL ASSESSMENT

The basis for continuing nutritional assessment should be established for each patient by her health care provider at the initial prenatal visit. Risk factors for nutritional deficiencies or generalized malnutrition begin by identifying

Table 5 Nutritional Risk Factors for Women of Reproductive Age

Low income	Adolescence
Cigarette smoking	Substance abuse
Frequent dieting, fasting, or meal skipping	Vegan (complete vegetarian) diet
Pica	High parity
Menorrhagia	Physical or mental illness, including depression
Use of certain medications, phenytoin	Mental retardation
Decreased sense of smell or taste	Problems with chewing, swallowing, or mobility
Elderliness	Disability
Cancer and treatment	Chronic diseases

Source: Ref. 4.

Table 6 Sample Questions for Basic Nutritional and Lifestyle History

What did you eat and drink yesterday?
Do you avoid any foods for religious reasons? For health reasons? Which ones?
Do you drink alcoholic beverages? How often? How much?
Do you take any vitamin, mineral, or food supplements? What kind? How much?
Do you exercise? What kind? How often?
Do you smoke cigarettes?
Has your weight changed in the past 5 years? How
Are you trying to lose (or gain) weight? How? Why?
How often do you skip meals?
Do you eat breakfast?
Does it bother you to know that you are going to be weighed?
Do you ever force yourself to vomit? Use laxatives or diuretics to lose weight?
Are you on a special diet? What kind? Why?
Do you have problems with planning and preparing meals for yourself and your family? If so, for what reasons:
    To little time?
    Poor access to shopping?
    Financial constraints?
    Lack of equipment and space for storing food or preparing means?
    Anything else?

Source: Ref. 4.

Table 7 Criteria for Referral for Nutritional Counseling

I. Weight or growth problems
   A. Infant
      1. Previous low-birth-weight infant
      2. Present intrauterine growth retardation or SGA
   B. Mother
      1. Overweight
         a. Pregravid obesity (>20% above ideal weight for height)
         b. Excessive weight gain (>7 lb/mo)
      2. Underweight
         a. Low pregravid weight (>10% below ideal weight for height)
         b. Inadequate weight gain (<2 lb/mo after first trimester)
         c. Excessive vomiting (sufficient to cause weight loss or ketonuria)
II. Diet-related anemias
   A. Iron-deficiency anemia
   B. Pica
   C. Vegetarian
III. Medical problems
   A. Gestational diabetes
   B. Lactose intolerance
   C. Alcoholism
   D. Drug use
   E.

Source: Ref. 4.

women with high-risk behaviors resulting from lifestyle, dietary concerns, and eating behavior, as illustrated in Table 5. A nutritional assessment questionnaire, easily incorporated into the routine prenatal visit, is illustrated in Table 6. [Tables 5 and 6 are endorsed by the American College of Obstetrics and Gynecology (4).] Once patients have been screened for nutritional history and special requirements, they should be referred to a nutritionist or registered dietician trained in maternal nutrition, as illustrated in Table 7. After assessing the nutritional high-risk patient, you can use Table 8 to determine the patient that requires hospital admission.

V. DIETARY GUIDELINES

During pregnancy, there is a change in nutritional requirements from the prepregnant state that necessitates changes in caloric intake and dietary supplement dosages. A good starting point for maintaining healthy maternal

Table 8 Guidelines for Admission for Maternal Malnutrition

1. Weight loss of 10% or more of pregravid weight during the first trimester
2. Inadequate net weight gain (less than 10 pounds) by 30 weeks' gestation
3. Hyperemesis gravidarum, as defined by meeting two of the following criteria:
   a. Inability to retain any solid or liquid food
   b. Abnormal electrolytes (especially chlorides); acidosis
   c. Acetonuria
   d. Weight loss or no gain by 12 weeks' gestation or later
   e. Failure of drug therapy
4. Discrepancy between size and dates of 2 weeks or more at 20 weeks gestation or later with weight loss or failure to gain

Source: Ref. 8.

nutritional status throughout pregnancy can be addressed with reference to the Food Guide Pyramid, supplemented with appropriate vitamins and minerals (5). Attention to the dietary principles listed that follow should accompany advice on avoidance of known teratogenic and/or toxic agents that might be consumed during pregnancy (alcoholic beverages or excessive Vitamin A intake).

There is justifiable concern that many women of reproductive age engage in suboptimal or poor dietary practices. Despite access to adequate nutrition, many patients also are hampered by lack of nutritional knowledge, limited resources, and social inequalities (6). Women under 18 years of age have greater pregnancy nutritional requirements, secondary to the growth and development of normal adolescence. Compounded by erratic eating patterns and lower dietary intake, these patients are very often nutritionally disadvantaged (7).

On a daily basis, women should be encouraged to eat a minimum of three servings from the dairy food group, two to four servings from the fruit food group, six to eleven servings from the grain products food group, two to three servings from the protein food group, and three to five servings from the vegetable food group (4). Typical servings and foodstuffs are shown in Table 9.

VI. RECOMMENDED DIETARY ALLOWANCES

The recommended dietary allowances (RDAs) are the current United States standards for prescribing a balanced diet during pregnancy (8). The Food and Nutrition Board of the National Academy of Sciences in its first edition of the recommended dietary allowances (1943) included only 10 nutrients, while the

Table 9 Daily Food Guide

Food group	Servings/day	Serving size
Dairy	3	1 cup milk or yogurt
		2 oz process cheese
		1 1/2 cup ice cream
		3 oz tofu
Fruits	2–4	6 oz fruit juice
		1 medium orange or 1/2 grapefruit
		1/4 cantaloupe or mango
Grain products	6–11	1 slice bread
		1 oz dry cereal
		1/2 cup cooked rice, cereal, or pasta
		1/2 bagel or roll
Protein foods	2–3	2–3 oz cooked lean meat, poultry or fish
		1 egg
		2 tbsp peanut butter
		1/2 cup cooked dry beans
Vegetables	3–5	1/2 cup cooked or 1 cup raw spinach
		6 oz vegetable juice
		1/2 cup cooked greens
		1/2 cup sliced vegetables

Source: Ref. 22.

1992 edition includes 19 nutrients. RDAs are based on the best evidence from indirect estimates and metabolic balance studies and have been calculated in the absence of environmental, lifestyle, or health factors. Nutrient requirements during pregnancy are set at slightly higher levels than standard RDAs to prevent nutritional deficiencies during pregnancy. These higher RDA levels encompass individual variations in digestion, absorption, and utilization of vitamins and minerals. It should be clearly recognized that certain of the nutrients, including vitamins A, B_6, C, and D, iron, and zinc, can exert toxic effects when consumed in excess (9).

A. Vitamins

The RDAs for the standard vitamin supplements are shown in Table 10.

1. Vitamin A

The RDA is unchanged during pregnancy. Vitamin A is obtained from animal sources as retinol and from vegetable sources as beta-carotene. Both sources

Table 10 Recommended Daily Allowances for Vitamins and Minerals

Nutrient	Nonpregnant	Pregnancy	Percent increase	Lactation
Vitamins				
Vitamin A (μg RE)[a]	800	800	No change	1,300
Vitamin D (μg)	5	10	+50	10
Vitamin E (mg TE)	8	10	+25	10
Vitamin C (mg)	60	70	+17	95
Vitamin B_{12} (μg)	2.0	2.2	+10	2.6
Vitamin B_6 (mg)	1.6	2.2	+38	2.2
Folate (μg)	180	400	+122	280
Minerals				
Calcium (mg)	800	1,200	+50	1,200
Iron (mg)	15	30	+50	15
Magnesium (mg)	280	320	+14	355
Zinc (mg)	12	15	+25	19
Iodine (μg)	150	175	+17	200
Selenium (μg)	55	65	+18	75

[a] RE = retinal equivalent.
Source: Ref. 12.

are converted to retinal in the gastrointestinal tract. Vitamin A activity in foods is expressed as retinal equivalents (RE). The RDA for vitamin A retinal is 800 (RE), or 2700 IU. The RDA for vitamin A beta-carotene is 4800 μg. Foods rich in vitamin A include liver, fish, milk, carrots, and dark green leafy vegetables. Beta-carotene has not been associated with toxicity and is the form contained in most multivitamin supplements. Toxic effects are associated with daily intakes exceeding 15,000 RE (retinal and retinyl esters). Isotretinoin, a synthetic derivative of vitamin A (Accutane) can cause facial, cardiac, and growth abnormalities. Routine supplementation is not recommended. In cases where vitamin A may not be adequate, as in strict vegetarians, supplementation should not exceed 5000 IU per day (10).

2. Vitamin B_6

The RDA increases 38% during pregnancy, from 1.6 mg to 2.2 mg during pregnancy and lactation. This vitamin is required for protein, carbohydrate, and lipid metabolism. Its placental transport results in fetal blood concentrations that are two to five times higher than those in the maternal blood. This vitamin is found in meats, liver, and enriched grains. Pregnant women who are substance abusers, adolescents, and/or carry multifetal gestations (4) should receive a multivitamin containing 2 mg of vitamin B_6. Toxic effects in the nonpregnant patient can result in sensory neuropathy with ingestions of >500 mg/d (10).

3. Vitamin B$_{12}$ (Cyanocobalamin)

The RDA increases from 2.0 µg (nonpregnant) to 2.2 µg during pregnancy and 2.6 µg during lactation. Vitamin B$_{12}$ is necessary for normal cell division and protein synthesis. This vitamin is found in animal products. It is recommended that strict vegetarians supplement with 2 µg/day (10). Deficiency of vitamin B$_{12}$ can cause megaloblastic anemia.

4. Vitamin C

The RDA increases from 60 mg/d in nonpregnant women to 70 mg/d during pregnancy and 95 mg/d during lactation. This vitamin functions as a chemical reducing agent and is essential for hydroxylation reactions that require molecular oxygen. Dietary sources include fruits and vegetables. Vitamin C deficiency can lead to newborn scurvy. Pregnant women who are cigarette smokers or alcohol abusers or who have multiple gestations (4) require higher amounts of vitamin C and should supplement with 50 mg/d (11).

5. Vitamin D (Calciferol)

The RDA increases from 5 µg (200 IU) to 10 µg (400 IU) during pregnancy. This vitamin is essential for proper formation of skeleton and mineral homeostasis. Exposure of skin to ultraviolet light catalyzes the synthesis of vitamin D$_3$ (cholecalciferol). Fortified foods like processed cow's milk are the major dietary source of vitamin D. Toxic effects have been documented with daily intakes of 45 µg (1800 IU) per day and include deposition of calcium in soft tissues and irreversible renal and cardiovascular damage (10).

6. Vitamin E (Alpha-Tocopherol)

The RDA increases from 8 mg to 10 mg during pregnancy. The main function of vitamin E is to prevent cellular membrane damage with subsequent neurologic manifestations. The main dietary sources are vegetable oils, wheat, nuts, and dark green leafy vegetables. No reports have linked toxic doses to congenital anomalies (10).

7. Folic Acid

The RDA increases from 180 µg to 400 µg during pregnancy. Folic acid is one of the B-complex vitamins that must be increased more than any other nutrient during pregnancy (10). This vitamin is necessary for amino acid metabolism, nucleic acid synthesis, cell division, and protein synthesis. Dietary sources include liver, leafy vegetables, legumes, and fruits. Low folic acid intake and maternal conditions leading to a low folic acid status are associated with an increased risk of neural-tube defects (NTDs). The average American consumes 0.2 mg of folic acid daily. The CDC recommends all women who are capable of becoming pregnant consume 0.4 mg of folic acid/day. It is recommended that a patient with a prior pregnancy complicated by NTD consume 4 mg daily of folic acid. This increase in folic acid should occur one month before conception through the first 3 months of gestation (4,10). This unscores the need for education among women of childbearing age. Fortification of foods that has been accomplished, by itself, will not satisfy this increased requirement.

B. Minerals

The RDAs for minerals are shown in Table 10.

1. Calcium

The RDA increases from 800 mg in the nonpregnant state to 1200 mg during pregnancy and lactation. Calcium is essential for nerve conduction, bone maintenance and formation, muscle contraction, and membrane permeability. Dietary sources include green leafy vegetables, fish (cooked salmon and sardines), and fortified foods. High intake may inhibit the absorption of iron and zinc and result in deterioration of renal function. Calcium supplements are available as calcium citrate or calcium carbonate in 200- to 500-mg tablets. Calcium-rich antacids contain 500 mg of calcium carbonate per tablet and can be taken two to three times per day with meals for maximum absorption (10).

During pregnancy the fetus accumulates 30 g of calcium at the rate of 1.5 g by 20 weeks, 10 g by 30 weeks, and 30 g by 40 weeks. Calcium is actively transported across a concentration gradient in the placenta. The large amount of calcium needed by the fetus is provided by increasing maternal calcium absorption, which doubles by 24 weeks and remains at this level until term (10).

2. Iron

The RDA increases from 15 mg in the nonpregnant state to 30 mg during pregnancy (Table 11). The average daily iron intake of American women is 10 mg. Iron, an essential nutrient, is a constituent in hemoglobin, myoglobin, and various enzyme systems. The iron requirement for a singleton pregnancy is approximately 1000 mg (500 mg for RBC mass, 300 mg for fetus, 200 mg for mother). Menstruating women have total body iron of 2–2.5 g and iron stores

Table 11 Maternal and Fetal Iron Balances

Input		Output	
Stores		Increased requirement	
Normal adult female iron stores (total)	2 g	Maternal red blood cell mass	450 mg
Red blood cells (60–70%)	1.2–1.4 g	Fetus (single), placenta, cord	360 mg
Liver, spleen, bone marrow (10–30%)	0.3 g	Total	810 mg
Other cell compounds (remainder)		Lactation (daily)	0.5–1.0 mg
Diet		Losses	
Average absorption (280 days)	1.3–2.6 mg/day	Gastrointestinal, renal, sweat (280 days)	0.5–1.0 mg/d
Supplementation		Delivery	
Daily iron supplement	30–60 mg	Vaginal	200–250 mg
Ferrous sulfate	12–25%	Cesarean	140 mg
Ferrous fumarate	33%		
Ferrous gluconate	11%		

Source: Ref. 1, p. 242.

of 300 mg. When body stores are normal, 10% of ingested iron is absorbed in the duodenum. Normal absorption in pregnancy is 3.5 mg/d and can reach 7 mg/d in iron-deficient patients (10). Iron metabolism is unique because no physiological mechanism for regulating its increases or decreases in its excretion exists.

C. Protein

Nonpregnant protein requirements of 50 gm/d increase to 60 g or 1 g/kg/day (Table 12). According to the U.S. Department of Agriculture's 1985 Con-

Table 12 RDA Recommendations for Protein

	Nonpregnant	Pregnancy	Percent increase	Lactation
Protein (g)	48–50	60	10	65

Source: Ref. 12.

tinuing Survey of Food Intake by Individuals (CSFII), the average protein intake is 59–62 g/day.

D. Milk

Milk and milk products are considered the primary sources of dietary calcium. It is recommended that 500 mL milk be consumed per day in skimmed or semiskimmed form in order to reduce the intake of energy in the form of lipids (Table 13).

A significant number of pregnant women may be unable to digest varying amounts of milk due to insufficient production of the enzyme lactase (10). Lactase is located on the brush border of the small intestine. Insufficient quantities allow lactose to enter the jejunum. Lactose is slowly hydrolyzed and absorbed, and the excess sugar is transported to the large intestine, where it increases the osmolarity of the intestinal fluid and draws water from the surrounding tissues into the intestinal lumen. The undigested lactose is also fermented by bacteria and produces carbon dioxide, hydrogen, and lactic, pyruvic, and acetic acids. These products, along with a large water load, lead to the symptoms of lactose intolerance: abdominal cramps, bloating, flatulence, and diarrhea. Lactose-reducing tablets and lactose-free products are available and should be incorporated into the diet of such patients.

E. Energy Requirements

Energy requirements are increased by 150 kcal/d during the first trimester, 350 kcal/d during the second and third trimesters, and 500 kcal/d during lactation (Table 14). It is important to consider the progressive increase in caloric requirements in normal pregnancy in dietary counseling of patients, for caloric insufficiencies in the last trimester of pregnancy have been shown to impair fetal somatic growth. In addition, special populations, such as adolescents, will have caloric requirements that may exceed these threshold levels per trimester.

Table 13 Fat Content in Milk

	Gram of fat/100 mL
Whole milk	3.2
Semiskimmed milk	1.6
Skimmed milk	0.5

Source: Ref. 23.

Table 14 Energy Requirements

	kcal/d
1st trimester	150
2nd and 3rd trimesters	350
Lactation	500

Source: Ref. 24.

VII. WEIGHT GAIN DURING PREGNANCY

In 1990 the Institute of Medicine established guidelines to assess weight gain in pregnancy. This expert panel reviewed large observational studies of weight gain during pregnancy and the epidemiologic data on prematurity, fetal death, and low birth weight. They concluded that poor maternal weight gain increases the risk for adverse perinatal outcomes (13). In 1993 the American College of Obstetrics and Gynecology issued Technical Bulletin 179 supporting these guidelines (shown in Table 15). While inadequate weight gain may be linked to low birth weight, it should be noted that excessive weight gain may predispose fetuses to overgrowth and the attendant complications of macrosomia.

VIII. EVALUATION OF FETAL GROWTH

Clinical determination of fetal size is evaluated at each prenatal care visit. The most common and objective method of making this assessment is to measure

Table 15 Weight Gain Recommendations in Pregnancy

Food and Nutrition Board (1985)	Institute of Medicine (1990) ACOG Technical Bulletin (1993)		
20–25 lb (9.1–11.3 kg)	BMI < 19.8	28–40 lb	(12.7–18.2 kg)
	BMI-19.8–26	25–35 lb	(11.3–15.9 kg)
	BMI-26.1–29	15–25 lb	(6.8–11.3 kg)
	BMI > 29	15 lb	(6.8 kg)

BMI = body mass index = [weight (kg)/height (m^2)] × 100 = [weight (lb)/height (in.^{2})] × 705.
Source: Refs. 13 and 24.

Table 16 Average Fetal Growth by
Gestational Age

Weeks of gestation	Grams per day
14–15	5–10
15–20	10–20
20–30	20–30
30–34	30–35

Source: Ref. 15, p. 507.

the distance between the symphysis pubis and the fundus of the uterus. This distance, known as the *fundal height*, correlates with the gestational age of the fetus, in weeks. Ultrasound examinations are performed when the fundal height measurements are more than or less than 3 cm from expected norms. Average fetal growth is shown in Table 16. Mean peak rate for fetal growth occurs at 32–34 weeks, reaching values of 230–285 g/wk. Growth rate declines after 34 weeks, with weight loss commonly occurring at approximately 40 weeks (Fig. 1).

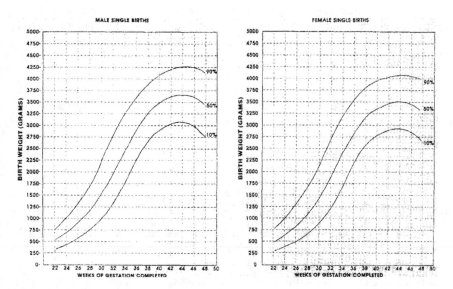

Figure 1 Fetal weight as a function of gestational age. (From Ref. 26; references in the art can be found in this original source.)

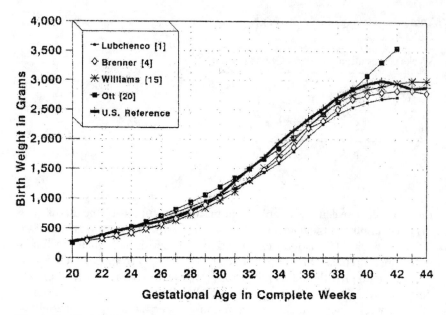

Figure 2 Birthweight percentiles for fixed gestations. (From Ref. 27.)

Fetal sonographic weight standards are estimated by evaluating multiple sonographic parameters. The most commonly used parameters are the biparietal diameter (BPD), head circumference (HC), abdominal circumference (AC), and femur length (FL).

Intrauterine growth restriction describes a fetus that is less than 10% for the estimated gestational age. Large for gestational age decribes a fetus that is under 90% for the estimated gestational age. Figure 2 presents mean birth weight curves for male and female single births, with the corresponding growth percentiles. Table 17 shows the estimated fetal weight by menstrual weeks, in percentiles.

IX. MICRONUTRIENTS AND ABNORMAL DEVELOPMENT

Several micronutrients have been linked to abnormal human prenatal development (Table 18). The review of the RDAs for most of these substrates were presented previously in this chapter. It is noteworthy that surveys conducted during pregnancy show that a significant number of women receive less than 70% of the RDAs for this category of dietary elements (14) (Table 19).

Table 17 Estimated Fetal Weight (in grams) by Gestational Age

Menstrual weeks	Percentile				
	3rd	10th	50th	90th	97th
10	26	29	35	41	44
11	34	37	45	53	56
12	43	48	58	68	73
13	55	61	73	85	91
14	70	77	93	109	116
15	88	97	117	137	146
16	110	121	146	171	183
17	136	150	181	212	226
18	167	185	223	261	279
19	205	227	273	319	341
20	248	275	331	387	414
21	299	331	399	467	499
22	359	398	478	559	598
23	426	471	568	665	710
24	503	556	670	784	838
25	589	652	785	918	981
26	685	758	913	1068	1141
27	791	876	1055	1234	1319
28	908	1004	1210	1416	1513
29	1034	1145	1379	1613	1724
30	1169	1294	1559	1824	1949
31	1313	1453	1751	2049	2189
32	1465	1621	1953	2285	2441
33	1622	1794	2162	2530	2703
34	1783	1973	2377	2781	2971
35	1946	2154	2595	3036	3244
36	2110	2335	2813	3291	3516
37	2271	2513	3028	3543	3785
38	2427	2686	3236	3786	4045
39	2576	2851	3435	4019	4294
40	2714	3004	3619	4234	4524

Source: Ref. 25.

Table 18 Micronutrient Deficiencies Postulated to Contribute to Abnormal Human Prenatal Development

Vitamin A	Vitamin B_6	Vitamin B_{12}	Vitamin D
Vitamin K	Folate	Copper	Iodine
Iron	Magnesium	Zinc	

Source: Ref. 14.

X. USE OF SUPPLEMENTS

Data from national surveys reveal that approximately 60% of pregnant women consume some form of vitamin–mineral supplements on a regular basis (10). A task force including representatives from the American Medical Association, the American Institute of Nutrition, the American Society for Clinical Nutrition, the Society for Nutrition Education, and the American Dietetic Association issued the following summary statement regarding the use of vitamin and mineral supplements in 1987 (10):

> Healthy children and adults should obtain adequate nutrient intakes from dietary sources. Meeting nutrient needs by choosing a variety of foods in moderation, rather than by supplementation, reduces the potential risk for both nutrient deficiencies and nutrient excesses. Individual recommendations regarding supplements and diets should come from physicians and registered dietitians. . . . Nutrients are potentially toxic when ingested in sufficiently large amounts. Safe intake levels vary widely from nutrient and may vary with the age and health of the individual. In addition, high-dosage vitamin and mineral supple-

Table 19 Proportion of Women Aged 19–50 Years with Intakes Below 70% of the 1989 RDA

Nutrient	RDA	<70% RDA (%)
Vitamin A	800 RE	54
Vitamin B_6	60 mg	62
Folate	180 µg	36
Calcium	800 mg	60
Iron	15 mg	70
Zinc	12 mg	57

RE = retinal equivalents.
Source: Ref. 14.

ments can interfere with the normal metabolism of other nutrients and with the therapeutic effects of certain drugs. The Recommended Dietary Allowances represent the best currently available assessment of safe and adequate intakes . . . and there are no demonstrated benefits of self-supplementation beyond these allowances.

XI. COMMON NUTRITIONAL COMPLICATIONS

A. Iron-Deficiency Anemia

Pregnancy imposes an iron demand on the mother. Iron deficiency anemia (IDA) is the most common nutritional disorder. The Pregnancy Nutrition Surveillance System of the Centers for Disease Control for 1987 indicated that the prevalence of IDA varied by race and trimester. Among white gravidas, the prevalence ranged from 3.5 to 18.8% and among black gravidas, from 12 to 38%. Decreased oxygen tension in the amniotic fluid and hypertrophy of the placenta leading to placental insufficiency may increase perinatal morbidity and mortality. Table 20 lists the cutoff values for IDA.

B. Neural-Tube Defects

Folate is the single nutrient that has been strongly implicated in neural-tube defects (10). Neural-tube defects range from anencephaly to lumbar meningocele with little or no neurological impairment. This defect results from failure of the neural tube to close within 28 days after conception (15). The incidence in the United States is 1.5–2.0 per 1000 births, 2–3% in a second child with one previous affected sibling, and 5% in a third child with two previous affected siblings (15). The outcome is poor, with high lumbar or thoracic defects, severe hydrocephalus, or other brain malformations and associated anomalies. Closure of the defect immediately results in 90% chance of survival.

Table 20 Cutoff Values for Anemia in Women

Pregnancy status	Hemoglobin (g/dL)	Hematocrit (%)
Nonpregnant	12.0	36
1st trimester	11.0	33
2nd trimester	10.5	32
3rd trimester	11.0	33

Source: Ref. 22.

XII. FETAL PROGRAMMING AND ADULT DISEASE

Maternal nutritional deficiencies that are associated with poor intrauterine growth have been shown to contribute to morbidity later in adult life. This effect, called *programming* by Lucas (16) "occurs when an early stimulus or insult, operating at a critical or sensitive period, results in a permanent or long-term change in the structure or function of the organism." Other literature (17) supports this hypothesis, linking fetal–placental development with the prediction of adult supports this hypothesis, linking fetal-placental development with the prediction of adult health and disease. Barker and colleagues have formulated a hypothesis linking coronary heart disease and other chronic adult diseases with an origin in fetal life (18).

The programming concept has shown that abnormal birth weight is associated with diabetes, hypertension, coronary heart disease, and obesity. Obesity is a persistent public health problem in the United States. The incidence of obesity among pregnant women ranges from 18.5% to 38.3% (19). With an increasing trend of obesity among U.S. women of reproductive ages comes concern regarding weight gain and weight retention following pregnancy. Several studies have linked postpartum weight retention and gestational weight gain with perinatal mortality. Obese women have a greater risk to develop carbohydrate intolerance, hypertension, and thromboembolic disorders (20). The rate of cesarean deliveries is one- to threefold higher than rates of control groups (19).

While other examples exist of linkages between prenatal development and the onset of disorders in adult life, it is clear that maternal nutrition can be an important modulator of fetal development and growth and the potential for acquiring disease propensities.

XIII. CONCLUSION

This chapter attempts to survey maternal dietary requirements during normal pregnancy. It summarizes some of the basic information on the roles of various dietary components and the complex maternal–placental–fetal inter- actions responsible for fetal growth and pregnancy outcome. While the tools for assessing the fetal impact of maternal nutrition are improving, there are many areas that require further study. For example, the measured dynamic of intrauterine fetal growth may not be as important as establishing the potential for fetal growth that is inherent in each pregnancy. The ability to know whether a fetus is achieving its growth potential is not yet possible.

Another important area for study is the actual dietary compliance of pregnant women who have been given specific dietary instruction and supplementation. Large population surveys indicate that this area remains problematic and that many patients receiving regular prenatal care do not maintain adequate nutritional programs.

Finally, the intimate and determining relationships between the timing of maternal nutritional events and pregnancy outcome are far from well established. With the exception of a limited number of teratogenic and/or toxic effects observed by timed deficiencies or excesses of macro- and micro-nutrients, the impact of shortfalls in other dietary components throughout pregnancy remain unclear. What is becoming apparent is that disturbed fetal development, which can have lifelong consequences, can be traced to inappropriate or inadequate maternal nutrition.

REFERENCES

1. Worthington-Roberts B, Williams S. Nutrition in Pregnancy and Lactation. 5th ed. St. Louis: Mosby, 1993:67.
2. Sastry BV. Techniques to study human placental transport. Adv Drug Deliv Rev 1998; 38:17–39.
3. McClellan R, Novak D. Fetal nutrition: how we become what we are. J Pediatric Gastroenterol Nutr 2001; 33(3):233–244.
4. American College of Obstetricians and Gynecologists. Nutrition and Women. ACOG Educational Bulletin 229, October 1996. Washington, DC: Compendium of Selected Publications, 2001:622–632.
5. Food Guide Pyramid from US Department of Agriculture, Human Nutrition Information Service, 1992.
6. Hally S. Nutrition in reproductive health. J Nurse Midwifery 1998; 43:459–470.
7. Berenson AB, Wiemann CM, Rowe TF, Rickert VI. Inadequate weight gain among pregnant adolescents: risk factors and relationship to infant birth weight. Am J Obstet Gynecol 1997; 176(6):1220–1227.
8. Reece E, Hobbins J, Mahoney M, Petrie R. Mother and Fetus Maternal Nutrition. Philadelphia: Lippincott, 1992:871.
9. Menard K. Vitamin and mineral supplement prior to and during pregnancy. Obstetr Gynecol Clin 1997; 24(3):480–498.
10. Luke B, Johnson T, Petrie R. Clinical Maternal–Fetal Nutrition. Boston: Little, Brown, 1993:123–142.
11. Institute of Medicine: Committee on Nutritional Status During Pregnancy and Lactation. Food and Nutrition Board. Nutrition during pregnancy: Part I, weight gain: Part II, nutrition supplements. Washington, DC: National Academy Press, 1990.
12. National Research Council. Recommended Dietary Allowances. 10th ed. Report of the Subcommittee on the Tenth Edition of the RDAs, Food and Nutrition Board, Commission on Life Sciences. Washington, DC: National Academy Press, 1989:284.

13. Johnson J. A critique of the new recommendations for weight gain in pregnancy. Am J Obstet Gynecol 1996; 174:254–258.
14. Keen CL. Toxicant exposure and trace element metabolism in pregnancy. Environ Toxicol Pharmacol 1997; 4:301–308.
15. Creasy R, Resnik R. Maternal–Fetal Medicine. 4th ed. Philadelphia: WB Saunders, 1999:1186–1187.
16. Lucas A. Programming by early nutrition in man. In: Bock GR, Whelan J, eds. The Childhood Environment and Adult Disease. Chichester, UK: Wiley, 1991: 38–55.
17. Curhan G, Willet W. Birth weight and adult hypertension, diabetes mellitus, and obesity in US men. Circulation 1996; 94:3246–3250.
18. Barker DJF, Hautvast J. Adequate nutrition in pregnancy does matter. Eur J Obstet Reproductive Biol 1997; 75:33–35.
19. Galtier-Dereure F, Boegner C, Bringer J. Obesity and pregnancy: complications and cost. Am J Clin Nutr 2000; 71:1242S–1248S.
20. Edwards L, Hellerstedt W, Alton I, Story M, Himes J. Pregnancy complications and birth outcomes in obese and normal-weight women: effects of gestational weight change. Obstet Gynecol 1996; 87(3):389–394.
21. Clark S, Cotton D, Lee W. Central hemodynamic assessment of normal term pregnancy. Am J Obstet Gynecol 1989; 161:1439.
22. Centers for Disease Control. Criteria for anemia in children and childbearing-aged women. MMWR 1989; 38:400–404.
23. Iams JD, Gabbe SG, Zuspan FP, Quilligan EG. Intrauterine growth retardation. Manual of Obstetrics and Gynecology. 2nd ed. St Louis: Mosby, 1990:165–172.
24. American College of Obstetricians and Gynecologists. Ultrasound in Pregnancy. Dec. 1993; ACOG Technical Bulletin 187. Washington, DC: Compendium of Selected Publications, 2001:846–854.
25. Hadlock FP, Harrist RB, Martinez-Poyer J. In utero analysis of fetal growth: a sonographic weight standard. Radiology 1991; 181:129–133.
26. Alexander GR, Himes JH, Kaufman R, Mor J, Kogan M. A United States national reference for fetal growth. Obstet Gynecol 1996; 87:163–168.
27. Williams RL, Creasy RK, Cunningham GC, Hawes W, Norris FD, Tashiro M. Fetal growth and perinatal viability in California. Obstet Gynecol 1982; 59:624–632.

4

Placenta as a Nutritional Unit

Puttur D. Prasad, Chandra R. Jones, and Vadivel Ganapathy
Medical College of Georgia, Augusta, Georgia, U.S.A.

I. INTRODUCTION

The major function of the placenta is the promotion of fetal growth and viability. One of the ways by which it achieves this goal is by ensuring adequate nutrient supply from the mother to the fetus, with the placenta representing the interface between the two. The exchange of nutrients, gases, and metabolic waste products between the maternal and fetal circulations occurs across this interface. In humans, the trophoblasts, which constitute the functional unit of the placenta, are not in direct contact with maternal blood during the early stages of placentation (until 10–12 weeks of gestation), and the nutrients for the fetal growth are obtained mainly from the secretions of the uterine glands in the endometrium (1–3). Thus, the fetus during early stages of development is said to have *histiotrophic* nutrition. With the completion of implantation and the development of the definitive placenta, direct contact between the trophoblasts and the maternal blood is established. From this stage onward, the fetus derives its nutrition directly from the maternal circulation and is thus said to have *hemotrophic* nutrition. Fetal growth and development are intimately linked to the transport functions of the placenta, which is a metabolically active tissue rather than a simple permeable barrier. While some nutrients are transported unaltered through the trophoblasts, the majority of the nutrients are either partially consumed or metabolized to other molecules by the placenta. In addition to the transcellular pathway of nutrient flux, the presence of extracellular/paracellular pathways for transplacental nutrient flux has also been reported (4–6). However, due to the lack of morphological evidence, the quantitative and qualitative importance of such pathways to overall nutrient flux is still a matter of debate. Transplacental transport can be classified into four groups: (1) *simple diffusion*: transport down a concentration gradient without participation of any transport protein and expenditure of metabolic energy; (2) *facilitated diffusion*: transport down a concentration gradient without the expense of metabolic energy but with participation of specific transport protein; (3) *active transport*: transport against a concentration gradient, mediated by specific transport proteins and driven by one or more forms of metabolic energy; and (4) *receptor-mediated endocytosis*: transport involving specific cell surface receptors and clathrin-coated pit- or caveolae-mediated endocytosis. Recent progress in molecular biology has yielded a wealth of new information on the mechanisms of transplacental nutrient transport and its regulation. The purpose of this chapter is to summarize the current understanding of the cellular, molecular, and regulatory mechanisms underlying the placental transport of important nutrients that are essential for optimal growth and development of the fetus.

II. PLACENTAL ARCHITECTURE AND ITS RELEVANCE TO NUTRIENT TRANSFER

The maternal–fetal flux of nutrients is greatly facilitated in the placenta due to the close approximity of the maternal and fetal vascular systems. The placenta is a highly vascularized tissue, with both the fetal and maternal blood currents traversing through it. The fetal blood flows through the capillary network of the umbilical vessels situated within the highly branched terminal chorionic villi, whereas the maternal blood flows through the intervillous space without participation of the capillary network. Uterine arterioles bring the maternal blood into the intervillous space, and uterine venules drain the blood from the intervillous space. These fetal and maternal blood circulations are separated from each other by chorionic villi, termed the *placental barrier* (7). Since the maternal blood directly bathes the chorionic trophoblast, the interface between the mother and the fetus in humans is of the hemochorial type. In humans, the "barrier" separating the fetal blood from the maternal blood consists of several layers of tissue, which include the trophoblast cell layer, the underlying basal lamina, the villous core containing extracellular matrix, the basement membrane, and the endothelial cells of the fetal capillaries (8). As gestation progresses due to the repeated branching of the villi, the trophoblast is placed very close to the fetal capillaries, resulting in the fusion of the basal lamina of the chorionic villi and the basement membrane of the fetal capillaries. This reduces the number of layers separating the two blood circulations to just three: the trophoblast, the basement membrane, and the capillary endothelium (7,8). Though the transplacental flux of nutrients involves transport across all of these layers, the flux across the villous trophoblast barrier constitutes the rate-limiting step. In the fully developed human placenta, the trophoblast barrier comprises a single layer of polarized multinucleated cells, the *syncytiotrophoblast* (7). It is a continuous epithelial layer directly lining the intervillous space of the placenta and is devoid of lateral cell boundaries, thus forming a multinucleated syncytium. The basal surface of the syncytiotrophoblast is loosely attached to the adjacent basement membrane and has clusters of irregular invaginations (8). The apical surface of the syncytiotrophoblast that faces the intervillous space has numerous microvilli and is therefore often referred to as the *brush-border membrane*. These microvilli increase the surface area available for maternal–fetal exchange and impede maternal blood flow over the trophoblast cells, thereby increasing the contact time available for the exchange (8). The syncytiotrophoblast is a polarized cell, and transport systems mediating the transport of various nutrients are localized to the apical and basal plasma membrane surfaces of the syncytiotrophoblast. The syncytiotrophoblast is formed by the proliferation, terminal differentiation, and fusion of cytotrophoblast, which form a continuous layer of cells immediately beneath the syncytiotrophoblast layer during early stages of placentation (9). However, by the third trimester, when the fetal growth is the maximum and transplacental flux is at its peak, the cytotrophoblast layer is no longer continuous. Thus, the placental architecture is greatly conducive to the efficient transplacental flux of nutrients, not only by bringing the two circulations to a close approximity, but also by increasing the surface area of the plasma membrane that is in contact with maternal blood and reducing the thickness of the barrier separating the maternal and fetal circulations.

III. METHODS USED IN THE STUDY OF TRANSPLACENTAL TRANSPORT

The mechanism by which the efficient transplacental transport of nutrients takes place has been a topic of intense investigation for several decades. The methods used to evaluate the nutrient flux across placenta include whole-animal studies that involve injection of tracer compounds into experimental animals followed by chronic maternal and fetal blood sampling (10–14), in vitro perfusion of placenta or its cotyledons (15–19), and incubation of placental fragments (20,21). These methodologies have made significant contributions to our current understanding of cellular processes that contribute to the transplacental transfer of nutrients. More recently, standardization of methods to isolate the maternal-facing apical membranes and the fetal-facing basal membranes from term placenta in the form of transport-competent vesicles have paved the way for the use of these vesicles for investigations of placental transfer of nutrients (22–25). Radiotracer uptake studies into these isolated membrane vesicles have made immense contributions to our current knowledge of the energetics and kinetics of several nutrient transport systems expressed in these two placental membranes. Availability of several human trophoblast-derived cell lines and standardization of techniques used in the isolation and culture of primary trophoblast cells have also helped to complement and confirm the studies done using placental perfusion and explant cultures (26–30). Finally, recent advances made in the cloning of various transporter proteins from placenta and trophoblast cell lines and functional characterization of these transporters in heterologous expression systems have led us to understand the mechanisms of placental transfer of nutrients at the molecular level.

IV. TRANSPORT MECHANISMS FOR MAJOR ORGANIC NUTRIENTS

A. Glucose and Other Monosaccharides

Of the several metabolically relevant monosaccharides, the transplacental transfer has been studied in great detail only with glucose (31–33). Transport of other hexoses (galactose, fructose, and mannose) and pentoses (e.g., ribose) across human placental membranes has been investigated to a limited extent, and these studies have shown that the transport of only aldohexoses is carrier mediated and that there is no carrier-mediated transport mechanism for sugars such as fructose (a ketohexose) and ribose (an aldopentose) in the placenta (34). Glucose is the primary substrate for placental and fetal metabolism and is thus one of the most important substances transferred across the placental barrier (35,36). The fetal requirement for glucose increases with increase in gestational age. In human pregnancy, the concentration of glucose in fetal circulation is a function of both gestational age and the concentration of glucose in maternal blood (37). The concentration of glucose in the maternal plasma is always higher than in the fetal plasma. Thus, there exists a positive concentration gradient for glucose in the maternal-to-fetal direction (37). Molecular studies have identified two different glucose transport processes in mammalian cells: a sodium-dependent active transport process driven by an electrochemical Na^+ gradient, and a sodium-independent facilitative diffusion process with no involvement of any form of metabolic energy (38,39). Studies using in vitro placental perfusion methods and isolated microvillous apical membrane vesicles of the syncytiotrophoblast indicate that the uptake of glucose into syncytiotrophoblast is Na^+ and energy independent but saturable and sterospecific (selective for the D isomer). This indicates that glucose uptake into the placenta occurs via a facilitative diffusion process (40–43). Similar studies with isolated basal membrane vesicles have shown that the transfer of glucose across this membrane is also a Na^+- and energy-independent process occurring via facilitative diffusion. There is no evidence of Na^+-dependent active transport of glucose in the brush border or in the basal membrane.

The facilitative glucose transporters in mammalian cells comprise a family of 13 members termed GLUTs (gene name SLC2A), which differ in their kinetic characteristics, localization, and tissue-specific expression (39). Though the expression of eight different members of the GLUT family has been documented in human placental tissue, available data indicate that GLUT1 is the predominant isoform contributing to the transplacental glucose transport (31,33). Immunohistochemical analyses and Western blot analyses have shown the presence of GLUT1 protein on both the apical membrane and the basal membrane of the syncytiotrophoblast (44–46). The expression in the apical membrane is, however, significantly higher as compared to that in the basal membrane (44,45). GLUT1, like other members of the GLUT family, is a facilitative transporter capable of bidirectional transport, and the direction of the transfer is determined by the direction of the transmembrane glucose gradient. Thus, GLUT1 in the maternal-facing apical membrane of the syncytiotrophoblast mediates the entry of glucose from maternal blood into trophoblast. Since GLUT1 is also located in the fetal-facing basal membrane, the role of this transporter in this membrane is to mediate the efflux of glucose from the syncytiotrophoblast into fetal circulation. This explains the positive glucose concentration gradient that exists in the maternal-to-fetal direction. Because the expression of GLUT1 in the basal membrane is less than that in the apical membrane, the efflux process across the basal membrane may constitute the rate-limiting step in the overall process of transplacental transfer of glucose (47).

There is also evidence for the presence of GLUT3 mRNA in human placenta (48). However, since no GLUT3 protein can be detected immuno-logically (45,46), this GLUT isoform is believed not to play a significant role in transplacental glucose transport. The reasons for the discrepancy between the GLUT3 mRNA and protein levels are not clear at present. Available evidence suggests that GLUT3 is not expressed in significant amounts in the trophoblasts but is the principal transporter in the vascular endothelial cells within the placenta (49). Insulin is the major hormone that regulates glucose transport, and GLUT4 is the major insulin-responsive glucose transporter. Though human placenta is rich in insulin receptors (50,51), transplacental glucose transport is not subject to regulation by insulin because the insulin-responsive GLUT isoform GLUT4 is not expressed in the syncytiotrophoblast (46). The lack of insulin sensitivity of placental glucose transport in syncytiotrophoblast has been demonstrated experimentally (52–54).

B. Amino Acids

Amino acids form a complex group of nutrients, which differ widely in their structure and ionic charge. This group consists of not only the 20 amino acids commonly found in proteins, but also the nonprotein amino acids, such as taurine. The plasma concentrations of all amino acids, with the notable exception of the two anionic amino acids glutamate and aspartate, are higher in the fetus than in the mother (55,56). This suggests active transport of most amino acids across the human placenta. Characterization of the amino acid transport mechanisms responsible for transplacental transfer has been the focus of research in many laboratories for more than three decades. These studies have identified in the placenta several classical amino acid transport systems that have been originally described in mammalian cells (57–59). Thus, a multitude of amino acid transport systems, with overlapping substrate specificities, are expressed differentially in the apical membrane and basal membrane of the syncytiotrophoblast. While some of these transport systems are passive, functioning either as uniporters or exchangers without the involvement of any driving force, others are active, energized by transmembrane ion gradients and membrane potential (60,61). The combined activity of these active and passive transport systems with their differential distribution in the maternal-facing apical membrane and fetal-facing basal membrane of the syncytiotrophoblast contributes to the net transfer of amino acids in the maternal-to-fetal direction. Recent advances in molecular techniques have significantly enhanced our knowledge of amino acid transport systems expressed in the placenta. Several recent reviews have attempted to put the process of transplacental amino acid transport into proper perspective by integrating the recent molecular information on mammalian amino acid transporters with the available functional data on placental amino acid transport systems (62–64). In spite of the significant progress made in this area, specifics of transplacental transfer of amino acids remain elusive because of the multiplicity of amino acid transport systems that are expressed in the placenta, the substrate overlap among these transport systems, and the differential location of these transport systems in the apical versus basal membrane of the syncytiotrophoblast.

1. Zwitterionic Amino Acids

The amino acid transport systems expressed in the placenta that recognize zwitterionic amino acids as substrates include the Na^+-dependent transport systems A, ASC, and B^0 and the Na^+-independent transport system 1. Of these, system A appears to play a major physiological role, based on the evidence for the regulation of this transport system by several hormones (65–67) and for a positive relationship between the activity of this transport system in the placenta and fetal birth weight (68–74). Functional studies using isolated apical and basal membrane vesicles have shown that system A is expressed on both membranes of the syncytiotrophoblast, though at much higher levels in the apical than in the basal membrane (75,76). Recent molecular cloning studies have identified three different isoforms of system A, ATA1–3 (77). Of these three isoforms, only ATA1 and ATA2 are expressed in the placenta. The localization of the system A isoforms on the apical and basal membrane of the syncytiotrophoblast and the differential role of these two isoforms to fetal growth and birth weight are not known at present. The other Na^+-dependent transport systems expressed in the placenta are ASC and B^0. Functional studies suggest that they are localized in the basal membrane (76). System ASC mediates the transport of alanine, serine, and cysteine. System B^0 mediates the transport of glutamine and asparagine in addition to alanine, serine, and cysteine. Both transport systems are obligatory exchangers capable of mediating the efflux of amino acids from the syncytiotrophoblast into fetal circulation (78). The transport proteins responsible for the activities of system ASC(ASCT1) and B^0 (ATB; also called ASCT2) have been cloned (79–81). Northern analysis indicates that while ATB^0 is highly expressed in the placenta, ASCT1 is expressed at low levels (80,81). Though a third Na^+-dependent transport system, system N, which transports histidine and glutamine, has been reported in the placenta at the functional level, molecular studies to confirm these findings are lacking.

System 1 is the predominant Na^+-independent neutral amino acid transporter in the placenta, where it functions as an amino acid exchange system. Functional studies have detected the expression of system 1 in both apical and basal membranes of the syncytiotrophoblast (75,76,82,83). Molecular cloning studies have identified two isoforms of system 1, LAT1 and LAT2, both highly expressed in the placenta (84,85). LAT1 and LAT2 independently complex with a second protein, called 4F2hc (CD98), to constitute the two different isoforms of system 1. Thus, the system L isoforms are called heterodimeric transporters, consisting of the heavy-chain 4F2hc and either LAT1 or LAT2 as the light chain (84,85). The functional activities of the LAT1/4F2hc and LAT2/4F2hc complexes can be differentiated based on their substrate specificity and pH sensitivity. Functional studies with purified apical and basal membrane vesicles indicate that the LAT1/4F2hc complex operates in the apical membrane, whereas the LAT2/4F2hc complex operates in the basal membrane (86). Recent studies have shown that additional Na^+-independent amino acid transport systems participate in the placental transfer of amino acids. These include systems t and asc. Functional studies with isolated brush-border membrane vesicles suggest system t is not expressed on the maternal side of the syncytiotrophoblast (83). However, the transcripts of TAT1, the gene which codes for system t, is highly expressed in the placenta (87). Likewise, northern analysis indicates robust placental expression of asc2, one of the two known isoforms of the transport system asc (88). Further studies are needed to show if these transport systems are actually expressed in the syncytiotrophoblast detectable by the presence of the corresponding proteins and transport function.

2. Cationic Amino Acids

Transport systems for cationic amino acids expressed in the placenta include y^+, y^+L, and $b^{0,+}$, all of which transport cationic amino acids in a Na^+-independent manner (64). The uphill transport of cationic amino acids mediated by these transporters is energized by the transcellular potential gradient (89). In addition to cationic amino acids, y^+L can mediate the transport of neutral amino acids in the presence of Na^+. The transport system $b^{0,+}$ is also capable of transporting neutral amino acids; but, unlike system y^+L, the transport of neutral amino acids via system $b^{0,+}$ is a Na^+-independent process. Transport systems for cationic amino acids are expressed on both membranes of the syncytiotrophoblast (89–93). Available functional evidence suggests that while y^+ is the predominant transporter in the apical membrane, the principal transporter in the basal membrane is y^+L. System y^+ consists of at least three subtypes, identifiable at the molecular and functional levels. These subtypes are known as CAT1–3 (94). Of these, CAT2 consists of two alternative splice variants, CAT2A and CAT2B. Transcripts of CAT1 and CAT2B have been detected in the placenta (95), and thus multiple genes may be responsible for the y^+ activity in the placenta. Expression studies using the cloned CAT cDNAs suggest that CAT2B is responsible for the y^+ activity on the apical membrane of the syncytiotrophoblast and CAT1 is responsible for the y^+ activity on the basal membrane (96). A fourth CAT (CAT4) has been identified that is highly similar to CAT1–3 (97). The transcripts for CAT4 are expressed abundantly in placenta, but the transport activity mediated by CAT4 has not been characterized. The amino acid transport system y^+L consists of two subtypes that are distinguishable at the molecular level (98). Both subtypes are heterodimeric transporters consisting of a common heavy chain (4F2hc) and a subtype-specific light chain (y^+LAT1 or y^+LAT2). Though y^+L activity is predominantly in the basal membrane of the syncytiotrophoblast, the heavy-chain 4F2hc is expressed predominantly in the apical membrane (92). This apparent discrepancy can be explained by the fact that 4F2hc is a common subunit not only for system y^+L but also for system 1. System $b^{0,+}$ is also a heterodimeric transporter protein consisting of the light-chain $b^{0,+}$ AT. In heterologous expression studies, the light-chain $b^{0,+}$ AT has been shown to complex independently with either 4F2hc or rBAT as the heavy chain, resulting in functional complexes with identifiable $b^{0,+}$ transport activity (99,100).

3. Anionic Amino Acids

The concentration of the anionic amino acids glutamate and aspartate is lower in fetal circulation than in maternal circulation (55,56). Perfusion studies have shown that anionic amino acids are not transferred from maternal to fetal circulation (17,101). Uptake studies using isolated apical and basal membrane vesicles have revealed that the Na^+- and K^+-dependent transport system X_{AG}^- is expressed in both membranes of the syncytiotrophoblast (102,103). Molecular cloning studies have identified a family of five genes, called EAATs (EAAT1–5), that code for X_{AG}^- like transport activity (104). Of these, transcripts of EAAT1–4 have been detected in placenta by Northern analysis (105,106). Since there is no evidence of net transfer of glutamate and aspartate from mother to fetus across the placenta, X_{AG}^- activity found in the apical and basal membranes of the syncytiotrophoblast mediate the uptake of these anionic amino acids from both maternal and fetal circulations for metabolic use within the placental tissue.

4. β-Amino Acids

Of all the amino acids, the concentration of the β-amino acid taurine is the highest in placenta, which is 100- to 200-fold higher than the concentration in maternal blood (56). A Na^+- and Cl^--dependent transporter expressed exclusively on the apical membrane of the syncytiotrophoblast is responsible for the highly concentrative uptake of taurine into the syncytiotrophoblast (107). This transport system accepts taurine and other β-amino acids, such as β-alanine, as substrates but does not interact with α-amino acids. Taurine enters the fetal circulation by diffusion down the concentration gradient across the basal membrane of the syncytiotrophoblast. The TAUT cDNA, which codes for the taurine transporter, has been cloned from human placenta (108). It is a member of the Na^+- and Cl^--dependent neurotransmitter transporter family.

C. Lipids

Although fetal tissues can actively synthesize fatty acids, the bulk of fetal lipid is derived from the maternal circulaton via transplacental transport (109). Early in gestation, the fetal lipids are derived largely from maternal circulation. But as gestation progresses, there is a gradual shift to de novo synthesis in fetal tissue (110). Knowledge of transplacental transport of lipids is scant. Triglycerides, as such, are poorly transferred across the placenta (111). In contrast, the concentrations of essential fatty acids (EFAs) and long-chain polyunsaturated fatty acids (LCPFAs), which are not synthesized by the fetal tissues, are higher in fetal than in maternal circulation (112,113). This indicates that there is a mechanism for preferential transfer of EFAs and LCPFAs across the placenta in the maternal-to-fetal direction. Recent progress made in the area of placental transfer of lipids in the placenta has been reviewed by Haggarty (112) and by Herrera (114). Available evidence indicates that maternal lipid and lipid metabolites may cross the placenta by three different mechanisms. The first of these mechanisms is the transfer of lipid metabolites as ketone bodies (acetoacetate and β-hydroxybutyrate). The concentration of ketone bodies in the fetal plasma is same as that in the mother, indicating that ketone bodies from maternal circulation are readily transferred across the placental barrier, where they may be used as metabolic fuel and for lipogenesis (115). One or more of the isoforms of the monocarboxylate transport systems, known as MCTs, are likely to be responsible for the transplacental transfer of ketone bodies. The second major pathway for lipid entry into the syncytiotrophoblast is via internalization of lipoproteins. Several members of the low-density lipoprotein receptor family, such as the LDL receptor, VLDL receptor, cubulin, and megalin, are expressed in the apical membrane of the syncytiotrophoblast (114). Lipoprotein lipase on the maternal surface of the syncytiotrophoblast acts on the triglycerides present in lipoproteins, releasing free fatty acids, which are taken up into the syncytiotrophoblast (114). Finally, fetal fatty acids are also derived from the direct uptake of free, nonesterified fatty acids in the maternal blood. Though fatty acids can freely cross the lipid bilayer by simple diffusion, recent studies have shown that proteins such as fatty acid–binding proteins and fatty acid transport proteins are involved in the uptake of free fatty acids into the cell (116). Campbell et al. (117–119) have identified a placenta-specific plasma membrane fatty acid–binding protein, which, unlike the ubiquitous fatty acid–binding protein, is expressed only in the apical membrane of the syncytiotrophoblast and binds preferentially EFAs and LCPFAs. This protein is likely to contribute to the accumulation of EFAs and LCPFAs in the fetus. The release of nonesterified free fatty acids from the syncytiotrophoblasts into fetal circulation is mediated by specific proteins present on the basal membrane (113).

V. TRANSPORT MECHANISMS FOR MINOR ORGANIC NUTRIENTS

A. Water-Soluble Vitamins

Water-soluble vitamins, which comprise a heterogeneous group of metabolic substrates and cofactors, cannot be synthesized in the human body. The fetus, therefore, depends on the maternal supply for its vitamin needs. There is sufficient evidence to show that placenta actively concentrates water-soluble vitamins and that the concentration of several of these vitamins is higher in the fetal circulation than in maternal circulation (60,120). In spite of the fact that vitamins are very essential for the normal growth and development of the fetus, the transport mechanisms for several of the water-soluble vitamins (e.g., riboflavin, niacin, and pyridoxine) have still not been clearly defined. In contrast, specific transport systems in placenta for vitamins such as ascorbic acid, biotin, pantothenate, folic acid, and thiamine have been characterized at the functional and molecular levels.

At physiological concentrations, ascorbic acid (vitamin C) has been shown to be transported by two different mechanisms. Dehydroascorbic acid, the oxidized form of ascorbate, is taken up into mammalian cells via facilitative glucose transporters, whereas ascorbate, the reduced form, is taken up via a Na^+-dependent transport mechanism (121). The circulating concentration of dehydroascorbate is very low, and GLUT3, the facilitaive glucose transporter, which accepts dehydroascorbate at a relatively higher affinity than do other GLUTs, is not expressed on the apical membrane of the syncytiotrophoblast. Therefore, the contribution by the GLUT-mediated uptake of vitamin C to the overall vitamin C uptake into fetus may be limited. On the other hand, the Na^+-dependent uptake of ascorbate is active, energized by an electrochemical Na^+ gradient across the plasma membrane. This transport system has an affinity for ascorbate in the low-micromolar range. Two different Na^+-dependent vitamin C transporters have been cloned and characterized (122,123). These are known as SVCT1 and SVCT2. Of these, only SVCT2 is expressed in the placenta, where it is located in the maternal-facing apical membrane. While SVCT2 mediates the entry of ascorbate into the syncytiotrophoblast from the maternal circulation, the mechanism of exit of ascorbate into the fetal circulation is not known.

The uptake of the vitamins biotin and pantothenate into the syncytio-trophoblast is also mediated by a Na^+-dependent, electrogenic mechanism (124). Uptake of biotin into apical membrane vesicles of the syncytiotropho-blast is inhibited by pantothenate (125). Similarly, uptake of pantothenate into these vesicles is inhibited by biotin, indicating that biotin and pantothen-ate are transported by a single transport system (126). Recently, Wang et al. (127) cloned a protein called sodium-dependent multivitamin transporter (SMVT) from the human placenta, which mediates the transport of biotin, pantothenate, and lipoate. Available evidence indicates the presence of an additional transporter that is specific for biotin in mammalian tissues (128), but the molecular identity of this transport system has not been established. Whether or not this biotin-specific transport system is expressed in the placenta is not known. The mechanism by which biotin and pantothenate exit from the syncytiotrophoblast into the fetal circulation has not yet been explored.

The transplacental transfer of folate involves at least two different proteins, a glycosylphosphatidylinositol-anchored folate receptor (FR), on the maternal surface of the apical membrane, and the reduced folate transporter (RFT), on the basal membrane. Of the three FR genes known to exist in humans, FR-α, the protein that interacts with folate with high affinity, has been shown to be expressed on the apical membrane of trophoblasts (129). FR-α binds folate and folate derivatives present in the maternal circulation and initiates the process of endocytosis. N^5-methyltetrahydrofolate is the predominant form of folate in the maternal blood. Once this folate derivative binds to FR-α on the apical membrane, it is internalized by endocytosis. Acidification of the endosomes results in the dissociation of the bound folate. The released folate is transported into the cytoplasm across the endosomal membrane by a transport mechanism that has not yet been identified. Folate then exits out of the syncytiotrophoblast into the fetal circulation via RFT. Both Fr-α and RFT have been shown to be expressed abundantly in human syncytiotrophoblast, and the cDNAs coding for the two proteins have been isolated from the human placental cDNA library (120).

Studies using the in vitro perfusion technique and isolated placental microvillous apical membrane vesicles have clearly demonstrated a carrier-mediated transport mechanism for thiamine in human placenta (130–132). Uptake of thiamine into placental apical membrane vesicles is stimulated by an outwardly directed H^+ gradient, suggesting that entry of thiamine into the vesicles is coupled to efflux of H^+ (132). Dutta et al. (133) in 1999 cloned a transporter from human placenta that exhibits thiamine transport activity in heterologous expression systems. The transport of thiamine via the cloned thiamine transporter (ThTr1) is stimulated by an outwardly directed H^+ gradient, as has been observed in the placental apical membrane vesicles. This suggests that the cloned transporter is likely to be responsible for the entry of thiamine into the syncytiotrophoblast from the maternal circulation. A second thiamine transporter (ThTr2), cloned more recently, is also expressed robustly in the human placenta (134). Since immunolocalization studies have not yet been carried out in human placenta for these two proteins, their exact role in the vectorial transfer of thiamine in the maternal-to-fetal direction is not known at present. Both ThTr1 and ThTr2 proteins share significant homology at the amino acid level to the reduced folate transporter, and thus all three proteins belong to the same gene family (135).

The concentration of cobalamin, also known as vitamin B12, is higher in the fetal blood than in the maternal blood, suggesting that B12 is actively transported across the transplacental barrier (136). Free B12 is impervious to plasma membrane. The mechanism of B12 uptake into the syncytiotropho-blast is similar to the mechanism involved in B12 uptake into other cells. This process involves receptor-mediated endocytosis of transcobalamin II (TCII), a 38-kDa plasma protein, which binds B12 with high affinity (137). A specific TCII receptor, which shows preference for the TCII–B12 complex over TCII, has been identified in placental membranes (138,139). In addition, megalin and cubulin, which also bind TCII along with other, unrelated ligands, are also expressed in the placenta (140). The TCII–B12 complex, internalized via receptor-mediated endocytosis is degraded within the endosomes, and the released B12 is transported into the cytoplasm by an unknown mechanism. B12 in the cytoplasm again complexes with TCII, and the TCII–B12 complex is then secreted into the fetal circulation across the basal membrane (141).

B. Lipid-Soluble Vitamins

The lipid-soluble vitamins, A, D, E, and K, are also not synthesized by the fetus and therefore have to be derived from the maternal circulation through transplacental transfer. However, unlike the water-soluble vitamins, the concentration of lipid-soluble vitamins in the fetal blood is generally lower than in the maternal blood, suggesting absence of active transport systems in the placenta for these vitamins. There are not many studies describing the transplacental transport of lipid-soluble vitamins. Vitamins E and K and, to a limited extent, vitamins A and D are constituents of serum lipoproteins, and therefore the same mechanism that operates for the entry of lipids into the placenta from these lipoprotein complexes may also operate for the entry of fat-soluble vitamins. Vitamins A and D are predominantly transported in blood complexed with specific plasma proteins called retinol-binding protein (RBP) (142) and vitamin D–binding protein (DBP), respectively. Megalin has been shown to bind and aid in the receptor-mediated internalization of these two proteins (140). Placental perfusion studies indicate that the placental uptake of retinol and 1,25-dihydroxy vitamin D_3 is enhanced in the presence of these binding proteins (143,144). The uptake of retinol in other cell types involves the binding of RBP–retinol complex to a specific cell surface receptor different from megalin, followed by the transfer of the retinol to cellular retinol-binding proteins (CRBPs) (145). This may provide an additional mechanism for the entry of vitamin A into the syncytiotrophoblast. The receptor for RBP (146) as well as CRBPs have been purified and characterized from human placental extracts (147,148). However, in immunohistochemical studies from 1999, though RBP was detected in syncytiotrophoblasts and maternal decidual cells in the basal plate, mRNA for RBP was detectable by in situ hybridization only in the maternal decidual cells and not in the trophoblasts (149). Similarly, immunoreactive CRBP I was detectable only in maternal decidual cells and villous stromal cells but not in the syncytio-trophoblast and cytotrophoblasts. Thus, though it is clear that the uptake of vitamin A into trophoblasts involves the interaction of the RBP–retinol complex in the maternal blood with RBP receptors on the microvillous apical membrane of the syncytiotrophoblast, subsequent steps involved in the entry process are not clear. Whatever the mechanism available in the syncytiotro-phoblast for the entry of lipid-soluble vitamins into the placenta from the maternal blood, there is evidence to indicate that the absorbed vitamins are packaged again to lipoproteins within the syncytiotrophoblast and are subsequently secreted into the fetal circulation.

C. Monocarboxylates and Dicarboxylates

Studies using isolated microvillous apical membrane vesicles indicate that the syncytiotrophoblast can take up both monocarboxylates, such as lactate, and dicarboxylates, such as the citric acid cycle intermediates succinate and α-ketoglutarate, from the maternal circulation (150,151). The lactate transport-er expressed on the apical membrane is Na^+ independent and energized by a transcellular H^+ gradient (151). A similar H^+-dependent lactate transporter has also been characterized in the basal membrane of the syncytiotrophoblast (152). Depending on the direction of the H^+ gradient and on lactate concen-tration, the transporter can mediate lactate transport in either direction. Since the fetus and placenta utilize glucose as the main energy source under moderately anaerobic conditions, a significant amount of lactate is generated by the fetus and placenta. Since the fetal blood is more acidic (pH 7.3) than maternal blood (pH 7.4), there is a H^+ gradient in the fetal-to-maternal di-rection (153). Since accumulation of excessive lactate in the fetus is detrimen-tal to the normal development of the fetus, the lactate transporters on the basal and apical membranes of the syncytiotrophoblast may actually mediate the elimination of lactate from the fetus to the mother (153). Recent molecular cloning studies have identified eight isoforms of monocarboxylate trans-porters (MCTs) that can mediate the H^+-dependent transport of lactate (154). Of these, isoforms MCT5 and MCT6 are expressed in the placenta. However, their differential distribution on the apical and basal membrane of the syncytiotrophoblast has not yet been determined (154).

The transporter for dicarboxylates expressed in the placental microvil-lous apical membrane is driven by a Na^+ gradient and can accept as substrates various intermediates of the citric acid cycle (150). At the molecular level, there are three distinct transporters that can mediate the transport of citric acid cycle intermediates (NaDC1, NaDC3, and NaCT); only NaDC3, the high-affinity dicarboxylate transporter, is expressed in the placenta (155). The transcripts of NaDC1 (the low-affinity dicarboxylate transporte) (156) and NaCT (the Na^+-dependent citrate transporter) (157) cannot be detected in the human placenta. Since the concentration of citric acid cycle intermediates in the maternal blood is in the range of 40–130 μM, and because of the favorable electrochemical Na^+ gradient across the microvillous membrane, dicarboxylates are actively taken up into the syncytiotrophoblast, where they are either metabolized or exported out into the fetal blood. The efflux of dicarboxylates into the fetal circulation from the placental syncytiotrophoblasts may be due to diffusion down the concentration gradient or may be mediated by organic anion transporters expressed in the basal membrane.

D. Carnitine

The concentration of carnitine, a metabolite that is obligatorily required for fatty acid oxidation, in the fetal blood is significantly higher than in maternal blood (158). This suggests that the placenta actively concentrates carnitine, despite the fact that the fetus and the placenta derive their energy predominantly from the oxidation of glucose rather than fat. However, immediately after birth, fatty acids become the primary metabolic fuel. Since the neonate has limited capacity for carnitine synthesis, the physiological importance of transplacental transfer of carnitine is to build up the tissue reserves of carnitine in preparation for the metabolic transition that occurs at birth. Studies done using purified brush-border membrane vesicles have demonstrated Na^+-dependent, high-affinity carnitine binding, suggesting the presence of a Na^+-dependent uptake process in the maternal-facing apical membrane of the syncytiotrophoblast (159). Subsequent studies done using JAR choriocarcinoma cells confirmed the presence of a Na^+-dependent carnitine transport system in the syncytiotrophoblasts (160). A protein called organic cation transporter N2 (OCTN2), which transports carnitine in a Na^+-dependent manner, was cloned in 1998 (161). Northern analysis shows the presence of OCTN2 transcripts in the placenta, which suggests that OCTN2 is the transport protein mediating the entry of carnitine at the apical membrane of the syncytiotrophoblast. The mechanism for the exit of carnitine from the syncytiotrophoblast to the fetal circulation across the basal membrane has not yet been explored.

VI. TRANSPORT MECHANISMS FOR INORGANIC NUTRIENTS

A. Calcium

The concentration of calcium (Ca^{2+}) in fetal plasma is higher than in maternal plasma (162), suggesting that Ca^{2+} is transported across the placental barrier by an active energy-dependent process. During pregnancy, the human placenta transfers about 30 g of Ca^{2+} from the mother to the fetus (163). The transplacental movement of Ca^{2+} during the late part of gestation is highest, coinciding with the time of maximal fetal skeletal mineralization, reaching rates of ~140 mg Ca^{2+}/kg body weight per day (163). Despite the magnitude and importance of transplacental Ca^{2+} transfer, the biochemical and molecular mechanisms of the transfer process are poorly understood. Ca^{2+} uptake studies using purified brush-border membrane vesicles have demonstrated that the Ca^{2+} entry at the maternal interface is a mediated process similar to that found in the intestine and kidney (60). The transport process is of the low-affinity and high-capacity type and is insensitive to inhibitors of the voltage-dependent Ca^{2+} channels, suggesting that the voltage-dependent Ca^{2+} channels are not involved in Ca^{2+} influx into syncytiotrophoblast. Members of another type of Ca^{2+} channel family, the L-type Ca^{2+} channels, have been shown to be expressed functionally in primary cultures of trophoblasts, indicating that the L-type Ca^{2+} channels may mediate the entry of Ca^{2+} in the placenta (164,165). In 2001, a new voltage-independent Ca^{2+} transporter/channel family (CaT channels) were identified (166). Two members of the family, CaT1 and CaT2, have so far been identified at the molecular level, both of which are expressed predominantly in Ca^{2+}-transporting epithelium, such as the kidney, intestine, and placenta. Therefore, available evidence suggests that both L-type Ca^{2+} channels and CaT channels play a role in the entry of Ca^{2+} into the syncytiotrophoblast. On the basal membrane, the high-affinity and low-capacity plasma membrane Ca^{2+} pump that is ubiquitously expressed in all mammalian cells has been identified as the predominant protein involved in the extrusion of Ca^{2+} from the trophoblasts into the fetal circulation (167). Of the four plasma membrane Ca^{2+} pump isoforms so far identified, isoforms 1 and 4 have been shown to be expressed in the human placenta by Northern (168) and Western analysis (169). In addition to the Ca^{2+} channels and transporters at the apical membrane and Ca^{2+} pumps at the basal membrane, intracellular calcium-binding proteins are also believed to play a role in the vectorial transfer of Ca^{2+} (170). Several calcium-binding proteins have been found to be expressed in the human placenta. These proteins have high affinity for Ca^{2+} and play an important role in keeping the levels of intracellular Ca^{2+} at low, nontoxic levels. To summarize, the current model of transplacental Ca^{2+} transfer involves the L-type calcium channel– and CaT-mediated entry of Ca^{2+} at the apical end, shuttling of cytosolic Ca^{2+} bound to intracellular calcium-binding proteins, and its extrusion through the basal membrane mediated by the ubiquitously expressed ATP-dependent plasma membrane Ca^{2+} pump.

B. Sodium

Na^+ is the main extracellular cation, and its transplacental transfer is a two-step process involving the entry at the apical membrane and its extrusion at the basal side. The concentration of Na^+ in the fetal blood is slightly lower than in the maternal blood, indicating that there is a weak gradient in the maternal-to-fetal direction (171). The entry of Na^+ into the syncytiotrophoblast occurs by three different mechanisms, all of which are present in both the maternal-facing apical membrane and the fetal-facing basal membrane, indicating that Na^+ entry into the syncytiotrophoblast can occur from both the maternal and fetal sides of the placental barrier. The first mode of Na^+ entry is as a cotransported substrate of Na^+-dependent solute transporters. There are several Na^+-dependent solute transporters, which utilize a transmembrane Na^+ gradient as the driving force, expressed on the apical and basal membranes of the syncytiotrophoblast. Significant amounts of Na^+ enter the trophoblast via these transporters. The second mechanism of Na^+ entry is mediated by the Na^+–H^+ exchanger (NHE), which mediates the exchange of intracellular H^+ with extracellular Na^+. In addition to a role in the entry of Na^+ into the fetal circulation, NHE also plays a role in the regulation of intracellular pH and volume of the syncytiotrophoblast and in the elimination of H^+ from the fetus. NHE activity has been shown to be present in both apical and basal membranes of the syncytiotrophoblast by functional as well as immunological methods (172). The NHE activity in the brush-border membrane, however, is several-fold higher than that in the basal membrane. There are several isoforms of NHE, of which NHE1, NHE2, and NHE3 have been shown to be expressed in the human placenta (172). While NHE1 is expressed predominantly in the apical membrane, NHE3 is the principal isoform in the basal membrane. The third mode of Na^+ entry into the syncytiotrophoblast is the conductive pathway in which Na^+ moves down its electrochemical gradient. The extrusion of Na^+ from the syncytiotrophoblast is mediated by the Na^+–K^+ pump, which is localized predominantly in the basal membrane (60).

C. Phosphate

Phosphate (P_i) is also an essential nutrient with important physiological functions. Its requirement in the fetus is highest during the third trimester of pregnancy, needed primarily for bone mineralization. The concentration of P_i in the fetal blood is higher than in the maternal blood, suggesting the presence of an active mediated transplacental transfer mechanism (60). Measurement of transplacental maternal–fetal flux of P_i using placental perfusion is complicated because of the high P_i content of the placental tissue. A limited number of studies have been carried out using isolated brush-border membrane vesicles, which indicate that the uptake of P_i at the maternal side is active and highly dependent on the presence of an inwardly directed Na^+ gradient (162). The affinity of this transport system for P_i is $\sim 250\,\mu M$, which is much lower than the concentration of P_i in the maternal serum. Under physiological conditions, the transporter is fully saturated and operates with maximal activity. Three different Na^+-coupled P_i transport systems, designated NaP_i-I, NaP_i-II, and NaP_i-III, have been identified at the molecular level (173). The expression of NaP_i-II is restricted to the intestine and kidney, where it plays a major role in the absorption of P_i. NaP_i-III, on the other hand, is ubiquitously expressed and therefore is believed to be involved in supplying the cells with P_i for the basic metabolic needs. The molecular identity of the Na^+-coupled P_i transporter that is expressed in the placenta is not known. There is little information in the literature on the mechanisms that participate in the entry of P_i from the syncytiotrophoblast into the fetal circulation. This process is likely to be passive, with the transfer occurring down the concentration gradient from the syncytiotrophoblast to the fetal circulation.

D. Chloride

Chloride (Cl^-), like Na^+, is the main extracellular ion, and it is transported into the syncytiotrophoblast by three distinct mechanisms (60,162). Based on studies using isolated membrane vesicles, a significant fraction of Cl^- flux into the syncytiotrophoblast is mediated by a 4,4′-diisothiocyanostilbene-2,2′-disulfonic acid–sensitive, electroneutral anion exchanger (60,162,174,175). The exchanger mediates the exchange of extracellular Cl^- with intracellular HCO_3^-, resulting in the coupling of the influx of Cl^- to the efflux of HCO_3^-. Though the exchanger has high affinity for Cl^-, other monovalent ions, such as Br^-, I^-, NO_3^-, and SCN^-, are known to be transportable substrates (175). The Cl^-/HCO_3^- exchanger, along with Na^+/H^+ exchanger, is believed to play an important role in the transfer of CO_2 from fetus to mother for elimination (176). The second pathway of Cl^- transfer across the brush-border membrane is voltage dependent and saturable, mediated by Cl^- channels (174,175). The third pathway of Cl^- entry is as a cotransported substrate of certain Na^+- and Cl–coupled solute transporters expressed in the apical membrane of the syncytiotrophoblast. Three such transporters—the serotonin transporter, the norepinephrine transporter, and the taurine transporter—have been functionally characterized in the placental brush-border membrane vesicles (60). The mechanism of Cl^- extrusion at the basal membrane is yet to be characterized.

E. Iron

The requirement for iron in the developing fetus is very high. At term, approximately 5 mg of iron per day is transferred unidirectionally across the placenta from the maternal side to the fetal side (177). The concentration of iron is higher in fetal circulation, especially during the third trimester, and thus maternal-to-fetal transport of iron takes place against a concentration gradient. Transplacental iron transport is not understood completely. While the mechanism by which iron is taken up at the maternal side of the syncytiotrophoblast is well described, the mechanism by which iron is extruded into the fetal circulation is poorly defined. In blood, iron is transported bound to the carrier protein transferrin. Transferrin receptor is known to be highly expressed in the apical membrane of the syncytiotrophoblast (177). Receptor-mediated endocytosis of iron-bound transferrin is the principal mechanism by which placenta takes up iron from the maternal blood (178). Acidification of the endosomes releases the bound iron, and the resulting maternal apotransferrin is recycled back into maternal circulation. Iron subsequently exits the syncytiotrophoblastic endosome into the cytoplasm by a carrier-mediated process. The divalent metal iron transporter-1 (DMT-1, also called DCT-1 and NRAMP-2) localized on the endosomal membrane is believed to mediate this transport process (179). How iron traverses the cytoplasm and crosses the basal membrane to get into the fetal circulation is largely unknown. Placenta is known to synthesize transferrin (177). One of the possible mechanisms of iron extrusion is the directional secretion of placental transferrin at the basal side of the syncytiotrophoblast. Transferrin receptors and DMT-1 have also been localized at the basal membrane, albeit at much lower levels than at the apical membrane (179). The role, if any, of basal membrane transferrin receptor and DMT-1 in iron extrusion is not understood at present. Transferrin-independent uptake of iron into syncytiotrophoblast has also been reported (177). The transmembrane enzyme NADH-dependent ferrireductase, which catalyzes the reduction of Fe^{3+} to Fe^{2+}, is believed to play a role in this transport mechanism. Since the ferrireducatse activity is highest in basal membranes, this enzyme is hypothesized to play a role in the extrusion of iron into the fetal circulation (177).

F. Sulfate

Sulfate is an essential nutrient utilized for the synthesis of sulfated mucopolysaccharides, proteins, and steroids and in the detoxification of drugs by sulfation (180). Measurement of serum inorganic sulfate in paired samples from mothers and fetuses at parturition indicate a small but significant gradient in the fetal-to-maternal direction (180). Uptake studies using human placental slices have shown that sulfate transport in placenta is mediated by a DIDS-sensitive anion exchanger (60). The exchanger has been functionally characterized in both apical membrane and the basal membrane using purified membrane vesicles. Uptake of sulfate into apical and basal membrane vesicles is not sensitive to the presence of Na^+ in the uptake buffer, is stimulated at low pH, and is electroneutral, with an approximate K_t of 2.5 mM for sulfate. The presence of an outwardly directed HCO_3^- gradient stimulates the uptake, suggesting that efflux of HCO_3^- may be coupled to the entry of SO_4^{2-}. Monovalent ions such as Cl^-, I^-, and SCN^- do not inhibit the transport of sulfate. Oxyanions of metals such as selenium, tungsten, molybdenum, and chromium inhibit sulfate transport by the exchanger, implying a role for this transport system in the transplacental transport of these physiologically important trace elements. Exchange of intracellular HCO_3^- with maternal sulfate at the apical membrane of the syncytiotrophoblast and the exchange of intracellular sulfate with the HCO_3^- in the fetal blood are believed to drive the transplacental transfer of sulfate. In 1999, a new Na^+-dependent sulfate transporter (SUT1) was identified, and SUT1 transcripts are expressed most abundantly in the placenta (181). The cellular localization and the physiological role of this transporter, if any, in transplacental sulfate transport are not known at present.

VII. GESTATIONAL-AGE DEPENDENCE OF PLACENTAL NUTRIENT TRANSFER

Fetal requirements for essential and nonessential nutrients increase with increasing gestational age to support growth. Changes in blood flow and placental size are insufficient to account for this gestational-age-dependent increase in nutrient transfer across the placenta. There is evidence to support the notion that the expression of various transporters for nutrients in the placenta may itself be regulated in a gestational-age-dependent manner. Since glucose is the primary substrate for fetal and placental metabolism, several studies have focused on the gestational-age dependence of the expression of GLUT1. Interestingly, the gestational-age-dependent changes in GLUT1 expression are evident only in the basal membrane, expression of this transporter in the brush-border membrane remaining unaltered throughout gestation (31). These studies have shown that the placental expression of GLUT1 increases with gestational age, suggesting that the enhanced transfer of glucose across the placenta with advancing gestational age is at least partly due to the increased expression of this transporter. Similar studies on the gestational-age-dependent changes in the expression of transporters for other major nutrients are sparse.

VIII. REGULATION OF PLACENTAL NUTRIENT TRANSFER

Studies on the regulation of the expression and function of various nutrient transporters in the placenta have been carried out only in vitro using primary cultures of trophoblasts, choriocarcinoma cells, and placental villous fragments. These studies suggest that many of these transporters are regulated by specific substrates, hormones, and signaling mechanisms (31,61). The expression of GLUT1 has been shown to be inhibitable by exposure of the placental cells to high levels of glucose. In contrast, insulin, IGF-I, and IGF-II enhance the expression of GLUT1, and this effect is associated with an increase in GLUT1 mRNA, GLUT1 protein, as well as glucose transport activity. In the case of amino acid transporters, substrate-dependent adaptive regulation seems to play a significant role in the regulation of system A. The transport system–specific substrates influence the function of system A by a protein synthesis–dependent mechanism and by transinhibition. This mode of regulation has been substantiated in nonplacental cell types, where amino acid deprivation leads to enhanced expression of ATA2 (one of the subtypes of system A) and amino acid supplementation suppresses its expression (182–184). Both the stimulation and inhibition of ATA2 are associated with appropriate changes in the steady-state levels of the transporter mRNA, protein, and transport function. The activity of system 1 in placenta is modulated by transstimulation and by calmodulin. Protein kinase C down-regulates the activity of the taurine transporter, most likely by a mechanism involving the phosphorylation of the transporter protein. Insulin, IGF-I, IGF-II, and epidermal growth factor enhance the expression and activity of system A. These data on the regulation of various nutrient transporters in placenta by substrates and hormones are certainly interesting, but the in vivo relevance of these data remains largely unknown.

IX. ABERRATIONS IN PLACENTAL NUTRIENT TRANSFER AND THEIR CLINICAL CONSEQUENCES

The capacity of the placenta to transfer nutrients from the mother to the fetus can be compromised by reduced uteroplacental blood flow as well as by decreased placental growth. Such changes are expected to have deleterious effects on fetal growth and development due to the decreased supply of nutrients. Apart from the changes in blood flow and placental size, alterations in the expression and activity of nutrient transporters under various pathological conditions may play an important role in the placental transfer of nutrients.

Diabetes has been shown to be associated with an increase in the expression and activity of GLUT1 in the placental basal membrane (185,186), suggesting that enhanced transfer of glucose across the placenta may underlie the macrosomic growth of the fetus often seen in diabetic pregnancy. Since the expression of GLUT1 in the brush-border membrane remains unaffected in diabetes, these data support the notion that the transfer across the basal membrane is most likely the rate-limiting step in the transplacental transfer of glucose. The findings on the influence of maternal diabetes on placental transfer of amino acids are conflicting. The activity of system A in placental brush-border membranes is increased in gestational diabetes mellitus (187), suggesting that enhanced transfer of not only glucose but also amino acids from the mother to the fetus contribute to the macrosomic growth of the fetus associated with maternal diabetes. However, Kuruvilla et al. (70) have reported that the activity of system A in the placental brush-border membrane was decreased in diabetic pregnancies, even though these pregnancies were found to be associated with enhanced fetal growth. Since the size of the placenta is significantly larger in diabetic pregnancies than in normal pregnancies, these investigators suggested that, despite the reduced expression of system A in the placenta, the transplacental transfer of amino acids is enhanced in diabetes due to the increased size of the placental tissue and thus contributes to the macrosomic growth of the fetus in maternal diabetes.

It has been generally assumed that decreased transfer of nutrients, due either to decreased uteroplacental blood flow or to maternal undernutrition, is sufficient to explain the decreased fetal growth in intrauterine growth retardation (IUGR). However, recent studies have shown that changes in the expression and activity of nutrient transporters in the placenta also contribute to the decreased transfer of nutrients to the fetus associated with IUGR (69,71–73,91,188). Interestingly, these changes are not generalized changes in all nutrient transporters. IUGR-associated decrease in the expression of nutrient transporters is specific, affecting only certain transport systems. The activities of system A and taurine transporter are reduced in placental brush-border membranes in IUGR (69,71,72,188), whereas the activity of glucose transporters remains unaffected (45).

There are several studies in humans and in laboratory animals that document the deleterious effects of abusable drugs on placental nutrient transfer. Maternal alcohol consumption compromises the transport of amino acids in the placenta, most likely by affecting the activity of system A (189). Similarly, tobacco smoking during pregnancy is associated with decreased placental transfer of amino acids (190). Direct exposure of placental villous fragments to nicotine also reduces the uptake of amino acids. Another abusable drug that has deleterious effects on placental transfer of amino acids is cocaine. Exposure of intact placental villous fragments or purified placental brush-border membranes to cocaine leads to a significant inhibition of amino acid transport (191). Ethanol consumption, tobacco smoking, and the use of cocaine by pregnant women are all associated with IUGR. The ability of these drugs to interfere with the placental transfer of amino acids may at least partly explain the deleterious effects of these drugs on fetal growth.

REFERENCES

1. Foidart JM, Hustin J, Dubois M, Schaaps JP. The human placenta becomes haemochroial at the 13th week of pregnancy. Int J Dev Biol 1992; 36:451–453.
2. Burton GJ, Hempstock J, Jauniaux E. Nutrition of the human fetus during the first trimester—a review. Placenta 2001; 22(suppl A):S70–S77.
3. Burton GJ, Watson AL, Hempstock J, Skepper JN, Jauniaux E. Uterine glands provide histiotrophic nutrition for the human fetus during the first trimester of pregnancy. J Clin Endocrinol Metab 2002; 87:2954–2959.
4. Stulc J. Extra-cellular transport pathways in the hemochorial placenta. Placenta 1989; 10:113–119.
5. Kertschanska S, Kosanke G, Kaufmann P. Pressure dependence of so-called transtrophoblastic channels during fetal perfusion of human placental villi. Microsc Res Tech 1997; 38:52–62.
6. Kertschanska S, Stulcova B, Kaufmann P, Stulc J. Distensible transtrophoblastic channels in the rat placenta. Placenta 2000; 21:670–677.
7. Benirschke K, Kaufmann P. Placental types. 3rd ed. Pathology of Human Placenta. New York: Springer-Verlag, 1995:1–13.
8. Enders AS. A comparative study of the fine structure of the trophoblast in several hemochorial placentas. Am J Anat 1965; 116:29–68.
9. Cunningham FG, MacDonald PC, Gant NF. The placenta and fetal membranes. 18th ed. Williams Obstetrics. East Norwalk, CT: Appleton-Lange, 1989:39–65.
10. Anderson AH, Fennessey PV, Meschia G, Wilkening RB, Battaglia FC. Placental transport of threonine and its utilization in the normal and growth-restricted fetus. Am J Physiol 1997; 272:E892–E900.
11. Bell AW, Kennaugh JM, Battaglia FC, Meschia G. Uptake of amino acids and ammonia at mid-gestation by the fetal lamb. Q J Exp Physiol 1989; 74:635–643.
12. Lemons JA, Adcock EW 3rd, Jones MD Jr, Naughton MA, Meschia G, Battaglia FC. Umbilical uptake of amino acids in the unstressed fetal lamb. J Clin Invest 1976; 58:1428–1434.
13. Li HQ, Gilbert M, Teng C, Jones RO, Murray RD, Battaglia FC. The uptake of amino acids and oxygen across the rabbit uterus in normal and postterm pregnancies. Biol Neonate 1990; 58:347–354.
14. Simmons MA, Battaglia FC, Meschia G. Placental transfer of glucose. J Dev Physiol 1979; 1:227–243.
15. Hibbard JU, Pridjian G, Whitington PF, Moawad AH. Taurine transport in the in vitro perfused human placenta. Pediatr Res 1990; 27:80–84.

16. Nandakumaran M, Harouny AK, Al-Yatama M, Al-Azemi MK, Sugathan TN. Effect of increased glucose load on maternal–fetal transport of alpha-aminoisobutyric acid in the perfused human placenta: in vitro study. Acta Diabetol 2002; 39:75–81.

17. Schneider H, Mohlen KH, Challier JC, Dancis J. Transfer of glutamic acid across the human placenta perfused in vitro. Br J Obstet Gynaecol 1979; 86:299–306.

18. Schneider H, Mohlen KH, Dancis J. Transfer of amino acids across the in vitro perfused human placenta. Pediatr Res 1979; 13:236–240.

19. Schneider H, Reiber W, Sager R, Malek A. Asymmetrical transport of glucose across the in vitro perfused human placenta. Placenta 2003; 24:27–33.

20. Kudo Y, Boyd CA. The role of L-tryptophan transport in L-tryptophan degradation by indoleamine 2,3-dioxygenase in human placental explants. J Physiol 2001; 531:417–423.

21. Enders RH, Judd RM, Donohue TM, Smith CH. Placental amino acid uptake. III. Transport systems for neutral amino acids. Am J Physiol 1976; 230:706–710.

22. Ganapathy V, Prasad PD, Leibach FH. Use of human placenta in studies of monoamine transporters. Meth Enzymol 1998; 296:278–290.

23. Booth AG, Olaniyan RO, Vanderpuye OA. An improved method for the preparation of human placental syncytiotrophoblast microvilli. Placenta 1980; 1:327–336.

24. Kelley LK, Smith CH, King BF. Isolation and partial characterization of the basal cell membrane of human placental trophoblast. Biochim Biophys Acta 1983; 734:91–98.

25. Illsley NP, Wang ZQ, Gray A, Sellers MC, Jacobs MM. Simultaneous preparation of paired, syncytial microvillous and basal membranes from human placenta. Biochim Biophys Acta 1990; 1029:218–226.

26. Prasad PD, Leibach FH, Mahesh VB, Ganapathy V. Relationship between thyroid hormone transport and neutral amino acid transport in JAR human choriocarcinoma cells. Endocrinology 1994; 134:574–581.

27. Brandsch M, Leibach FH, Mahesh VB, Ganapathy V. Calmodulin-dependent modulation of pH sensitivity of the amino acid transport system L in human placental choriocarcinoma cells. Biochim Biophys Acta 1994; 1192:177–184.

28. Jones CR, Srinivas SR, Devoe LD, Ganapathy V, Prasad PD. Inhibition of system A amino acid transport activity by ethanol in BeWo choriocarcinoma cells. Am J Obstet Gynecol 2002; 187:209–216.

29. Eaton BM, Sooranna SR. In vitro modulation of L-arginine transport in trophoblast cells by glucose. Eur J Clin Invest 1998; 28:1006–1010.

30. Nelson DM, Smith SD, Furesz TC, Sadovsky Y, Ganapathy V, Parvin CA, Smith CH. Hypoxia reduces expression and function of system A amino acid transporters in cultured term human trophoblasts. Am J Physiol 2003; 284:C310–C315.

31. Illsley NP. Glucose transporters in the human placenta. Placenta 2000; 21:14–22.

32. Takata K, Hirano H. Mechanism of glucose transport across the human and rat placental barrier: a review. Microsc Res Tech 1997; 38:145–152.
33. Baumann MU, Deborde S, Illsley NP. Placental glucose transfer and fetal growth. Endocrine 2002; 19:13–22.
34. Quraishi AN, Illsley NP. Transport of sugars across human placental membranes measured by light scattering. Placenta 1999; 20:167–174.
35. Morriss FHJ, Boyd RDH. Placental transport. In: Knobil E, Neill JD, eds. The Physiology of Reproduction. New York: Raven Press, 1988:2043–2083.
36. Battaglia FC, Meschia G. An Introduction to Fetal Physiology. Orlando, FL: Academic Press, 1986.
37. Marconi AM, Paolini C, Buscaglia M, Zerbe G, Battaglia FC, Pardi G. The impact of gestational age and fetal growth on the maternal-fetal glucose concentration difference. Obstet Gynecol 1996; 87:937–942.
38. Longo N, Elsas LJ. Human glucose transporters. Adv Pediatr 1998; 45:293–313.
39. Stuart Wood I, Trayhurn P. Glucose transporters (GLUT and SGLT): expanded families of sugar transport proteins. Brit J Nutr 2003; 89:3–9.
40. Johnson LW, Smith CH. Monosaccharide transport across microvillous membrane of human placenta. Am J Physiol 1980; 238:C160–C168.
41. Johnson LW, Smith CH. Glucose transport across the basal plasma membrane of human placental syncytiotrophoblast. Biochim Biophys Acta 1985; 815:44–50.
42. Rice PA, Rourke JE, Nesbitt EL Jr. In vitro perfusion studies of the human placenta. IV. Some characteristics of the glucose transport system in the human placenta. Gynecol Invest 1976; 7:213–221.
43. Rice PA, Rourke JE, Nesbitt RE Jr. In vitro perfusion studies of the human placenta. VI. Evidence against active glucose transport. Am J Obstet Gynecol 1979; 133:649–655.
44. Tadokoro C, Yoshimoto Y, Sakata M, Fujimiya M, Kurachi H, Adachi E, Maeda T, Miyake A. Localization of human placental glucose transporter 1 during pregnancy. An immunohistochemical study. Histol Histopathol 1996; 11:673–681.
45. Jansson T, Wennergren M, Illsley NP. Glucose transporter protein expression in human placenta throughout gestation and in intrauterine growth retardation. J Clin Endocrinol Metab 1993; 77:1554–1562.
46. Barros LF, Yudilevich DL, Jarvis SM, Beaumont N, Baldwin SA. Quantitation and immunolocalization of glucose transporters in the human placenta. Placenta 1995; 16:623–633.
47. Illsley NP, Hall S, Stacey TE. The modulation of glucose transfer across the human placenta by intervillous flow rates: an in vitro perfusion study. Trophoblast Res 1987; 2:539–548.
48. Kayano T, Fukumoto H, Eddy RL, Fan YS, Byers MG, Shows TB, Bell GI. Evidence for a family of human glucose transporter-like proteins. Sequence and gene localization of a protein expressed in fetal skeletal muscle and other tissues. J Biol Chem 1988; 263:15245–15248.

49. Hauguel-de Mouzon S, Challier JC, Kacemi A, Cauzac M, Malek A, Girard J. The GLUT3 glucose transporter isoform is differentially expressed within human placental cell types. J Clin Endocrinol Metab 1997; 82:2689–2694.
50. Desoye G, Hartmann M, Jones CJ, Wolf HJ, Kohnen G, Kosanke G, Kaufmann P. Location of insulin receptors in the placenta and its progenitor tissues. Microsc Res Tech 1997; 38:63–75.
51. Desoye G, Hartmann M, Blaschitz A, Dohr G, Hahn T, Kohnen G, Kaufmann P. Insulin receptors in syncytiotrophoblast and fetal endothelium of human placenta. Immunohistochemical evidence for developmental changes in distribution pattern. Histochemistry 1994; 101:277–285.
52. Challier JC, Hauguel S, Desmaizieres V. Effect of insulin on glucose uptake and metabolism in the human placenta. J Clin Endocrinol Metab 1986; 62:803–807.
53. Urbach J, Mor L, Ronen N, Brandes JM. Does insulin affect placental glucose metabolism and transfer? Am J Obstet Gynecol 1989; 161:953–959.
54. Brunette MG, Lajeunesse D, Leclerc M, Lafond J. Effect of insulin on D-glucose transport by human placental brush border membranes. Mol Cell Endocrinol 1990; 69:59–68.
55. Lindblad BS, Baldesten A. The normal venous plasma free amino acid levels of nonpregnant women and of mother and child during delivery. Acta Paediatr Scand 1967; 56:37–48.
56. Philipps AF, Holzman IR, Teng C, Battaglia FC. Tissue concentrations of free amino acids in term human placentas. Am J Obstet Gynecol 1978; 131:881–887.
57. Christensen HN. Organic ion transport during seven decades. The amino acids. Biochim Biophys Acta 1984; 779:255–269.
58. Christensen HN. Exploiting amino acid structure to learn about membrane transport. Adv Enzymol 1979; 49:41–101.
59. Riggs TR, Christensen HN. Use of labeled nonmetabolized amino acids in biochemical research. Adv Tracer Methodol 1965; 2:183–188.
60. Smith CH, Moe AJ, Ganapathy V. Nutrient transport pathways across the epithelium of the placenta. Annu Rev Nutr 1992; 12:183–206.
61. Moe AJ. Placental amino acid transport. Am J Physiol 1995; 268:C1321–C1331.
62. Kudo Y, Boyd CA. Human placental amino acid transporter genes: expression and function. Reproduction 2002; 124:593–600.
63. Regnault TR, de Vrijer B, Battaglia FC. Transport and metabolism of amino acids in placenta. Endocrine 2002; 19:23–41.
64. Jansson T. Amino acid transporters in the human placenta. Pediatr Res 2001; 49:141–147.
65. Shotwell MA, Kilberg MS, Oxender DL. The regulation of neutral amino acid transport in mammalian cells. Biochim Biophys Acta 1983; 737:267–284.
66. Kilberg MS, Stevens BR, Novak DA. Recent advances in mammalian amino acid transport. Annu Rev Nutr 1993; 13:137–165.
67. McGivan JD, Pastor-Anglada M. Regulatory and molecular aspects of mammalian amino acid transport. Biochem J 1994; 299:321–334.
68. Sibley C, Glazier J, D'Souza S. Placental transporter activity and expression in relation to fetal growth. Exp Physiol 1997; 82:389–402.

69. Mahendran D, Donnai P, Glazier JD, D'Souza SW, Boyd RD, Sibley CP. Amino acid (system A) transporter activity in microvillous membrane vesicles from the placentas of appropriate- and small-for-gestational-age babies. Pediatr Res 1993; 34:661–665.

70. Kuruvilla AG, D'Souza SW, Glazier JD, Mahendran D, Maresh MJ, Sibley CP. Altered activity of the system A amino acid transporter in microvillous membrane vesicles from placentas of macrosomic babies born to diabetic women. J Clin Invest 1994; 94:689–695.

71. Glazier JD, Sibley CP, Carter AM. Effect of fetal growth restriction on system A amino acid transporter activity in the maternal facing plasma membrane of rat syncytiotrophoblast. Pediatr Res 1996; 40:325–329.

72. Glazier JD, Cetin I, Perugino G, Ronzoni S, Grey AM, Mahendran D, Marconi AM, Pardi G, Sibley CP. Association between the activity of the system A amino acid transporter in the microvillous plasma membrane of the human placenta and severity of fetal compromise in intrauterine growth restriction. Pediatr Res 1997; 42:514–519.

73. Dicke JM, Henderson GI. Placental amino acid uptake in normal and complicated pregnancies. Am J Med Sci 1988; 295:223–227.

74. Harrington B, Glazier J, D'Souza S, Sibley C. System A amino acid transporter activity in human placental microvillous membrane vesicles in relation to various anthropometric measurements in appropriate and small for gestational age babies. Pediatr Res 1999; 45:810–814.

75. Johnson LW, Smith CH. Neutral amino acid transport systems of microvillous membrane of human placenta. Am J Physiol 1988; 254:C773–C780.

76. Hoeltzli SD, Smith CH. Alanine transport systems in isolated basal plasma membrane of human placenta. Am J Physiol 1989; 256:C630–C637.

77. Ganapathy V, Inoue K, Prasad PD, Ganapathy ME. Cellular uptake of amino acids: systems and regulation. In: Cynober LA, ed. Metabolic and Therapeutic Aspects of Amino Acids in Clinical Nutrition. Boca Raton, FL: CRC Press, 2004:63–78.

78. Torres-Zamorano V, Leibach FH, Ganapathy V. Sodium-dependent homo- and hetero-exchange of neutral amino acids mediated by the amino acid transporter ATB^0. Biochem Biophys Res Commun 1998; 245:824–829.

79. Arriza JL, Kavanaugh MP, Fairman WA, Wu YN, Murdoch GH, North RA, Amara SG. Cloning and expression of a human neutral amino acid transporter with structural similarity to the glutamate transporter gene family. J Biol Chem 1993; 268:15329–15332.

80. Shafqat S, Tamarappoo BK, Kilberg MS, Puranam RS, McNamara JO, Guadano-Ferraz A, Fremeau RT Jr. Cloning and expression of a novel Na^+-dependent neutral amino acid transporter structurally related to mammalian Na^+/glutamate cotransporters. J Biol Chem 1993; 268:15351–15355.

81. Kekuda R, Prasad PD, Fei YJ, Torres-Zamorano V, Sinha S, Yang-Feng TL, Leibach FH, Ganapathy V. Cloning of the sodium-dependent, broad-scope, neutral amino acid transporter Bo from a human placental choriocarcinoma cell line. J Biol Chem 1996; 271:18657–18661.

82. Kudo Y, Boyd CA. Characterization of amino acid transport systems in human placental basal membrane vesicles. Biochim Biophys Acta 1990; 1021:169–174.

83. Ganapathy ME, Leibach FH, Mahesh VB, Howard JC, Devoe LD, Ganapathy V. Characterization of tryptophan transport in human placental brush-border membrane vesicles. Biochem J 1986; 238:201–208.

84. Prasad PD, Wang H, Huang W, Kekuda R, Rajan DP, Leibach FH, Ganapathy V. Human LAT1, a subunit of system L amino acid transporter: molecular cloning and transport function. Biochem Biophys Res Commun 1999; 255:283–288.

85. Rajan DP, Kekuda R, Huang W, Devoe LD, Leibach FH, Prasad PD, Ganapathy V. Cloning and functional characterization of a Na^+-independent, broad-specific neutral amino acid transporter from mammalian intestine. Biochim Biophys Acta 2000; 1463:6–14.

86. Kudo Y, Boyd CA. Characterisation of L-tryptophan transporters in human placenta: a comparison of brush border and basal membrane vesicles. J Physiol 2001; 531:405–416.

87. Kim DK, Kanai Y, Chairoungdua A, Matsuo H, Cha SH, Endou H. Expression cloning of a Na^+-independent aromatic amino acid transporter with structural similarity to H^+/monocarboxylate transporters. J Biol Chem 2001; 276:17221–17228.

88. Chairoungdua A, Kanai Y, Matsuo H, Inatomi J, Kim DK, Endou H. Identification and characterization of a novel member of the heterodimeric amino acid transporter family presumed to be associated with an unknown heavy chain. J Biol Chem 2001; 276:49390–49399.

89. Eleno N, Deves R, Boyd CA. Membrane potential dependence of the kinetics of cationic amino acid transport systems in human placenta. J Physiol 1994; 479:291–300.

90. Furesz TC, Moe AJ, Smith CH. Lysine uptake by human placental microvillous membrane: comparison of system y^+ with basal membrane. Am J Physiol 1995; 268:C755–C761.

91. Jansson T, Scholtbach V, Powell TL. Placental transport of leucine and lysine is reduced in intrauterine growth restriction. Pediatr Res 1998; 44:532–537.

92. Ayuk PT, Sibley CP, Donnai P, D'Souza S, Glazier JD. Development and polarization of cationic amino acid transporters and regulators in the human placenta. Am J Physiol 2000; 278:C1162–C1171.

93. Furesz TC, Smith CH. Identification of two leucine-sensitive lysine transport activities in human placental basal membrane. Placenta 1997; 18:649–655.

94. Palacin M, Estevez R, Bertran J, Zorzano A. Molecular biology of mammalian plasma membrane amino acid transporters. Physiol Rev 1998; 78:969–1054.

95. Kamath SG, Furesz TC, Way BA, Smith CH. Identification of three cationic amino acid transporters in placental trophoblast: cloning, expression, and characterization of hCAT-1. J Membr Biol 1999; 171:55–62.

96. Furesz TC, Heath-Monnig E, Kamath SG, Smith CH. Lysine uptake by cloned hCAT-2B: comparison with hCAT-1 and with trophoblast surface membranes. J Membr Biol 2002; 189:27–33.

97. Pfeiffer R, Rossier G, Spindler B, Meier C, Kuhn L, Verrey F. Amino acid transport of y^+L-type by heterodimers of 4F2hc/CD98 and members of the glycoprotein-associated amino acid transporter family. Embo J 1999; 18:49–57.

98. Torrents D, Estevez R, Pineda M, Fernandez E, Lloberas J, Shi YB, Zorzano A, Palacin M. Identification and characterization of a membrane protein (y^+L amino acid transporter-1) that associates with 4F2hc to encode the amino acid transport activity y^+L. A candidate gene for lysinuric protein intolerance. J Biol Chem 1998; 273:32437–32445.

99. Rajan DP, Kekuda R, Huang W, Wang H, Devoe LD, Leibach FH, Prasad PD, Ganapathy V. Cloning and expression of a $b^{0,+}$-like amino acid transporter functioning as a heterodimer with 4F2hc instead of rBAT. A new candidate gene for cystinuria. J Biol Chem 1999; 274:29005–29010.

100. Rajan DP, Huang W, Kekuda R, George RL, Wang J, Conway SJ, Devoe LD, Leibach FH, Prasad PD, Ganapathy V. Differential influence of the 4F2 heavy chain and the protein related to $b^{0,+}$ amino acid transport on substrate affinity of the heteromeric $b^{0,+}$ amino acid transporter. J Biol Chem 2000; 275:14331–14335.

101. Stegink LD, Pitkin RM, Reynolds WA, Filer LJ Jr, Boaz DP, Brummel MC. Placental transfer of glutamate and its metabolites in the primate. Am J Obstet Gynecol 1975; 122:70–78.

102. Moe AJ, Smith CH. Anionic amino acid uptake by microvillous membrane vesicles from human placenta. Am J Physiol 1989; 257:C1005–C1011.

103. Hoeltzli SD, Kelley LK, Moe AJ, Smith CH. Anionic amino acid transport systems in isolated basal plasma membrane of human placenta. Am J Physiol 1990; 259:C47–C55.

104. Gegelashvili G, Schousboe A. Cellular distribution and kinetic properties of high-affinity glutamate transporters. Brain Res Bull 1998; 45:233–238.

105. Fairman WA, Vandenberg RJ, Arriza JL, Kavanaugh MP, Amara SG. An excitatory amino-acid transporter with properties of a ligand-gated chloride channel. Nature 1995; 375:599–603.

106. Arriza JL, Fairman WA, Wadiche JI, Murdoch GH, Kavanaugh MP, Amara SG. Functional comparisons of three glutamate transporter subtypes cloned from human motor cortex. J Neurosci 1994; 14:5559–5569.

107. Miyamoto Y, Balkovetz DF, Leibach FH, Mahesh VB, Ganapathy V. Na^+ + Cl^- –gradient-driven, high-affinity, uphill transport of taurine in human placental brush-border membrane vesicles. FEBS Lett 1988; 231:263–267.

108. Ramamoorthy S, Leibach FH, Mahesh VB, Han H, Yang-Feng T, Blakely RD, Ganapathy V. Functional characterization and chromosomal localization of a cloned taurine transporter from human placenta. Biochem J 1994; 300:893–900.

109. Hull D, Elphick MC. Evidence for fatty acid transfer across the human placenta. Ciba Foundation Symposium 1979; 63:75–91.

110. Van Aerde JE, Feldman M, Clandinin MT. Accretion of lipid in the fetus and newborn. In: Polin RA, Fox WW, eds. Fetal and Neonatal Physiology. Philadelphia: WB Saunders, 1998:447–458.

111. Herrera E, Bonet B, Lasuncion MA. Maternal–fetal transfer of lipid metabolites. In: Polin RA, Fox WW, eds. Fetal and Neonatal Physiology. Philadelphia: WB Saunders, 1998:447–458.

112. Haggarty P. Placental regulation of fatty acid delivery and its effect on fetal growth—a review. Placenta 2002; 23(suppl A):S28–S38.

113. Dutta-Roy AK. Transport mechanisms for long-chain polyunsaturated fatty acids in the human placenta. Am J Clin Nutr 2000; 71:315S–322S.

114. Herrera E. Implications of dietary fatty acids during pregnancy of placental, fetal and postnatal development—a review. Placenta 2002; 23(suppl A):9–19.

115. Herrera E. Lipid metabolism in pregnancy and its consequences in the fetus and newborn. Endocrine 2002; 19:43–55.

116. Stremmel W, Kleinert H, Fitscher BA, Gunawan J, Klaassen-Schluter C, Moller K, Wegener M. Mechanism of cellular fatty acid uptake. Biochem Soc Trans 1992; 20:814–817.

117. Campbell FM, Gordon MJ, Dutta-Roy AK. Placental membrane fatty acid–binding protein preferentially binds arachidonic and docosahexaenoic acids. Life Sci 1998; 63:235–240.

118. Campbell FM, Dutta-Roy AK. Plasma membrane fatty acid–binding protein (FABPpm) is exclusively located in the maternal facing membranes of the human placenta. FEBS Lett 1995; 375:227–230.

119. Campbell FM, Taffesse S, Gordon MK, Dutta-Roy AK. Plasma membrane fatty-acid-binding protein in human placenta: identification and characterization. Biochem Biophys Res Commun 1995; 209:1011–1017.

120. Prasad PD, Leibach FH, Ganapathy V. Transplacental transport of water-soluble vitamins. A review. Trophoblast Res 1998; 11:243–257.

121. Prasad PD, Huang W, Wang H, Leibach FH, Ganapathy V. Transport mechanisms for vitamin C in the JAR human placental choriocarcinoma cell line. Biochim Biophys Acta 1998; 1369:141–151.

122. Wang H, Dutta B, Huang W, Devoe LD, Leibach FH, Ganapathy V, Prasad PD. Human Na^+-dependent vitamin C transporter 1 (hSVCT1): primary structure, functional characteristics and evidence for a nonfunctional splice variant. Biochim Biophys Acta 1999; 1461:1–9.

123. Rajan DP, Huang W, Dutta B, Devoe LD, Leibach FH, Ganapathy V, Prasad PD. Human placental sodium-dependent vitamin C transporter (SVCT2): molecular cloning and transport function. Biochem Biophys Res Commun 1999; 262:762–768.

124. Prasad PD, Ramamoorthy S, Leibach FH, Ganapathy V. Characterization of a sodium-dependent vitamin transporter mediating the uptake of pantothenate, biotin and lipoate in human placental choriocarcinoma cells. Placenta 1997; 18:527–533.

125. Grassl S. Human placental brush-border membrane Na^+-biotin cotransport. J Biol Chem 1992; 267:17760–17765.

126. Grassl S. Human placental brush-border membrane Na^+-panthothenate cotransport. J Biol Chem 1992; 267:22902–22906.

127. Wang H, Huang W, Fei YJ, Zia H, Yang-Feng TL, Leibach FH, Devoe LD, Ganapathy V, Prasad PD. Human placental Na^+-dependent multivitamin

transporter. Cloning, functional expression, gene structure, and chromosomal localization. J Biol Chem 1999; 274:14875–14883.

128. Mardach R, Zempleni J, Wolf B, Cannon MJ, Jennings ML, Cress S, Boylan J, Roth S, Cederbaum S, Mock DM. Biotin dependency due to a defect in biotin transport. J Clin Invest 2002; 109:1617–1623.

129. Prasad PD, Ramamoorthy S, Moe AJ, Smith CH, Leibach FH, Ganapathy V. Selective expression of the high-affinity isoform of the folate receptor (FR-alpha) in the human placental syncytiotrophoblast and choriocarcinoma cells. Biochim Biophys Acta 1994; 1223:71–75.

130. Schenker S, Johnson RF, Hoyumpa AM, Henderson GI. Thiamine-transfer by human placenta: normal transport and effects of ethanol. J Lab Clin Med 1990; 116:106–115.

131. Dancis J, Wilson D, Hoskins IA, Levitz M. Placental transfer of thiamine in the human subject: in vitro perfusion studies and maternal-cord plasma concentrations. Am J Obstet Gynecol 1988; 159:1435–1439.

132. Grassl SM. Thiamine transport in human placental brush border membrane vesicles. Biochim Biophys Acta 1998; 1371:213–222.

133. Dutta B, Huang W, Molero M, Kekuda R, Leibach FH, Devoe LD, Ganapathy V, Prasad PD. Cloning of the human thiamine transporter, a member of the folate transporter family. J Biol Chem 1999; 274:31925–31929.

134. Eudy JD, Spiegelstein O, Barber RC, Wlodarczyk BJ, Talbot J, Finnell RH. Identification and characterization of the human and mouse SLC19A3 gene: a novel member of the reduced folate family of micronutrient transporter genes. Mol Genet Metab 2000; 71:581–590.

135. Ganapathy V, Smith SB, Prasad PD. The Folate Transporter Gene Family, SLC19. Pflugers Arch 2004; 447:641–646.

136. Allen LH. Vitamin B12 metabolism and status during pregnancy, lactation and infancy. Adv Exp Med Biol 1994; 352:173–186.

137. Seetharam B, Li N. Transcobalamin II and its cell surface receptor. Vitam Horm 2000; 59:337–366.

138. Seligman PA, Allen RH. Characterization of the receptor for transcobalamin II isolated from human placenta. J Biol Chem 1978; 253:1766–1772.

139. Friedman PA, Shia MA, Wallace JK. A saturable high-affinity binding site for transcobalamin II–vitamin B12 complexes in human placental membrane preparations. J Clin Invest 1977; 59:51–58.

140. Christensen EI, Birn H. Megalin and cubilin: multifunctional endocytic receptors. Nat Rev Mol Cell Biol 2002; 3:256–266.

141. Perez-D'Gregorio RE, Miller RK. Transport and endogenous release of vitamin B12 in the dually perfused human placenta. J Pediatr 1998; 132:S35–S42.

142. Soprano DR, Blaner WS. Plasma retinol-binding protein. In: Sporn MB, Roberts AB, Goodman DS, eds. The Retinoids. New York: Raven Press, 1994:257–281.

143. Dancis J, Levitz M, Katz J, Wilson D, Blaner WS, Piantedosi R, Goodman DS. Transfer and metabolism of retinol by the perfused human placenta. Pediatr Res 1992; 32:195–199.

144. Ron M, Levitz M, Chuba J, Dancis J. Transfer of 25-hydroxyvitamin D_3 and

1,25-dihydroxyvitamin D$_3$ across the perfused human placenta. Am J Obstet Gynecol 1984; 148:370–374.

145. Bavik CO, Peterson A, Eriksson U. Retinol-binding protein mediates uptake of retinol to cultured human keratinocytes. Exp Cell Res 1995; 216:358–362.

146. Sivaprasadarao A, Boudjelal M, Findlay JB. Solubilization and purification of the retinol-binding protein receptor from human placental membranes. Biochem J 1994; 302:245–251.

147. Green T, Ford HC. Intracellular binding proteins for retinol and retinoic acid in early and term human placentas. Br J Obstet Gynaecol 1986; 93:833–838.

148. Okuno M, Kato M, Moriwaki H, Kanai M, Muto Y. Purification and partial characterization of cellular retinoic acid–binding protein from human placenta. Biochim Biophys Acta 1987; 923:116–124.

149. Johansson S, Gustafson AL, Donovan M, Eriksson U, Dencker L. Retinoid-binding proteins—expression patterns in the human placenta. Placenta 1999; 20:459–465.

150. Ganapathy V, Ganapathy ME, Tiruppathi C, Miyamoto Y, Mahesh VB, Leibach FH. Sodium-gradient-driven, high-affinity, uphill transport of succinate in human placental brush-border membrane vesicles. Biochem J 1988; 249:179–184.

151. Balkovetz DF, Leibach FH, Mahesh VB, Ganapathy V. A proton gradient is the driving force for uphill transport of lactate in human placental brush-border membrane vesicles. J Biol Chem 1988; 263:13823–13830.

152. Inuyama M, Ushigome F, Emoto A, Koyabu N, Satoh S, Tsukimori K, Nakano H, Ohtani H, Sawada Y. Characteristics of L-lactic acid transport in basal membrane vesicles of human placental syncytiotrophoblast. Am J Physiol 2002; 283:C822–C830.

153. Piquard F, Schaefer A, Dellenbach P, Haberey P. Lactate movements in the term human placenta in situ. Biol Neonate 1990; 58:61–68.

154. Halestrap AP, Price NT. The proton-linked monocarboxylate transporter (MCT) family: structure, function and regulation. Biochem J 1999; 343:281–299.

155. Wang H, Fei YJ, Kekuda R, Yang-Feng TL, Devoe LD, Leibach FH, Prasad PD, Ganapathy V. Structure, function, and genomic organization of human Na$^+$-dependent high-affinity dicarboxylate transporter. Am J Physiol 2000; 278:C1019–C1030.

156. Pajor AM. Molecular cloning and functional expression of a sodium-dicarboxylate cotransporter from human kidney. Am J Physiol 1996; 270:F642–F648.

157. Inoue K, Zhuang L, Ganapathy V. Human Na$^+$-coupled citrate transporter: primary structure, genomic organization, and transport function. Biochem Biophys Res Commun 2002; 299:465–471.

158. Novak M, Wieser PB, Buch M, Hahn P. Acetylcarnitine and free carnitine in body fluids before and after birth. Pediatr Res 1979; 13:10–15.

159. Roque AS, Prasad PD, Bhatia JS, Leibach FH, Ganapathy V. Sodium-dependent high-affinity binding of carnitine to human placental brush-border membranes. Biochim Biophys Acta 1996; 1282:274–282.

160. Prasad PD, Huang W, Ramamoorthy S, Carter AL, Leibach FH, Ganapathy V. Sodium-dependent carnitine transport in human placental choriocarcinoma cells. Biochim Biophys Acta 1996; 1284:109–117.

161. Wu X, Prasad PD, Leibach FH, Ganapathy V. cDNA sequence, transport function, and genomic organization of human OCTN2, a new member of the organic cation transporter family. Biochem Biophys Res Commun 1998; 246:589–595.

162. Stulc J. Placental transfer of inorganic ions and water. Physiol Rev 1997; 77:805–836.

163. Lafond J, Goyer-O'Reilly I, Laramee M, Simoneau L. Hormonal regulation and implication of cell signaling in calcium transfer by placenta. Endocrine 2001; 14:285–294.

164. Robidoux J, Simoneau L, Masse A, Lafond J. Activation of L-type calcium channels induces corticotropin-releasing factor secretion from human placental trophoblasts. J Clin Endocrinol Metab 2000; 85:3356–3364.

165. Cemerikic B, Zamah R, Ahmed MS. Identification of L-type calcium channels associated with kappa opioid receptors in human placenta. J Mol Neurosci 1998; 10:261–272.

166. Peng JB, Brown EM, Hediger MA. Structural conservation of the genes encoding CaT1, CaT2, and related cation channels. Genomics 2001; 76:99–109.

167. Fisher GJ, Kelley LK, Smith CH. ATP-dependent calcium transport across basal plasma membranes of human placental trophoblast. Am J Physiol 1987; 252:C38–C46.

168. Howard A, Legon S, Walters JR. Plasma membrane calcium pump expression in human placenta and small intestine. Biochem Biophys Res Commun 1992; 183:499–505.

169. Strid H, Powell TL. ATP-dependent Ca^{2+} transport is up-regulated during third trimester in human syncytiotrophoblast basal membranes. Pediatr Res 2000; 48:58–63.

170. Belkacemi L, Simoneau L, Lafond J. Calcium-binding proteins: distribution and implication in mammalian placenta. Endocrine 2002; 19:57–64.

171. Sibley CP, Boyd RD. Control of transfer across the mature placenta. Oxf Rev Reprod Biol 1988; 10:382–435.

172. Sibley CP, Glazier JD, Greenwood SL, Lacey H, Mynett K, Speake P, Jansson T, Johansson M, Powell TL. Regulation of placental transfer: the Na^+/H^+ exchanger—a review. Placenta 2002; 23(suppl A):S39–S46.

173. Werner A, Dehmelt L, Nalbant P. Na^+-dependent phosphate cotransporters: the NaPi protein families. J Exp Biol 1998; 201:3135–3142.

174. Illsley NP, Glaubensklee C, Davis B, Verkman AS. Chloride transport across placental microvillous membranes measured by fluorescence. Am J Physiol 1988; 255:C789–C797.

175. Shennan DB, Davis B, Boyd CA. Chloride transport in human placental microvillus membrane vesicles. I. Evidence for anion exchange. Pflugers Arch 1986; 406:60–64.

176. Grassl SM. Cl/HCO3 exchange in human placental brush border membrane vesicles. J Biol Chem 1989; 264:11103–11106.

177. Verrijt CE. Vectorial aspects of iron transfer in human term placenta. Eur J Obstet Gynecol Reprod Biol 1999; 83:125–126.
178. Harris ED. New insights into placental iron transport. Nutr Rev 1992; 50:329–331.
179. Georgieff MK, Wobken JK, Welle J, Burdo JR, Connor JR. Identification and localization of divalent metal transporter-1 (DMT-1) in term human placenta. Placenta 2000; 21:799–804.
180. Mulder GJ. Sulfation of Drugs and Related Compounds. Boca Raton, FL: CRC Press, 1981.
181. Girard JP, Baekkevold ES, Feliu J, Brandtzaeg P, Amalric F. Molecular cloning and functional analysis of SUT-1, a sulfate transporter from human high endothelial venules. Proc Natl Acad Sci (USA) 1999; 96:12772–12777.
182. Ling R, Bridges CC, Sugawara M, Fujita T, Leibach FH, Prasad PD, Ganapathy V. Involvement of transporter recruitment as well as gene expression in the substrate-induced adaptive regulation of amino acid transport system A. Biochim Biophys Acta 2001; 1512:15–21.
183. Gazzola RF, Sala R, Bussolati O, Visigalli R, Dall'Asta V, Ganapathy V, Gazzola GC. The adaptive regulation of amino acid transport system A is associated to changes in ATA2 expression. FEBS Lett 2001; 490:11–14.
184. Hyde R, Christie GR, Litherland GJ, Hajduch E, Taylor PM, Hundal HS. Subcellular localization and adaptive up-regulation of the system A (SAT2) amino acid transporter in skeletal muscle cells and adipocytes. Biochem J 2001; 355:563–568.
185. Gaither K, Quraishi AN, Illsley NP. Diabetes alters the expression and activity of the human placental GLUT1 glucose transporter. J Clin Endocr Metab 1999; 84:695–701.
186. Jansson T, Wennergren M, Powell TL. Placental glucose transport and GLUT1 expression in insulin-dependent diabetes. Am J Obstet Gynecol 1999; 180:163–168.
187. Jansson T, Ekstrand Y, Bjorn C, Wennergren M, Powell TL. Alterations in the activity of placental amino acid transporters in pregnancies complicated by diabetes. Diabetes 2002; 51:2214–2219.
188. Norberg S, Powell TL, Jansson T. Intrauterine growth restriction is associated with a reduced activity of placental taurine transporters. Pediatr Res 1998; 44:233–238.
189. Henderson GI, Schenker S. Alcohol, placental function, and fetal growth. In: Rama Sastry BV, ed. Placental Toxicology. Boca Raton, FL: CRC Press, 1995:27–44.
190. Rama Sastry BV, Janson VE. Smoking, placental function, and fetal growth. In: Rama Sastry BV, ed. Placental Toxicology. Boca Raton, FL: CRC Press, 1995:45–81.
191. Rama Sastry BV. Cocaine addiction, placental function, and fetal growth. In: Rama Sastry BV, ed. Placental Toxicology. Boca Raton, FL: CRC Press, 1995:133–160.

5

Intrauterine Growth Restriction

William W. Hay, Jr.
University of Colorado School of Medicine, Denver, Colorado, U.S.A.

I. INTRODUCTION

Intrauterine growth restriction (IUGR) represents fetal growth that is less than the potential, and presumably optimal, rate of growth of a specific fetus. Intrauterine growth restriction is highly variable and depends on the severity, duration, and time of occurrence during gestation of disorders that cause growth failure. Because growth is fundamental in the fetus, nearly any aberration in fetal condition can lead to growth failure. Growth failure also occurs after birth, particularly in preterm infants who are not nourished sufficiently to produce normal growth and who experience many disorders that interfere with normal nutritional metabolism that supports growth.

IUGR fetuses must be distinguished from "small-for-gestational-age" (SGA) fetuses who did not experience IUGR. SGA infants are those with anthropometric measurements of weight, length, and head circumference that are less than the 10th percentile of normal population values. An infant also can be considered "relatively" SGA when its weight/length ratio (or the Ponderal index = [weight, g]/[length, cm]^3) is less than normal (1) (Fig. 1). SGA infants also can be the result of normal but slower-than-average rates of fetal growth, such as constitutionally small but normal infants whose parents, siblings, and more distant relatives are small (2). SGA infants also can be the result of abnormally slow fetal growth caused by genetic disorders (e.g., extra or insufficient chromosomes) or diseases (e.g., intrauterine infection). Thus, small size at birth indicates either a normal outcome or a result of intrinsic or extrinsic factors that restricted fetal growth.

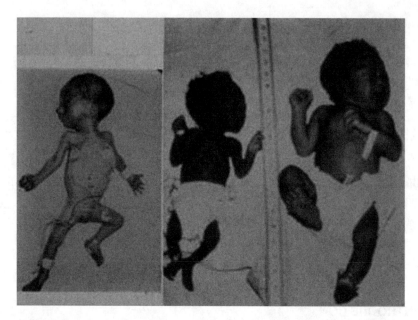

Figure 1 Preterm, small-for-gestational-age infant at 34 weeks of gestation (left), severely small-for-gestational-age infant at 39 weeks (middle), and average-for-gestational-age infant at 40 weeks (right). (From Ref. 205.)

II. BIRTHWEIGHT CLASSIFICATION OF GROWTH

Newborns can have normal birthweight (greater than 2500 grams), low birthweight (LBW, less than 2500 grams), very low birthweight (VLBW, less than 1500 grams), or extremely low birthweight (ELBW, less than 1000 grams). Classification by weight alone does not define normal or aberrant growth, because most infants with less-than-normal birthweights are the result of a shorter-than-normal gestation; i.e., they are preterm. Similarly, classifying newborns as preterm or term on the basis of birthweight alone also is erroneous, because infants with IUGR can be smaller than normal at any gestational age. Although population-specific data indicate that "normal" fetal growth varies almost twofold, from as low as 2400 g for neonates born in New Guinea (3) to as high as 4000 g (4) among newborns of women who eat extremely high-carbohydrate diets during pregnancy, such extremes probably are the result of under- and overnutrition and are not necessarily examples of "optimal" fetal growth for humans.

A. Symmetrical and Asymmetrical Growth Restriction

Intrauterine growth restriction has been divided into symmetrical IUGR and asymmetrical IUGR. Symmetrical IUGR implies that the growth of head circumference (i.e., brain), length, and body weight is similarly limited. Patterns of symmetrical growth restriction usually start early during fetal life, reflecting their intrinsic nature (5). Symmetrical IUGR may involve normal growth processes but often is associated with hereditary or congenital disorders. Factors that limit growth of both fetal brain and fetal body include chromosomal anomalies, congenital infections, dwarf syndromes, some inborn errors of metabolism, and some drugs.

Asymmetrical IUGR implies that the growth of body length and weight is restricted to a greater extent than growth of the head circumference. Moderately to severely affected IUGR infants have restrictions in both brain and body growth, but to varying degrees that depend on the duration and severity of the insults that inhibit growth (Fig. 2). This is the most prevalent form of IUGR, accounting for between 70% and 80% of IUGR babies and, in some reports, increased perinatal mortality of up to 12 times that of appropriate-for-gestational-age (AGA) infants (6). Asymmetrical growth restriction classically has been considered to develop during the late second and third trimesters in response to decreased fetal nutrient supply (7). In this situation, decreased energy substrate supply to the fetus limits fat and glycogen storage and the growth of skeletal muscle but allows for continued bone and brain growth. More extreme limitations of energy substrates for longer periods affect both growth and energy storage. Decreased amino acid supply at any gestational age will limit growth, since new tissue cannot be synthesized at normal rates.

Mechanisms that allow brain growth to continue at a faster rate than adipose tissue and skeletal muscle are not completely known, but they may include an increased rate of cerebral blood flow relative to the umbilical and systemic circulations (8) and, in some experimental models, preservation of cerebral glucose transporter concentrations and cerebral glucose uptake capacity (9). The heart can be large for body weight in asymmetrical IUGR infants, indicating preserved growth similar to that of the brain. The liver, however, usually is reduced in size, representing deficits in both growth and glycogen content. The thymus also is reduced in size, perhaps indicating a response to stress but also indicating potential immunological inadequacy. Within this group of fetuses, easily definable subgroups exist whose pathological alterations are related to the severity of their IUGR (10–12). The combined use of umbilical artery velocimetry and fetal heart rate monitoring has demonstrated that approximately two-thirds of IUGR infants display an increased umbilical arterial pulsatility index, with 50% of these fetuses having

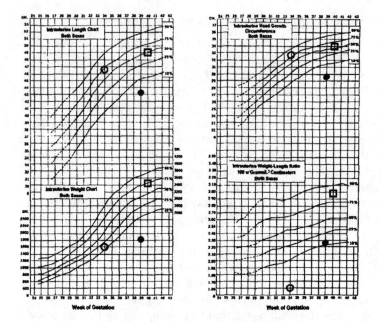

Figure 2 Colorado Intrauterine Growth Charts, including symbols that define the anthropometric measurements for the three infants in Fig. 1. (○) preterm infant at 34 weeks' gestation, showing asymmetry of weight (15th percentile) vs. length and head circumference (75th percentile), producing a weight–length ratio ≪ 10th percentile; (●) severely but symmetrically SGA infant at 39 weeks, showing weight, length, and head circumference all about equally and markedly less than 10th percentile, with the weight–length ratio of about the 10th percentile because the weight was still most reduced; (□) symmetric AGA infant at 40 weeks, showing weight, length, head circumference, and weight–length ratio about the 65th–75th percentile. (Growth charts from Ref. 206.)

an increased fetal heart rate. Those fetuses not displaying alterations in umbilical arterial velocimetry or heart rate are still classified as IUGR and not SGA, because they still have reduced umbilical blood flow per unit fetal weight (10). In addition to decreased umbilical blood flow, IUGR fetuses also have diminished hepatic perfusion (12). Measurements of ductus venosus blood flow in IUGR fetuses have demonstrated an increased percentage of umbilical blood flow entering the ductus venous associated with decreased umbilical blood flow and hepatic perfusion (13). Hypoperfusion of fetal hepatic tissue results in a reduced liver mass and possibly hepatic function. This weight reduction, together with a relative increase in brain mass, increases the brain/liver ratio. These increased indices, together with reduced fat deposition, result in a reduced Ponderal index in IUGR fetuses.

A more recent appraisal of fetal growth restriction has shown that, compared with non-growth-restricted infants of the same gestational age, growth-restricted infants have substantially lower lengths, head circumferences, and proportionality ratios and that the magnitude of the deficits increases significantly with increasing degrees of growth retardation. When the comparison is based on birthweight rather than gestational age, however, growth-restricted infants have slightly but significantly greater lengths and head circumferences, with increased variability in body proportions, but no evidence of the bimodality that would characterize two distinct subtypes. This analysis suggests that proportionality among intrauterine growth-restricted infants represents a continuum, with progressive disproportionality as severity of growth retardation increases. Moreover, despite evidence of some "sparing," the absolute magnitudes of the deficits in length and head growth remain substantial (14).

III. DETECTION OF INTRAUTERINE GROWTH RESTRICTION

IUGR is best detected in a specific fetus by comparing serial ultrasound anthropometric measurements with similar serial ultrasound measurements of fetuses that subsequently were born at term in healthy condition with normal anthropometric measurements (Fig. 3). Fetal growth standards are even better measures of IUGR and its consequences among infants born prematurely. When fetal growth standards are used, preterm SGA infants have increased risk of neonatal mortality, respiratory distress syndrome, bronchopulmonary dysplasia, intraventricular hemorrhage, retinopathy of prematurity (ROP), and necrotizing enterocolitis (NEC), whereas only increased risk of neonatal mortality, ROP, and NEC are detected when neonatal growth standards are used (15).

Markers that can accurately differentiate the more severe IUGR subpopulation of SGA infants are limited. Recent studies indicate that these IUGR neonates can be suspected based on fetal surveillance evidence of placental insufficiency with associated progressive growth failure in utero and abnormal in utero umbilical blood flow patterns (16). Subsequent studies have shown that the severity of these abnormalities in utero correlates with the severity of a variety of fetal metabolic abnormalities, including increased lactate concentrations and hypoxia (16–19), decreased placental amino acid transporter activity (17), and increased fetal protein breakdown (19).

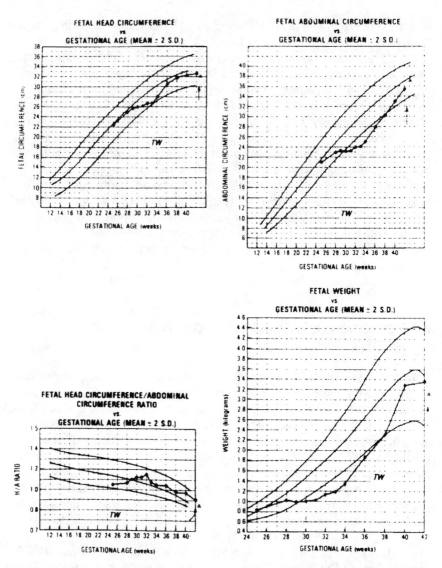

Figure 3 Normative intrauterine fetal growth curves (solid lines) representing the mean ± 2 S.D. of a reference population of human fetuses with normal fetal growth rates according to ultrasound measurements, plus serial fetal body measurements in a mother with severe ulcerative colitis. Note that fetal growth (–●–●–) begins to decrease markedly in midgestation but returns to normal following the initiation of central hyperalimentation at approximately 28–30 weeks. (From Ref. 207.)

IV. INTRAUTERINE GROWTH RESTRICTION AND PRETERM BIRTH

Most cases of fetal growth restriction occur in late gestation, involve only minimal growth delay, and are not major causes of preterm delivery. In cases of severe IUGR, the pathophysiological processes causing the IUGR are stressful and can lead to preterm labor and preterm delivery. Thus, up to 10% of infants are classified as SGA/IUGR at term, while up to 30–40% may be SGA/IUGR at less than 28–30 weeks' gestational age (20). Several maternal conditions associated with both IUGR and preterm delivery are listed in Table 1 (21–24).

V. REGULATION OF FETAL GROWTH

A. Epidemiological Considerations

The major maternal risk factors for IUGR (Table 2) include small maternal size (height and prepregnancy weight) and low maternal weight gain during pregnancy. Low maternal body mass index (the degree of thinness or fatness, defined as [weight (kg)]/[height (cm)]^2), is a major predictor of IUGR. This characteristic interacts with other risk factors, such as diet, smoking, and many illnesses, to affect fetal growth. For example, smoking has only half the

Table 1 Maternal Conditions Associated with Both IUGR and Preterm Delivery

Both young and advanced maternal age
Maternal prepregnancy short stature and thinness
Poor maternal weight gain during the last third of pregnancy
Maternal illness during pregnancy
Nulliparity
Failure to obtain normal medical care during pregnancy
Lower socioeconomic status
Black race (in the United States)
Multiple gestation
Uterine and placental anomalies
Polyhydramnios
Preeclampsia
Diabetes
Intrauterine infections
Cigarette smoking, cocaine use, and other substance abuse

Source: Adapted from Ref. 21.

Table 2 Factors Determining Variance in Birth
Weight

	Percent of total variance
Fetal	
Genotype	16
Sex	2
	—
	18
Maternal	
Genotype	20
Maternal environment	24
Maternal age	1
Parity	7
	—
	52
Unknown	30

Source: Derived from Penrose LS. Proc 9th Int Congr Genetics
Part 1, 1954, p. 520. From Ref. 29, p. 285.

impact on fetal growth in obese versus thin women and in black versus white
women (25). Low blood pressure has a detrimental impact on fetal growth,
mostly in thin women (26). Moderate obesity, therefore, protects against most
growth-inhibiting risk factors except for black race and female gender.

B. Genetic Factors

Maternal genotype is more important than fetal genotype in the overall
regulation of fetal growth. However, the paternal genotype is essential for
trophoblast development, which secondarily regulates fetal growth by the
provision of nutrients (27). Furthermore, normal fetal and placental growth
in mice require that the IGF-II gene be paternal (28) and the IGF-II receptor
gene be maternal, while maternal disomy producing IGF-II underexpression
results in fetal dwarfism (29). Such cases represent gene imprinting, or the
expression of genes from only one of the parental chromosomes (30,31).

C. Nongenetic Maternal Factors

Maternal constraint represents a relatively limited uterine size, including
placental implantation surface area and uterine circulation, and thus the
capacity to support placental growth and nutrient supply to the fetus. A clear
example of maternal constraint is the reduced rate of fetal growth of multiple

fetuses in a species—human—that optimally supports only one fetus (Fig. 4) (32). Furthermore, although it has been assumed that small fetuses of small parents do not reflect fetal growth restriction (they are considered and called "constitutionally" small), it is not known whether such fetuses would grow faster or to a larger size if more nutrients were provided. Animal studies indicate that they might. For example, a small-breed embryo transplanted into a large-breed uterus will grow larger than a small-breed embryo remaining in a small-breed uterus (33). Furthermore, partial reduction in fetal number in a polytocous species such as the rat produces greater-than-normal birthweights in the remaining offspring. Conversely, embryo transfer of a large-breed embryo into a small-breed uterus will result in a newborn that is smaller than in its natural large-breed environment. Such evidence supports the concept that fetal growth is normally constrained and that this constraint comes from the maternal environment, i.e., the size of the uterus.

D. Maternal Nutrition

Normal variations in maternal nutrition have relatively little impact on fetal growth and the severity of IUGR. This is because changes in maternal nutrition, unless extreme and prolonged, do not markedly alter maternal plasma concentrations of nutrient substrates or blood oxygenation, the principal determinants of nutrient substrate transport to the fetus by the

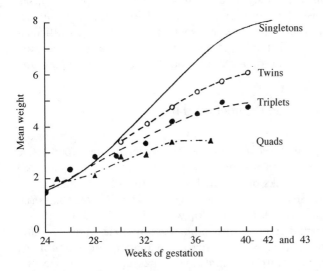

Figure 4 Mean birthweight of single and multiple fetuses related to duration of gestation. (Adapted from Ref. 32, p. 386.)

placenta and the utilization of nutrients for fetal protein accretion (34). Human epidemiological data from conditions of prolonged starvation, as well as nutritional deprivation in experimental animals, indicate that severe limitations in maternal nutrition limit fetal growth only by 10–20% (35,36). Restriction of calorie and protein intakes to less than 50% of normal for a considerable portion of gestation is needed before marked reductions in fetal growth are observed. For example, attempts to limit weight gain in pregnancy with a 1200-kcal diet, 50% of recommended caloric intake, to prevent preeclampsia increased the incidence of fetal growth restriction up to tenfold (37).

Attempts to increase fetal weight gain with maternal nutritional supplements have produced mixed results. Maintaining good nutrition in pregnant woman who otherwise would experience undernutrition tends to prevent IUGR. Among lower-socioeconomic class women without clear evidence of undernutrition or among normally nourished pregnant women, higher-caloric feeding usually increases fetal adiposity, not growth of muscle mass or gain in length or head circumference. In contrast, high protein supplements to such women tend to produce delayed fetal growth (38); the mechanisms responsible for this phenomenon are not known.

E. Maternal Chronic Diseases

Chronic hypertension, pregnancy-induced hypertension, and preeclampsia, like other vascular disorders, including severe and long-standing diabetes mellitus and serious autoimmune disease associated with the lupus anticoagulant, have a common effect of limiting trophoblast invasion, placental growth and development, uteroplacental blood flow, and fetal oxygen and nutrient supply and uptake (39).

1. Hypertension-Associated Disorders and IUGR

Gestational hypertension, preeclampsia, eclampsia, chronic hypertension, and preeclampsia superimposed on chronic hypertension are hypertensive disorders that may occur during pregnancy. Chronic hypertension and preeclampsia increase the risks of low birthweights and IUGR (40,41). The most common hypertensive condition associated with IUGR is preeclampsia. In preterm preeclampsia, IUGR may develop when, despite normal maternal oxygenation, the placental and fetal circulations are hypoxic. Similarly, late-gestation preeclampsia often is associated with inadequate trophoblast invasion, leading to reduced intraplacental oxygen pressure, or uteroplacental hypoxia. Both preplacental and uteroplacental hypoxia are associated with increased placental angiogenesis, leading to the development of a reduced capillary-mediated impedance within the fetal placental vasculature (42,43).

Preeclampsia represents a heterogeneous outcome in fetal growth. Two groups represent the extreme changes, one displaying an asymmetrical growth restriction associated with impaired placental growth, perfusion, and transport function most commonly found starting in early pregnancy, and a second group characteristic of later onset during gestation in which the fetus grows at a more normal rate and displays normal weight indices (44). Morphological examination of placentas affected by preeclampsia reveals pathological changes similar to those found in placentas from women who were pregnant at high altitude and those with marked anemia. Characteristic pathological changes include thinning of the trophoblast and stromal tissue layers and reduced villous surface area (45,46). Interestingly, other studies have reported an increase in the incidence of preeclampsia at high altitude (47,48).

2. Postplacental Hypoxia and Severe IUGR

The most severely affected IUGR fetuses develop with marked fetal hypoxia that occurs in conjunction with normal maternal oxygenation (43,49,50). Severe early-onset IUGR with reduced, absent, or even reversed umbilical end diastolic flow (EDF) is associated with increased intraplacental oxygen partial pressure, or relative *placental hyperoxia* (51,52). In this situation, reduced villous development leads to diminished angiogenesis of the intermediate and terminal villi, resulting in the development of increased fetal vascular impedance (53–55). Progressive embolization of the sheep placenta can replicate absent EDF, as observed in severely growth-restricted human fetuses (56). Embolization reportedly decreases the number of perfused villi and the area available for gas exchange (56). However, further stereological studies and studies using plastic cast and scanning electron microscope techniques indicate that increased placental vascular impedance is associated with a more global reduction in vascularity (52,53,57). Reduced villous tree arborization and maternal arteriovenous thrombosis surrounding peripheral villi could contribute to reduced surface areas and impeded oxygen and nutrient substrate exchange.

3. Other Maternal Conditions That Limit Oxygen Supply to the Placenta and Fetus

Maternal cyanotic congenital heart disease also can limit fetal oxygen supply, which can limit fetal growth (58). Severe sickle cell crises can damage uterine vasculature, leading to placental growth and transport capacities (59,60).

4. Pregnancy at Altitude and Preplacental Hypoxia

High-altitude hypoxia also can limit fetal growth (61), but usually this is clinically significant only for nonindigenous women who move to altitudes above 10,000 feet (62,63). In these situations, maternal hypoxemic hypoxia results in intervillous blood hypoxia, or what can be termed preplacental hypoxia, and subsequent fetal hypoxia. The low birthweights observed in well-adapted high-altitude populations are due to physiological adaptation rather than a higher number of pathologically IUGR babies (64). The growth restriction of these fetuses also is characterized by an increased head circumference: body weight ratio and impaired cardiac circulation, reflecting more asymmetric IUGR (65,66). High-altitude pregnancies are characterized by low umbilical artery flow impedance values, indicating increased villous capillary diameter (49,51), proposed to be the result of increased branching angiogenesis (43). In addition, decreased uterine artery flow resistance, possibly due to improved trophoblast invasion, may be a compensatory mechanism in response to reduced oxygen tension at altitude; such differences are not observed at altitudes less than 1600 meters (67). Where changes in flow are observed, thinner tissue layers are observed within the placenta, leading to improved diffusion capacity of the tissue layers (68). Thinner tissue layers also are related to increased villous capillary diameter (69,70).

Maternal glucose concentrations appear to be reduced in pregnant women who are genetically adapted to high altitude (61), possibly due to an increased utilization of glucose per mole of O_2. Such hypoglycemia might, along with the hypoxia, account for reduced fetal birthweight. In addition, elevated maternal IGFBP-1 in late gestation can impair fetal IGF-I-mediated growth, another example of an adaptation to a reduced-oxygen environment that limits fetal growth (71). Additional changes in the maternal neural–immune axis may predispose women at altitude to IUGR (72).

5. Other Maternal Conditions That Lead to Uteroplacental Hypoxia

Maternal anemia and asthma are associated with an IUGR outcome as a result of a preplacental hypoxia. Maternal anemia can be controlled with iron supplementation, but it still remains a contributing factor to IUGR outcome in developing countries with inadequate medical service distribution. Maternal asthma also is treatable, but there remains debate about whether controlled asthma results in a favorable perinatal outcome (73). For example, steroid-dependent asthmatic women are at an increased risk of gestational diabetes, preterm delivery, and admission of the infant to a neonatal intensive care unit (74).

F. Maternal Drugs

Specific effects of drugs on fetal growth (Table 3) are often difficult to sort out, because many women take many drugs, intermittently, at different doses, and at different periods of fetal vulnerability. Women who abuse drugs also frequently suffer from other disorders that could lead to poor fetal growth, such as poor nutrition, recurrent acute illnesses, and chronic diseases (75). Fetal growth restriction does appear to be a major part of the fetal alcohol syndrome. Alcohol may exert its nonteratogenic effects by limiting placental-to-fetal amino acid transport (76). Cocaine may contribute to fetal growth restriction by causing uterine and perhaps umbilical vasoconstriction and reduced placental perfusion, resulting in fetal hypoxia (77). The most consistent drug effect that reduces fetal growth is cigarette smoking (78). Deficits of at least 300 g (about 10% of normal term weight) are not uncommon. Likely common mechanisms include the effect of nicotine and of catecholamines released in response to nicotine to constrict the uterine and perhaps the umbilical vasculature, reducing placental perfusion. Carbon monoxide, cyanide, and other cellular toxins may limit oxygen transport to fetal tissues as well as cellular respiration.

Table 3 Drugs Associated with IUGR

Amphetamines
Antimetabolites (e.g., aminopterin, busulfan, methotrexate)
Bromides
Cocaine
Ethanol
Heroin and other narcotics such as morphine and methadone
Hydantoin
Isotretinoin
Metals such as mercury and lead
Phencyclidine
Polychlorinated biphenyls (PCBs)
Propranalol
Steroids
Tobacco (carbon monoxide, nicotine, thiocyanate)
Toluene
Trimethadione
Warfarin

Source: Adapted from Ref. 205.

G. The Placenta

The size of the placenta and its directly related nutrient transport functions are the principal regulators of nutrient supply to the fetus and thus the rate of fetal growth (79,80). Nearly all cases of IUGR are associated with a smaller-than-normal placenta. Variable limitations in placental nutrient transfer capacity modulate this primary effect of placental size on fetal growth (81,82). A variety of placental pathological conditions are associated with IUGR (Table 4). In most of these cases, the placenta is simply smaller than normal. In many there also is abnormal trophoblast development, including abnormal vascular growth in the trophoblast villi, frequently associated with limited uterine vascular perfusion of the intervillous spaces. At more advanced stages of placental growth failure, placental production of growth factors and growth regulating hormones are decreased, particularly placental lactogen, which is synthesized and secreted by the syncytiotrophoblast cells of the placenta (83) and mediates fetal growth process by stimulation of IGF production in the fetus and by increasing the availability of nutrients to fetal tissues (84).

A major contributor to placental insufficiency is abnormal development of the placental vascular bed through alterations in vasculogenesis and angiogenesis. Placental blood vessel development is divided into two phases,

Table 4 Placental Growth Disorders That Lead to or Are Associated with IUGR

Abnormal umbilical vascular insertions (circumvallate, velamentous)
Abruption (chronic, partial)
Avascular villi
Decidual arteritis
Fibrinosis, atheromatous changes, cytotrophoblast hyperplasia, basement
   membrane thickening
Infectious villitis (as with TORCH infections)
Ischemic villous necrosis and umbilical vascular thromboses
Multiple gestation (limited endometrial surface area, vascular anastomoses)
Multiple infarcts
Partial molar pregnancy
Placenta previa
Single umbilical artery
Spiral artery vasculitis, failed or limited erosion into intervillous space
Syncytial knots
Tumors including chorioangioma and hemangiomas

Source: Adapted from Ref. 205.

branching and nonbranching angiogenesis. *Branching angiogenesis* occurs during early gestation under relatively hypoxic conditions and is responsible for the expansion of the preexisting vascular bed, a process postulated to be driven by vascular endothelial growth factor (VEGF). *Nonbranching angiogenesis* promotes the elongation of preexisting capillary loops and occurs later in gestation under the influence of placental IGF (PIGF) (42). Recently, a number of different villous morphologies have been documented in association with altered states of placental oxygenation. For example, villous structure observed from IUGR placentas that developed under maternal hypoxia, as in pregnancy at altitude, is characterized by increased branching angiogenesis and reduced vascular impedance (51,85). In contrast, placentas of severe IUGR characterized by absent end diastolic flow in the umbilical artery and increased vascular impedance are associated with a predominance of nonbranching angiogenesis (49,86). Villous development with excessive branching-type angiogenesis, as a result of elevated VEGF concentrations in relation to PIGF, develops in situations of intraplacental hypoxia. Nonbranching angiogenesis predominates when there is an increase in intraplacental oxygen concentration; PIGF appears to regulate this form of angiogenesis (51,85).

VI. FETAL NUTRIENT UPTAKE, METABOLISM, AND GROWTH

In general, decreased rates of fetal growth represent an "adaptation" to inadequate nutrient supply. IUGR that results from decreased nutrient supply can be interpreted, therefore, as a successful, if not perfect, adaptation to maintain fetal survival. Fetal undernutrition also appears to affect rapidly growing fetuses more than slow-growing fetuses, who may have been programmed to grow more slowly for genetic or embryonic and early fetal pathological reasons (87).

A. Water

Fetal water content as a fraction of body weight decreases over gestation due to relative increases in protein and mineral accretion (88) and development of adipose tissue in the third trimester. Fetuses with marked IUGR, who have decreased body fat content, have even higher fractional contents of body water, but extracellular space in IUGR infants usually is normal for gestational age, for adipose tissue, skeletal muscle, and mineral accretion are similarly decreased (89).

B. Minerals

Fetal calcium content increases exponentially with a linear increase in length and thus is similar in normally grown and IUGR infants, because bone density, area, and circumference increase exponentially in relation to linear growth (90). Accretion of other minerals varies more directly with body weight and according to the distribution of the minerals into extracellular (e.g., sodium) or intracellular (e.g., potassium) spaces.

C. Glucose Uptake, Metabolism, and Fetal Growth

A common characteristic of IUGR fetuses is a relatively lower plasma glucose concentration as compared with normally grown fetuses (91,92). Such relative fetal "hypoglycemia" is an important compensatory mechanism that helps maintain the maternal-to-fetal glucose concentration gradient and thus the transport of glucose across the placenta to the fetus (93). Despite this compensation, lower fetal glucose concentration limits tissue glucose uptake directly by diminished mass action and also indirectly by limiting fetal insulin secretion and thus the effect of insulin to promote tissue glucose uptake. Insulin also normally suppresses hepatic glucose production and release and acts as an anabolic hormone that increases net protein balance by inhibiting protein breakdown. Thus, a decrease in fetal plasma insulin concentration initially may allow fetal glucose production to take place, thereby providing glucose for both fetal and placental needs, but subsequently, combined with lower glucose concentration, results in increased protein breakdown and decreased protein accretion (94,95).

Circulating concentrations and tissue-specific expression of growth factors such as IGF-I and IGF-II also are decreased directly with lower fetal glucose concentrations (96), which may contribute to increased fetal protein breakdown and decreased rates of fetal growth. Thus, the relative hypoglycemia in the IUGR fetus maintains fetal glucose supply, but it also leads to lower anabolic hormone concentrations, which limit the rate of fetal growth, thereby decreasing fetal nutrient needs.

D. Glycogen

Many tissues in the fetus, including brain, liver, lung, heart, and skeletal muscle, produce glycogen over the second half of gestation (97). Liver glycogen content, which increases with gestation (Fig. 5), is the most important store of carbohydrate for systemic glucose needs (98), because only the liver contains sufficient glucose-6-phosphatase for release of glucose

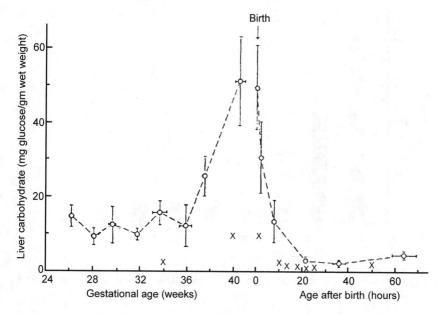

Figure 5 Liver glycogen content (as carbohydrate) in normal human fetuses and newborn infants with normal birthweights for gestational age (O----O; mean ± sem) and infants of low birthweight for gestational age (**X**). (From Ref. 208.)

into the circulation. Glycogen content is markedly reduced in IUGR infants, both in the liver and in the skeletal muscles (97,99), due to lower fetal plasma concentrations of glucose and insulin. Repeated episodes of hypoxemia in the IUGR fetus induce epinephrine and cortisol secretion, leading to further depletion of glycogen by increasing glycogenolysis.

E. Adipose Tissue

Fetal fat content, expressed as a fraction of fetal weight, varies markedly among species (100) (Fig. 6), from 1–3% in most land mammals to 15–20% in human newborns at term (51). Fat content may be less than 10% of body weight (100) in IUGR infants, due to decreased fatty acid, triglyceride, glucose, and glycerol supply to the fetus. Secondary insulin deficiency in the IUGR fetus also limits fat synthesis by decreasing activation of peripheral lipoprotein lipase, which normally is necessary to release fatty acids from circulating lipoproteins for adipocyte uptake and triglyceride synthesis and stimulation of fatty acid synthase within adipocytes.

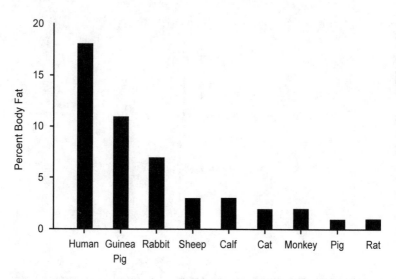

Figure 6   Fetal fat content at term as a percent of fetal body weight among species. (From Ref. 100, p. 376.)

F. Amino Acid Uptake, Metabolism, and Protein Accretion

The placenta contains a large variety of amino acid transporters, most of which use energy to actively concentrate amino acids in the trophoblast, which then diffuse into the fetal plasma, producing higher concentrations than in the maternal plasma (101). With small placentas, fetal amino acid supply is reduced, as are fetal amino acid concentrations, leading to decreased rates of fetal protein synthesis, protein and nitrogen balance, and growth rate. Reduced energy supply to the placenta also reduces amino acid transport to the fetus. This is especially the case for oxygen deficit from maternal hypoxemia and glucose deficit from chronic maternal and fetal hypoglycemia (102,103). Of course, hypoxemia and hypoglycemia could reduce fetal growth, independent of reduced amino acid transport, by limiting anabolic hormone and growth factor production or by decreasing energy supply, both of which are necessary to produce protein synthesis and limit protein breakdown in fetal tissues.

The reason why amino acid and energy supplies are so important for fetal protein and nitrogen balance and for fetal growth is illustrated in Fig. 7 (104), which shows that fractional protein synthetic rate and growth rate are several-fold higher at 50–60% of term gestation in fetal sheep (equivalent to about 20–24 weeks of human gestation). Such high rates of protein turnover require a much greater rate of amino acid supply and energy

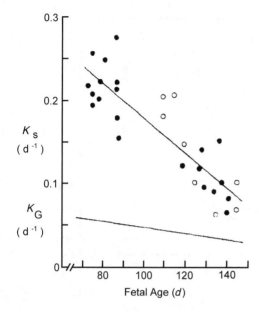

Figure 7 Fractional rate of protein synthesis (K_s) over gestation in fetal sheep studied with leucine (●) and lysine (○) radioactive tracers compared with the fractional rate of growth (K_G) in the lower portion of the figure (—). (From Ref. 102, p. 629. Adapted from Refs. 46, 80, and 104.)

than at term, when fetal protein turnover rate is much lower. Indeed, in midgestation fetal sheep, glucose utilization rates per whole fetal weight and oxygen consumption rates per dry fetal weight are much higher in the early fetus than at term (105). These conditions result in a 50% higher rate of net protein accretion and fractional rate of fetal growth at midgestation than at term. Approximately 25% of fetal oxygen consumption is used for normal protein synthetic and growth rates (34).

G. Nitrogen and Protein

Nonfat dry weight and nitrogen content, predictors of protein content, show a linear relationship with fetal weight and an exponential relationship with gestational age (Fig. 8) (90,106). Among IUGR infants, nitrogen and protein contents are reduced for body weight, primarily due to deficient production of muscle mass, often below that of fat as a fraction of body weight (99–101).

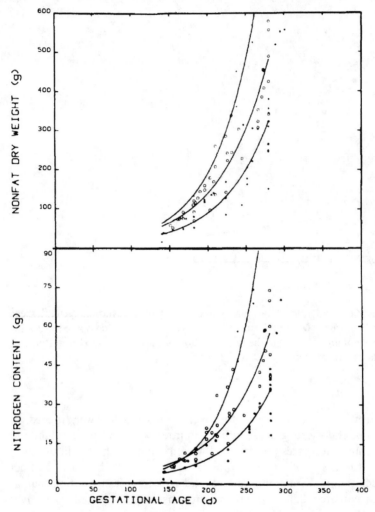

Figure 8 Nonfat dry weight (top) and nitrogen content (bottom) vs. gestational age. Top curve, LGA infants (●); middle curve, AGA infants (○); bottom curve, SGA infants (●). (From Ref. 90, p. 272.)

H. Altered Fetal Organ Development

1. Pancreas

Abnormal pancreatic growth and/or dysfunction have been observed in three pregnant rat models of IUGR. Maternal calorie restriction (50%) during late gestation reduces β-cell mass and insulin content as well as fetal weight by 18% (107). Decreased β-cell mass in these models is not due to β-cell replication; rather, it appears to result from reduced β-cell formation (108). Maintaining the offspring of calorie-restricted females until weaning augments the reduction in β-cell mass, which persists into adulthood (109). In addition, offspring of IUGR dams have significant reductions in β-cell mass and reductions of β-cell and epithelial cell expression of Pdx-1, an essential growth-regulating transcription factor. Glucose homeostasis in the IUGR offspring in this malnutrition model, however, was not affected (111,112). These data are an example of generational persistence of abnormal β-cell development in a model of IUGR. A second model, created by feeding the pregnant mother an isocaloric low-protein diet (8% vs. 20% protein) during gestation, reduces fetal weight (8%), pancreas weight, β-cell mass, and fetal islet insulin secretion responsiveness (112–114). A specific deficit in this model appears to be low fetal concentrations of taurine (115). As adults, these IUGR offspring exhibit decreased endocrine cell volume and impaired glucose tolerance (116). In a third model, the uterine artery was ligated at E19; pups delivered are 15% growth restricted (117). These IUGR rats have no differences in β-cell mass, islet size, or pancreas size at 1 or 7 weeks of age; however, β-cell mass at 15 weeks is 50% of normal and decreases to 33% of normal by 26 weeks. Additionally, acute pancreas responsiveness to glucose progressively diminished in the uterine artery ligation rats, and they developed an NIDDM phenotype (118). Performing the uterine artery ligations at E17 results in a reduced β-cell population at postnatal day 1 (119). Comparatively, these reports indicate that there are unique programming windows for subsequent β-cell formation versus postnatal β-cell function.

Pancreatic dysfunction in other mammalian models of human IUGR has not been characterized to the same extent as the rat models, but data from sheep are beginning to parallel those of human IUGR infants, in that both have decreased endocrine mass (118) and reduced insulin secretion in vivo (119). An ovine model of placental insufficiency at 135 days (92%) of gestation had significantly reduced plasma glucose and insulin concentrations and exhibited a 51% reduction in fetal weight at autopsy (120). Pancreas insulin content was 36% lower per gram of pancreas in the IUGR fetuses as compared to control fetuses, and fetal β-cell mass was reduced approximately 78% (120). These data indicate that IUGR has a significant impact on the developing endocrine pancreas. Additionally, chronic hypoglycemia for 2 weeks during late gestation produced a 19% reduction in fetal weight, and these fetuses displayed blunted insulin secretion responsiveness to glucose and arginine (121). Interestingly, when these fetuses were returned to normal glucose concentrations for as few as 5 days, the maximum concentrations of insulin were regained, but the insulin secretion responsiveness remained blunted (122). These data from ovine models of IUGR demonstrate that islet function in vivo can be permanently altered with hypoglycemic insults for as short as 10% of gestation.

2. Kidney

Another long-term pathological outcome related to IUGR is hypertension, which has been associated with impaired development of the kidney and the renin–angiotensin system (123–125). In IUGR human infants, nephron number is reduced and associated with aberrant kidney development and hypertension in adult life (126–128). In rat models of IUGR created by maternal low-protein diet, sodium restriction, or reduced uterine perfusion all exhibited elevated mean arterial blood pressures in postnatal life (128–131). A reduction in the number of glomeruli was observed for low-protein diet and uterine artery ligation pregnant rat models (132,133). In another model, reduced glomerular number and development were observed in fetuses exposed to cortisol during organogenesis of the kidney, and these animals exhibited an increased mean arterial blood pressure in adulthood (134). Among ovine models of IUGR, not all exhibit postnatal hypertension. In fact, in late-gestation fetal sheep made IUGR by placental embolization, the mean arterial pressure actually decreased in the lambs after birth (135). Nevertheless, these data together indicate that altered fetal organ development at critical times during organogenesis can result in adverse effects during postnatal life.

I. Fetal Endocrine and Autocrine-/Paracrine-Acting Growth Factors and Fetal Growth

Several hormones lead to a reduction in fetal growth when they are deficient (136). These fetal hormones promote growth (and development) in utero by altering both the metabolism and gene expression of fetal tissues. These hormonal actions ensure that fetal growth rate is commensurate with nutrient supply.

1. Insulin

Insulin has direct mitogenic effects on cellular development and thus can regulate cell number. Increased insulin concentrations in the fetus activate the insulin signal transduction pathway, promoting GLUT4 translocation to the cell surface of skeletal muscle myocytes, thereby enhancing glucose uptake and utilization (137). Insulin also activates the mitogen-activated protein (MAP) kinase pathway, which could lead to cellular hyperplasia (138) and also activates those proteins in its signal transduction pathway that promote amino acid incorporation into protein synthesis (139,140). Physiological studies also show that increased insulin concentrations limit fetal protein breakdown (96). Opposite effects are associated with reduced fetal growth when insulin concentrations are low (141,142) or absent (143). A significant portion of the growth reduction with hypoinsulinemia also could be caused by a release of insulin's normal inhibitory role on glucose production, resulting in fetal hyperglycemia, a secondary decrease in the maternal–fetal glucose concentration gradient, and thus a decrease in glucose transport to the fetus (144). Fetal amino acid uptake decreases under the same circumstances. Thus, insulin deficiency, directly and indirectly, results in a decrease in fetal nutrient supply.

2. Insulin-Like Growth Factor-I (IGF-I)

IGF-I is positively regulated by glucose supply in the fetus. Infusion of IGF-I into fetal sheep decreases protein breakdown, especially when protein breakdown is increased by fasting-induced hypoglycemia. Metabolic effects of a decreased plasma concentration of IGF-I have not been made, although, as for insulin, such effects might be difficult to separate from simultaneous changes in nutrient substrate supply and concentration. Plasma IGF-I concentrations are positively related to fetal size at birth. Transgenic mouse models have shown that decreased expression of IGF-I results in markedly reduced rates of fetal growth. Other transgenic models with increased expression of IGF-I have been associated with increased brain growth (145,146), and this growth can be inhibited by overexpression of IGF binding protein-1 (IGFBP-1) (147). IGF-I stimulates an increase in oligodendrocytes and neuronal number as well as neuronal outgrowth with increased dendritic arborization and axon terminal fields (148). Because IGF-I is decreased directly by reduced nutrient supply, particularly glucose, and IGFBP-1 is decreased under the circumstances, the smaller, more densely packed neuronal structure of the undernourished brain that is seen in some infants with severe IUGR may have been mediated by nutrient regulation of IGF-I and IGFBP-1 expression. Such developmental limitations might underlie the poorer neurodevelopmental outcome of severely SGA infants who have relative microcephaly.

3. IGF-II, IGFBP-2, and IGFBP-3

Although serum concentrations of IGF-II do not correlate with fetal size at birth in human infants, it has been shown conclusively that targeted mutation of the IGF-II gene reduces fetal size in mice (149,150). Furthermore, IGF-II is the predominant IGF expressed in the tissues of embryos and fetuses of all species. As with IGF-I and IGFBP-1, transgenic overexpression of IGF-II and IGFBP-2 shows that cellular growth is dependent on the balance between the binding protein and the IGF molecule itself. IGFBP-3 is the predominant IGF-binding protein in several mammalian species, including humans (151,152), and is reduced in cord blood of infants with intrauterine growth restriction (153).

4. Thyroid Hormones

Fetal thyroid hormone deficiency produces developmental abnormalities in several tissues. When maternal thyroid hormones cannot compensate, fetal growth restriction develops, primarily reflecting deficient carcass growth (skin, bone, and muscle) (136). This growth restriction results from both hypoplasia (in muscle) and hypotrophy (in lung). More generally, fetal hypothyroidism decreases oxygen consumption and the oxidation of glucose, potentially decreasing fetal energy supply for growth. Hypothyroidism also decreases circulating and tissue concentrations of IGF-I.

5. Glucocorticoids

Glucocorticoids do not have strong effects on fetal growth rate, but they are important in the maturation of many fetal enzymatic pathways (29,136). These include glycogen deposition, gluconeogenesis, fatty acid oxidation, induction of surfactant production and release, structural maturation of alveoli, structural maturation of the gastrointestinal tract, increased expression of digestive enzymes, increased adrenal function, switch from fetal to adult hemoglobin synthesis, and others. Many IUGR fetuses have increased cortisol concentrations that appear to result from intermittent hypoxic stress. This may account for much of the apparent increased maturation of IUGR fetuses, even when born preterm.

VII. METABOLIC AND NUTRITIONAL PROBLEMS RELATED TO IUGR IN SGA/IUGR INFANTS

A. Hypoglycemia: Causes

Hypoglycemia is extremely common in SGA/IUGR infants, increasing with the severity of intrauterine growth restriction (154–157). The risk of hypoglycemia is greatest during the first 3 days of life, but fasting hypoglycemia, with or without ketonemia, can occur repeatedly up to weeks after birth. Early hypoglycemia usually is due to diminished hepatic and skeletal muscle glycogen contents (158). Early hypoglycemia is aggravated by diminished alternative energy substrates, including fatty acids and lactate. Hyperinsulinemia, increased sensitivity to insulin, or both may contribute to a greater incidence of hypoglycemia (155). These infants also demonstrate decreased gluconeogenesis (159), and resolution of persistent hypoglycemia is coincident with improved capacity for and rates of gluconeogenesis. Deficient counterregulatory hormones, particularly catecholamines, also contribute to the pathogenesis of hypoglycemia in SGA/IUGR infants (160). In contrast, basal glucagon levels may be elevated, but its effect to enhance glycemia is limited because of the decreased hepatic glycogen stores.

B. Hypoglycemia: Prevention and Management

Fasting hypoglycemia is now less common in SGA/IUGR infants because conventional nutritional treatment now involves earlier enteral and intravenous feeding as well as a more liberal use of intravenous glucose (161). Early and frequent measurements of plasma glucose concentration can be used to adjust initial IV glucose rates of 4–8 mg/kg/min to keep plasma glucose concentration over 45 mg/dL (preventing concern for the relatively undetermined issues of whether lower glucose concentrations, how low, for how long, with what associated problems, etc., can cause irreversible neuronal injury). Less frequently repeated glucose measurements should be continued until the infant is tolerating reasonably full enteral feedings. Infants at greatest risk of having severe hypoglycemia are those who have been asphyxiated and those are the thinnest according to the Ponderal index, representing those infants with the least amount of body glycogen content.

C. Hyperglycemia

Most very preterm SG/IUGR infants have developmentally low insulin secretion rates and plasma insulin concentrations, which may underlie the relatively common problem of hyperglycemia in ELBW SGA infants (162). Unnecessarily high rates of glucose infusion (>14 mg/min per kg) also contribute to this hyperglycemia (163). Higher concentrations of counterregulatory hormones, such as epinephrine, glucagon, and cortisol, also may contribute, although there is only limited evidence to support this commonly held assumption. In contrast, administration of insulin to even preterm SGA infants usually produces prompt decreases in glucose concentration, indicating at least normal and perhaps greater-than-normal insulin sensitivity (164).

D. Lipid Metabolism and Lipid Nutrition

SGA/IUGR infants have lower plasma free fatty acid concentrations than normally grown infants. Fasting blood glucose levels in these infants correlate directly with plasma free fatty acid and ketoacid concentrations. In addition, once fed, SGA/IUGR infants have deficient utilization and oxidation of intravenous triglyceride-derived fatty acids (165,166). Fatty acid oxidation is important because it spares peripheral tissue use of glucose, whereas the hepatic oxidation of fatty acids may contribute the reducing equivalents and energy required for hepatic gluconeogenesis. Deficient provision and/or oxidation of fatty acids may be partly responsible for the development of fasting hypoglycemia in these infants.

E. Energy Metabolism and Energy Nutrition

Most studies show increased resting and total energy expenditure per kilogram of body weight in SGA/IUGR infants (167,168), although the magnitude of such increases is highly variable, ranging from 6.3% to 44% (167–170). Such hypermetabolism in the SGA/IUGR infant is in part the product of a large brain-to-body weight ratio (171) and an increased protein metabolic rate. Partly because of enhanced caloric intake and because metabolic rate and oxygen consumption are related more to gestational age than to birthweight, SGA/IUGR infants have a higher oxygen consumption rate and a higher rate of total energy expenditure (due primarily to increased resting energy expenditure) than less mature neonates (172). This also reflects an increase in cell number relative to total mass and greater heat production in response to increased heat loss.

F. Amino Acid and Protein Metabolism and Nutrition

SGA/IUGR infants are particularly deficient in muscle mass. There is conflicting information from a limited number of studies, however, about how well SGA infants tolerate aggressive amino acid and protein nutrition, from a 20–30% increase in rates of protein synthesis and breakdown compared with AGA infants (173) to a 20% decrease in such rates of protein turnover (169,170,173,174). Several study design problems were behind such divergent results. Most importantly, these studies included heterogeneous groups of infants. Some studies compared AGA and SGA groups of infants who were of comparable gestational age and presumably metabolic maturity, while others compared groups of similar weight but at different gestational ages and therefore of different "maturity." Feeding schedules and food composition among studies were not always comparable. Even the definitions of SGA and IUGR have varied, mixing "mildly" SGA with those who were markedly growth restricted.

VIII. NUTRITIONAL PREVENTION OF POSTNATAL GROWTH RESTRICTION

From 54% to 92% (depending on the study) of preterm infants are small for gestational age at birth, representing the result of IUGR, and the fraction of preterm infants who are SGA increases with increasingly preterm delivery (175–177). Despite overall improved medical care, such prenatal growth restriction is augmented by postnatal growth failure that is not reversed by the time of hospital discharge (178,179). Presumably, this additional postnatal growth restriction is caused by inadequate nutritional support. In general, better rates of weight gain occur in such infants among those who received early parenteral nutrition after birth, were started earlier after birth on enteral nutrition, and reached full enteral nutrition sooner (180).

The consequences of adding postnatal growth restriction to prenatal growth restriction may have marked impact on future development. Both human and animal investigations indicate that malnutrition at sensitive periods during the late prenatal and early postnatal period can have long-term adverse growth and developmental consequences (181,182). In humans, the most critical developmental period of brain growth and function occurs during the last trimester of pregnancy and the first 2 years of postnatal life. Outcome studies after malnutrition in the neonatal period, however, have produced ambiguous results, because undernourished neonatal populations often grow up in environments with multiple other adverse social and economic factors that may affect long-term outcome. Autopsy studies of infants who died of severe malnutrition in the first 12 months of life demonstrate significant reductions in brain weight and cell number and protein, DNA, and RNA contents (183). In a British study of preterm infants who received different nutrient intakes over the first month of life, long-term follow-up indicated that a higher protein intake earlier in life conferred a developmental advantage at 7.5–8 years of life (184).

IX. CATCH-UP GROWTH AND OUTCOME IN SGA INFANTS

Population studies of catch-up growth in SGA/IUGR infants indicate highly variable growth outcomes (185). Furthermore, the slower the rate of intrauterine growth, the less likely it is that the infant will continue to catch up and eventually grow normally (186). Thus less growth-restricted and healthier SGA/IUGR infants are more likely to respond to nutritional intervention. Regardless of the severity of the growth restriction and the overall response to nutritional treatment, several studies indicate that SGA/IUGR infants are prone to persistent deficits in muscle mass but normal or excessive gain in fat (187,188).

There is increasing evidence that early diet can have long-term effects on developmental outcome (189,190), although there have been few prospective trials of nutrient interventions on growth outcomes (191,192). The majority of SGA/IUGR infants achieve catch-up growth over the first 2 years of life, but a failure to demonstrate early compensatory growth may be associated with permanently decreased growth (193,194). Whether this is due to inadequate early nutrition or to permanent programming of decreased growth capacity is unknown.

There also is concern from recent animal and epidemiological studies in human infants that aggressive feeding producing catch-up growth that includes primarily fat (induction of relative obesity, or rapid positive crossing of weight-for-age centiles) is most strongly associated with subsequent development of obesity, insulin resistance, and diabetes in later life (195). This phenomenon has been called the *catch-up growth* hypothesis (196). Considerable data now indicate that the opposite, in terms of low nutrient intake and reduced growth rates among infants who were previously growth restricted, can actually lead to increased insulin sensitivity (197).

X. POSSIBLE ADULT DISORDERS RESULTING FROM IUGR

Recent epidemiological evidence indicates that obesity, insulin resistance, diabetes, and cardiovascular disease are more common among adults who were smaller than normal at birth and very likely SGA secondary to intra-uterine growth restriction, particularly those who had a high placental-to-fetal-weight ratio (198). A variety of animal studies support this concept, including the greater incidence of obesity, glucose intolerance, plasma lipid abnormalities, and hypertension in offspring whose mothers were fed a low-protein diet during pregnancy (199–202). These examples indicate that certain adult pathologies may be unavoidable consequences of environmentally imposed conditions, such as severe and prolonged fetal undernutrition, that lead to fetal growth restriction in order to ensure successful fetal survival. These conditions may represent an example of "programming," in which an insult, when applied at a critical or sensitive stage in development, may result in a lasting, even lifelong, effect on the structure or function of the organism (203). IUGR, therefore, is increasingly seen as an adaptive physiological process, even though it can produce adverse fetal, neonatal, and potentially adult consequences (204). Mechanisms responsible for these later-life morbidities in adults who were growth restricted in utero are not yet established. There is some evidence of diminished pancreatic growth and development, which might manifest in later life as pancreatic insufficiency when the adult starts and then continues eating a diet rich in simple carbohydrates and lipids. Peripheral insulin resistance may develop in the same way, and hypertension in adulthood may be the result of altered adrenal development in response to IUGR.

REFERENCES

1. Chard T, Costeloe K, Leaf A. Evidence of growth retardation in neonates of apparently normal weight. Eur J Obstet Gynecol Reprod Endocrinol 1992; 45:59–62.
2. Chard T, Yoong A, Macintosh M. The myth of fetal growth retardation at term. Br J Obstet Gynaecol 1993; 100:1076–1981.
3. Wark L, Malcolm LA. Growth and development of the Lumi child in the Sepik district of New Guinea. Med J Aust 1969; 2:129–138.
4. Ashcroft MT, Buchanan IC, Lovell HG, Welsh B. Growth of infants and preschool children in St Christopher-Nevis-Anguilla West Indies. Am J Clin Nutr 1966; 19:37–59.
5. Sabbagha RE. Intrauterine growth retardation. In: Sabbagha RE, ed. Ultrasound Applied to Obstetrics and Gynecology. Philadelphia: Lippincott, 1987: 112–131.
6. Rosso P. Morbidity and mortality in intrauterine growth retardation. In: Santerre J, ed. Intrauterine Growth Retardation. Nestlé Nutrition Workshop Series. Vol. 18. Nestlé Ltd., New York: Vevey/Raven Press, 1989: 123–142.
7. Hill RDG. Insulin as a growth factor. Pediatr Res 1985; 19:879–886.
8. Evans MI, Mukherjee AB, Schulman JD. Animal models of intrauterine growth retardation. Obstet Gynecol Surv 1983; 38:183–192.
9. Simmons RA, Gounis AS, Bangalore SA, Ogata ES. Intrauterine growth retardation: fetal glucose transport is diminished in lung but spared in brain. Pediatr Res 1992; 32:59–63.
10. Pardi G, Cetin I, Marconi AM, Lanfranchi A, Bozzetti P, Ferrazzi E, et al. Diagnostic value of blood sampling in fetuses with growth retardation. N Engl J Med 1993; 328(10):692–696.
11. Tchirikov M, Rybakowski C, Huneke B, Schroder HJ. Blood flow through the ductus venosus in singleton and multifetal pregnancies and in fetuses with intrauterine growth retardation. Am J Obstet Gynecol 1998; 178(5):943–949.
12. Jansson T, Ylven K, Wennergren M, Powell TL. Glucose transport and system A activity in syncytiotrophoblast microvillous and basal plasma membranes in intrauterine growth restriction. Placenta 2002; 23(5):392–399.
13. Rigano S, Bozzo M, Ferrazzi E, Bellotti M, Battaglia FC, Galan HL. Early and persistent reduction in umbilical vein blood flow in the growth-restricted fetus: a longitudinal study. Am J Obstet Gynecol 2001; 185(4):834–838.
14. Kramer MS, McLean FH, Olivier M, Willis DM, Usher RH. Body propor-

tionality and head and length "sparing" in growth-retarded neonates: a critical reappraisal. Pediatrics 1989; 84(4):717–723.

15. Zaw W, Gagnon R, da Silva O. The risks of adverse neonatal outcome among preterm small-for-gestational-age infants according to neonatal versus fetal growth standards. Pediatrics 2003; 111:1273–1277.

16. Pardi G, Cetin I, Marconi AM, et al. Diagnostic value of blood sampling in fetuses with growth retardation. N Engl J Med 1993; 328:692–696.

17. Glazier JD, Cetin I, Perugino G, et al. Association between the activity of the system A amino acid transporter in the microvillous plasma membrane of the human placenta and severity of fetal compromise in intrauterine growth restriction. Pediatr Res 1997; 42:514–519.

18. Marconi AM, Cetin I, Ferrazzi E, Ferrari MM, Pardi G, Battaglia FC. Lactate metabolism in normal and growth retarded human fetuses. Pediatr Res 1990; 28:652–656.

19. Marconi A, Paolini C, Stramare L, et al. Steady state maternal–fetal leucine enrichments in normal and intrauterine growth-restricted pregnancies. Pediatr Res 1999; 46:114–119.

20. Lucas A, Gore SM, Cole TJ, Bamford MF, Dossetor JF, Barr I, Dicardo L, Cork S, Lucas PJ. A multicenter trial on feeding low-birthweight infants: effects of diet on early growth. Arch Dis Child 1984; 59:722–730.

21. Kramer MS. Intrauterine growth and gestational duration determinants. Pediatrics 1987; 80:502–511.

22. Virgi SK, Cottington E. Risk factors associated with preterm deliveries among racial groups in a national sample of married mothers. J Perinatol 1991; 8:347–353.

23. Klebanoff MA, Schulsinger C, Mednick BR, Secher NJ. Preterm and small-for-gestational-age birth across generations. Am J Obstet Gynecol 1997; 176:521–526.

24. Abrams B, Newman V. Small-for-gestational-age birth: maternal predictors and comparison with risk factors of spontaneous preterm delivery in the same cohort. Am J Obstet Gynecol 1991; 164:785–790.

25. Cliver SP, Goldenberg RL, Cutter GR, Hoffman HJ, Davis RO, Nelson KG. The effect of cigarette smoking on neonatal anthropometric measurements. Obstet Gynecol 1995; 85:630–635.

26. Goldenberg RL, Cliver SP, Cutter GR, Davis RO, Hoffman HJ, Wen SW. Blood pressure, growth retardation, and preterm delivery. Int J Technol Assess Health Care 1992; 8:82–90.

27. Constância M, Hemberger M, Hughes J, Dean W, Ferguson-Smith A, Fundele R, Stewart F, Kelsey G, Fowden A, Sibley C, Reik W. Placental-specific IGF-II is a major modulator of placental and fetal growth. Nature 2002; 417:945–948.

28. DeChiara TM, Robertson EJ, Efstratiadis A. Parental imprinting of the mouse insulin-like growth factor II gene. Cell 1991; 64:849–859.

29. Milner RDG, Gluckman PD. Regulation of Intrauterine Growth. In: Gluckman PD, Heymann MA, eds. Pediatrics and Perinatology: The Scientific Basis. 2d ed. London: Arnold, 1993:284–289.

30. Reik W, Walter J. Genomic imprinting: parental influence on the genome. Nature Rev Genet 2001; 2:21–32.
31. Ferguson-Smith A, Surani MA. Imprinting and the epigenetic asymmetry between parental genomes. Science 2001; 293:1086–1089.
32. McKeown T, Record RG. Observations on foetal growth in multiple pregnancy in man. J Endocrinol 1952; 8:386–401.
33. Ounsted M, Ounsted C. On Fetal Growth Rate. Clinics in Developmental Medicine No. 46. Philadelphia: Lippincott, 1973.
34. Battaglia FC, Meschia G. An Introduction to Fetal Physiology. Orlando, FL: Academic Press, 1986.
35. Lumey LH. Decreased birthweights in infants after maternal in utero exposure to the Dutch famine of 1944–1945. Paediatr Perinat Epidemiol 1992; 6:240–253.
36. Antonov AM. Children born during the siege of Leningrad in 1942. J Pediatr 1947; 30:250–259.
37. Hickey CA, Cliver SP, Goldenberg RL, Kohatsu J, Hoffman HJ. Prenatal weight gain, term birthweight, and fetal growth retardation among high-risk multiparous black and white women. Obstet Gynecol 1993; 81:529–535.
38. Rush D, Stein Z, Susser M. A randomized controlled trial of prenatal nutritional supplementation in New York City. Pediatrics 1980; 68:683–697.
39. Sibai B, Anderson GD. Pregnancy outcome of intensive therapy in severe hypertension in first trimester. Obstet Gynecol 1986; 67:517–522.
40. Xiong X, Mayes D, Demianczuk N, Olson DM, Davidge ST, Newburn-Cook C, et al. Impact of pregnancy-induced hypertension of fetal growth. Am J Obstet Gynecol 1999; 180(1 Pt 1):207–213.
41. Eskenazi B, Fenster L, Sidney S, Elkin EP. Fetal growth retardation in infants of multiparous and nulliparous women with preeclampsia. Am J Obstet Gynecol 1993; 169(5):1112–1118.
42. Benirschke K, Kaufmann P. Architecture of normal villous trees. In: Benirschke K, Kaufmann P, eds. Pathology of the Human Placenta. London: Springer Verlag, 2000:116–154.
43. Ong S, Lash G, Baker PN. Angiogenesis and placental growth in normal and compromised pregnancies. Best Pract Res Clin Obstet Gynaecol 2000; 14(6):969–980.
44. Rasmussen S, Irgens LM. Fetal growth and body proportion in preeclampsia. Obstet Gynecol Mar 2003; 101(3):575–583.
45. Mayhew TM. Thinning of the intervascular tissue layers of the human placenta is an adaptive response to passive diffusion in vivo and may help to predict the origins of fetal hypoxia. Eur J Obstet Gynaecol Reprod Biol 1998; 81(1):101–109.
46. Teasdale F. Histomorphometry of the human placenta in preeclampsia associated with severe intrauterine growth retardation. Placenta 1987; 8(2):119–128.
47. Zamudio S, Palmer SK, Dahms TE, Berman JC, McCullough RG, McCullough RE, et al. Blood volume expansion, preeclampsia, and infant birthweight at high altitude. J Appl Physiol 1993; 75(4):1566–1573.
48. Palmer SK, Moore LG, Young D, Cregger B, Berman JC, Zamudio S. Altered

blood pressure course during normal pregnancy and increased preeclampsia at high altitude (3100 meters) in Colorado. Am J Obstet Gynecol 1999; 180 (5):1161–1168.

49. Kingdom J, Huppertz B, Seaward G, Kaufmann P. Development of the placental villous tree and its consequences for fetal growth. Eur J Obstet Gynaecol Reprod Biol 2000; 92(1):35–43.

50. Regnault TRH, de Vrijer B, Galan HL, Davidsen ML, Trembler KA, Battaglia FC, et al. The relationship between transplacental O_2 diffusion and placental expression of P1GF, VEGF and their receptor in a placental insufficiency model of fetal growth restriction. J Physiol 2003; 550:641–656.

51. Kingdom JCP, Kaufmann P. Oxygen and placental villous development—origins of fetal hypoxia. Placenta 1997; 18(8):613–621.

52. Krebs C, Macara LM, Leiser R, Bowman AW, Greer IA, Kingdom JC. Intrauterine growth restriction with absent end-diastolic flow velocity in the umbilical artery is associated with maldevelopment of the placental terminal villous tree. Am J Obstet Gynecol 1996; 175(6):1534–1542.

53. Jackson MR, Walsh AJ, Morrow RJ, Mullen JB, Lye SJ, Ritchie JW. Reduced placental villous tree elaboration in small-for-gestational-age pregnancies: relationship with umbilical artery Doppler waveforms. Am J Obstet Gynecol 1995; 172(2 Pt 1):518–525.

54. Giles WB, Trudinger BJ, Baird PJ. Fetal umbilical artery flow velocity waveforms and placental resistance: pathological correlation. Br J Obstet Gynaecol 1985; 92(1):31–38.

55. Trudinger BJ, Stevens D, Connelly A, Hales JR, Alexander G, Bradley L, et al. Umbilical artery flow velocity waveforms and placental resistance: the effects of embolization of the umbilical circulation. Am J Obstet Gynecol 1987; 157 (6):1443–1448.

56. Morrow RJ, Adamson SL, Bull SB, Ritchie JW. Effect of placental embolization on the umbilical arterial velocity waveform in fetal sheep. Am J Obstet Gynecol 1989; 161(4):1055–1060.

57. Macara L, Kingdom JC, Kaufmann P, Kohnen G, Hair J, More IA, et al. Structural analysis of placental terminal villi from growth-restricted pregnancies with abnormal umbilical artery Doppler waveforms. Placenta 1996; 17 (1):37–48.

58. Novy MJ, Peterson EN, Metcalfe J. Respiratory characteristics of maternal and fetal blood in cyanotic congenital heart disease. Am J Obstet Gynecol 1968; 100:821–828.

59. Brown AK, Sleeper LA, Pegelow CH, Miller ST, Gill FM, Waclawisn MA. The influence of infant and maternal sickle cell disease on birth outcome and neonatal course. Arch Pediatr Adolesc Med 1994; 148:1156–1162.

60. Lichty JA, Ting RY, Bruns PD, Dyar E. Studies of babies born at high altitude. Am J Dis Child 1957; 93:666–678.

61. Krampl E, Kametas NA, Cacho Zegarra AM, Roden M, Nicolaides KH. Maternal plasma glucose at high altitude. BJOG 2001; 108(3):254–257.

62. Krampl E. Pregnancy at high altitude. Ultrasound Obstet Gynecol 2002; 19(6):535–539.
63. Moore LG, Armaza F, Villena M, Vargas E. Comparative aspects of high-altitude adaptation in human populations. Adv Exp Med Biol 2000; 475:45–62.
64. Zamudio S, Droma T, Norkyel KY, Acharya G, Zamudio JA, Niermeyer SN, et al., Protection from intrauterine growth retardation in Tibetans at high altitude. Am J Phys Anthropol 1993; 91(2):215–224.
65. Giussani DA, Phillips PS, Anstee S, Barker DJ. Effects of altitude versus economic status on birthweight and body shape at birth. Pediatr Res 2001; 49 (4):490–494.
66. Garcia FC, Stiffel VM, Gilbert RD. Effects of long-term high-altitude hypoxia on isolated fetal ovine coronary arteries. J Soc Gynecol Invest 2000; 7(4):211–217.
67. Galan HL, Rigano S, Chyu J, Beaty B, Bozzo M, Hobbins J, et al. Comparison of low- and high-altitude Doppler velocimetry in the peripheral and central circulations of normal fetuses. Am J Obstet Gynecol 2000; 183(5):1158–1161.
68. Mayhew TM. Thinning of the intervascular tissue layers of the human placenta is an adaptive response to passive diffusion in vivo and may help to predict the origins of fetal hypoxia. Eur J Obstet Gynecol Reprod Biol 1998; 81(1):101–109.
69. Espinoza J, Sebire NJ, McAuliffe F, Krampl E, Nicolaides KH. Placental villus morphology in relation to maternal hypoxia at high altitude. Placenta 2001; 22(6):606–608.
70. Zhang EG, Burton GJ, Smith SK, Charnock-Jones DS. Placental vessel adaptation during gestation and to high altitude: changes in diameter and perivascular cell coverage. Placenta 2002; 23(10):751–762.
71. Krampl E, Kametas NA, McAuliffe F, Cacho-Zegarra AM, Nicolaides KH. Maternal serum insulin-like growth factor binding protein-1 in pregnancy at high altitude. Obstet Gynecol 2002; 99(4):594–598.
72. Coussons-Read ME, Mazzeo RS, Whitford MH, Schmitt M, Moore LG, Zamudio S. High-altitude residence during pregnancy alters cytokine and catecholamine levels. Am J Reprod Immunol (Copenhagen) 2002; 48(5):344–354.
73. Sobande AA, Archibong EI, Akinola SE. Pregnancy outcome in asthmatic patients from high altitudes. Int J Gynaecol Obstet 2002; 77(2):117–121.
74. Perlow JH, Montgomery D, Morgan MA, Towers CV, Porto M. Severity of asthma and perinatal outcome. Am J Obstet Gynecol 1992; 167:963–967.
75. Goldenberg RL, Merkatz IR, thompson JE, Mullen PD. Intrauterine growth retardation. In: Merkatz IR, et al., ed. New Perspectives on Prenatal Care. New York: Elsevier, 1990:461–478.
76. Abel EL. Consumption of alcohol during pregnancy: a review of effects on growth and development of offspring. Hum Biol 1982; 54:421–453.
77. Woods JR, Plessinger MA, Clark KE. Effect of cocaine on uterine blood flow and fetal oxygenation. JAMA 1986; 257:957–961.
78. Yau K-IT, Chang M-H. Growth and body composition of preterm, small-for-

gestational-age infants at a postmenstrual age of 37–40 weeks. Early Hum Dev 1993; 33:117–131.

79. Hay WW, Jr. Glucose metabolism in the fetal–placental unit. In: Cowett RM, ed. Principles of Perinatal–Neonatal Metabolism. 2d ed. New York: Springer-Verlag, 1998:337–368.

80. Molteni RA, Stys SJ, Battaglia FC. Relationship of fetal and placental weight in human beings: fetal/placental weight ratios at various gestational ages and birthweight distributions. J Reprod Med 1978; 21:327–334.

81. Owens JA, Falconer J, Robinson JS. Effect of restriction of placental growth on fetal and utero-placental metabolism. J Dev Physiol 1987; 9:225–238.

82. Beischer NA, Sivasamboo R, Vohra S, Silpisornkosal S, Reid S. Placental hypertrophy in severe pregnancy anaemia. J Obstet Gynaecol Br Commonwealth 1970; 77:398–409.

83. Handwerger S. The physiology of placental lactogen in human pregnancy. Endocr Rev 1992; 12:329–336.

84. Freemark M, Handwerger S. The role of placental lactogen in the regulation of fetal metabolism. J Pediatr Gastroenterol Nutr 1989; 8:281–287.

85. Ali KZ, Burton GJ, Morad N, Ali ME. Does hypercapillarization influence the branching pattern of terminal villi in the human placenta at high altitude? Placenta 1996; 17(8):677–682.

86. Ahmed A, Perkins J. Angiogenesis and intrauterine growth restriction. Best Pract Res Clin Obstet Gynaecol 2000; 14(6):981–998.

87. Harding JE, Johnston BM. Nutrition and fetal growth. Reprod Fert Dev 1995; 7:539–547.

88. Ziegler EE, O'Donnell AM, Nelson SE, Fomon SJ. Body composition of the reference fetus. Growth 1976; 40:329–341.

89. Nimrod CA. The biology of normal and deviant fetal growth. In: Reece EA, Hobbins JC, Mahoney MJ, Petrie RH, eds. Medicine of the Fetus and Mother. Philadelphia: Lippincott, 1992:285–290.

90. Sparks JW, Ross JR, Cetin I. Intrauterine growth and nutrition. In: Polin RA, Fox WW, eds. Fetal and Neonatal Physiology. 2d ed. Philadelphia: Saunders, 1998:267–289.

91. Thureen PJ, Trembler KA, Meschia G, Makowski EL, Wilkening RB. Placental glucose transport in heat-induced fetal growth retardation. Am J Physiol 1992; 263:R578–R585.

92. Marconi AM, Cetin I, Davoli E, Baggaini AM, Fanelli R, Fennessey PV, Battaglia FC, Pardi G. An evaluation of fetal gluconeogenesis in intrauterine growth retarded pregnancies. Metabolism 1993; 42:860–864.

93. Molina RD, Meschia G, Battaglia FC, Hay WW Jr. Gestational maturation of placental glucose transfer capacity in sheep. Am J Physiol 1991; 261:R697–R704.

94. Ross JC, Fennessey PV, Wilkening RB, Battaglia FC, Meschia G. Placental transport and fetal utilization of leucine in a model of fetal growth retardation. Am J Physiol 1996; 270:E491–E503.

95. Milley JR. Effects of insulin on ovine fetal leucine kinetics and protein metabolism. J Clin Invest 1994; 93:1616–1624.

96. Townsend SF, Briggs KK, Carver TD, Hay WW Jr, Wilkening RB. Altered fetal liver and kidney insulin-like growth factor II mRNA in the sheep after chronic maternal glucose or nutrient deprivation. Clin Res 1992; 40:91A.

97. Shelley HJ. Glycogen reserves and their changes at birth. Br Med Bull 1961; 17:137.

98. Philipps AF. Carbohydrate metabolism of the fetus. In: Polin RA, Fox WW, eds. Fetal and Neonatal Physiology. 2d ed. Philadelphia: Saunders, 1998:560–573.

99. Lapillonne A, Brailon P, Claris O, Chatelain PG, Delmas PD, Salle BL. Body composition in appropriate and in small-for-gestational-age infants. Acta Paediatr 1997; 86:196–200.

100. Hay WW Jr. Nutrition and development of the fetus: carbohydrate and lipid: metabolism. In: Walker WA, Watkins JB, eds. Nutrition in Pediatrics. 2d ed. Hamilton: BC Dekker, 1996:364–378.

101. Hay WW Jr. Fetal requirements and placental transfer of nitrogenous compounds. In: Polin RA, Fox WW, eds. Fetal and Neonatal Physiology. 2d ed. Philadelphia: Saunders, 1998:619–635.

102. Milley JR. Ovine fetal leucine kinetics and protein metabolism during decreased oxygen availability. Am J Physiol 1998; 274:E618–E626.

103. Milley JR. Ovine fetal protein metabolism during decreased glucose delivery. Am J Physiol 1993; 265:E525–E531.

104. Meier PR, Peterson RG, Bonds DR, Meschia G, Battaglia FC. Rates of protein synthesis and turnover in fetal life. Am J Physiol 1981; 240:E320–E324.

105. Bell AW, Kennaugh JM, Battaglia FC, Makowski EL, Meschia G. Metabolic and circulatory studies of the fetal lamb at mid gestation. Am J Physiol 1986; 250:E538–E544.

106. Widdowson EM. Changes in body proportions and composition during growth. In: Davis JA, Dobbing J, eds. Scientific Foundations of Paediatrics. Philadelphia: Saunders, 1974:155–163.

107. Garofano A, Czernichow P, Breant B. In utero undernutrition impairs rat beta-cell development. Diabetologia 1997; 40(10):1231–1234.

108. Garofano A, Czernichow P, Breant B. In utero undernutrition impairs rat beta-cell development. Diabetologia 1997; 40(10):1231–1234.

109. Garofano A, Czernichow P, Breant B. Beta-cell mass and proliferation following late fetal and early postnatal malnutrition in the rat. Diabetologia 1998; 41(9):1114–1120.

110. Blondeau B, Avril I, Duchene B, Breant B. Endocrine pancreas development is altered in foetuses from rats previously showing intrauterine growth retardation in response to malnutrition. Diabetologia 2002; 45(3):394–401.

111. Avril I, Blondeau B, Duchene B, Czernichow P, Breant B. Decreased beta-cell proliferation impairs the adaptation to pregnancy in rats malnourished during perinatal life. J Endocrinol 2002; 174(2):215–223.

112. Snoeck A, Remacle C, Reusens B, Hoet JJ. Effect of a low-protein diet during pregnancy on the fetal rat endocrine pancreas. Biol Neonate 1990; 57(2):107–118.

113. Berney DM, Desai M, Palmer DJ, Greenwald S, Brown A, Hales CN, et al. The effects of maternal protein deprivation on the fetal rat pancreas: major structural changes and their recuperation. J Pathol 1997; 183(1):109–115.

114. Petrik J, Reusens B, Arany E, Remacle C, Coelho C, Hoet JJ, et al. A low-protein diet alters the balance of islet cell replication and apoptosis in the fetal and neonatal rat and is associated with a reduced pancreatic expression of insulin-like growth factor-II. Endocrinology 1999; 140(10):4861–4873.

115. Cherif H, Reusens B, Ahn MT, Hoet JJ, Remacle C. Effects of taurine on the insulin secretion of rat fetal islets from dams fed a low-protein diet. J Endocrinol 1998; 159(2):341–348.

116. Dahri S, Snoeck A, Reusens-Billen B, Remacle C, Hoet JJ. Islet function in offspring of mothers on low-protein diet during gestation. Diabetes 1991; 40(2):115–120.

117. Simmons RA, Templeton LJ, Gertz SJ. Intrauterine growth retardation leads to the development of type 2 diabetes in the rat. Diabetes 2001; 50(10):2279–2286.

118. De Prins FA, Van Assche FA. Intrauterine growth retardation and development of endocrine pancreas in the experimental rat. Biol Neonate 1982; 41(1–2):16–21.

119. Van Assche FA, De Prins F, Aerts L, Verjans M. The endocrine pancreas in small-for-dates infants. Br J Obstet Gynaecol 1977; 84(10):751–753.

120. Nicolini U, Hubinont C, Santolaya J, Fisk NM, Rodeck CH. Effects of fetal intravenous glucose challenge in normal and growth retarded fetuses. Horm Metab Res 1990; 22(8):426–430.

121. Limesand SW, Hay WW Jr. A placental insufficiency ovine model of intra-uterine growth restriction (PI-IUGR) exhibits reduced beta-cell mass [abstr]. Pediatr Res 2003; 53(6):125.

122. Limesand SW, Hay WW Jr. Adaptation of ovine fetal pancreatic insulin secretion to chronic hypoglycaemia and euglycaemic correction. J Physiol 2002; 547:95–105.

123. Wadsworth ME, Cripps HA, Midwinter RE, Colley JR. Blood pressure in a national birth cohort at the age of 36 related to social and familial factors, smoking, and body mass. Br Med J (Clin Res Ed) 1985; 291(6508):1534–1538.

124. Law CM, de Swiet M, Osmond C, Fayers PM, Barker DJ, Cruddas AM, et al. Initiation of hypertension in utero and its amplification throughout life. BMJ 1993; 306(6869):24–27.

125. Barker DJ. The fetal origins of hypertension. J Hypertens (suppl) 1996; 14(5):S117–S120.

126. Hinchliffe SA, Lynch MR, Sargent PH, Howard CV, Van Velzen D. The effect of intrauterine growth retardation on the development of renal nephrons. Br J Obstet Gynaecol 1992; 99(4):296–301.

127. Manalich R, Reyes L, Herrera M, Melendi C, Fundora I. Relationship between weight at birth and the number and size of renal glomeruli in humans: a histomorphometric study. Kidney Int 2000; 58(2):770–773.

128. Mackenzie HS, Lawler EV, Brenner BM. Congenital oligonephropathy: the fetal flaw in essential hypertension? Kidney Int 1996; 55(suppl):S30–S34.

129. Alexander BT. Placental insufficiency leads to development of hypertension in growth-restricted offspring. Hypertension 2003; 41(3):457–462.

130. Battista MC, Oligny LL, St Louis J, Brochu M. Intrauterine growth restriction in rats is associated with hypertension and renal dysfunction in adulthood. Am J Physiol Endocrinol Metab 2002; 283(1):E124–E131.

131. Vehaskari VM, Aviles DH, Manning J. Prenatal programming of adult hypertension in the rat. Kidney Int 2001; 59(1):238–245.

132. Merlet-Benichou C, Gilbert T, Muffat-Joly M, Lelievre-Pegorier M, Leroy B. Intrauterine growth retardation leads to a permanent nephron deficit in the rat. Pediatr Nephrol 1994; 8(2):175–180.

133. Wintour EM, Moritz KM, Johnson K, Ricardo S, Samuel CS, Dodic M. Reduced nephron number in adult sheep, hypertensive as a result of prenatal glucocorticoid treatment. J Physiol 2003; 549(Pt 3):929–935.

134. Dodic M, Hantzis V, Duncan J, Rees S, Koukoulas I, Johnson K, et al. Programming effects of short prenatal exposure to cortisol. FASEB J 2002; 16(9):1017–1026.

135. Louey S, Cock ML, Stevenson KM, Harding R. Placental insufficiency and fetal growth restriction lead to postnatal hypotension and altered postnatal growth in sheep. Pediatr Res 2000; 48(6):808–814.

136. Fowden A. Endocrine regulation of fetal growth. Reprod Fertil Dev 1995; 7:469–477.

137. Anderson MS, Thamotharan M, Kao D, Devaskar SU, Friedman JE, Hay WW Jr. Effects of hyperinsulinemia on fetal ovine signal transduction proteins and glucose transporters in skeletal muscle. Pediatric Res 2003; 53(2209):390A.

138. Stephens E, Thureen PJ, Goalstone ML, Anderson MS, Leitner JW, Hay WW Jr, Draznin B. Fetal hyperinsulinemia increases farnesylation of p21 Ras in fetal tissues. Am J Physiol Endocrinol Metab 2001; 281:E217–E223.

139. Shen W, Wisniowski P, Ahmed L, Boyle DW, Denne SC, Liechty EA. Protein anabolic effects of insulin and IGF-I in the ovine fetus. Am J Physiol Endocrinol Metab 2003; 284:E748–E756.

140. Shen W, Mallon D, Boyle DW, Liechty EA. IGF-I and insulin regulate eIF4F formation by different mechanisms in muscle and liver in the ovine fetus. Am J Physiol Endocrinol Metab 2002; 283:E593–E603.

141. Fowden AL, Hay WW Jr. The effects of pancreatectomy on the rates of glucose utilization, oxidation and production in the sheep fetus. Q J Exp Physiol 1988; 73:973–984.

142. Hay WW Jr, Meznarich HK, Fowden AL. The effects of streptozotocin on rates of glucose utilization, oxidation and production in the sheep fetus. Metabolism 1988; 38:30–37.

143. Sherwood WG, Chance GW, Hill DE. A new syndrome of pancreatic agenesis. The role of insulin and glucagon in cell and cell growth. Pediatr Res 1974; 8:360.

144. Carver TD, Anderson SM, Aldoretta PW, Esler AL, Hay WW Jr. Glucose suppression of insulin secretion in chronically hyperglycemic fetal sheep. Pediatr Res 1995; 38:754–762.

145. Mathews LS, Hammer RE, Behringer RR, D'Ercole AJ, Bell GI, Brinster RL,

Palmiter RD. Growth enhancement of transgenic mice expressing human insulin-like growth factor I. Endocrinology, 1988; 123:2827–2833.

146. Behringer RR, Lewin TM, Quaife CJ, Palmiter RD, Brinster RL, D'Ercole AJ. Expression of insulin-like growth factor I stimulates normal somatic growth in growth hormone-deficient transgenic mice. Endocrinology 1990; 127:1033–1040.

147. D'Ercole AJ, Dai Z, Xing Y, Boney C, Wilkie MB, Lauder JM, Han VKM, Clemmons DR. Brain growth retardation due to the expression of human insulin like growth factor binding protein 1 (IGFBP-1) in transgenic mice: an in vivo model for the analysis of IGF function in the brain. Dev Brain Res 1994; 82:213–222.

148. Ye P, Carson J, D'Ercole AJ. In vivo actions of insulin-like growth factor-I (IGF-I) on brain myelination: studies of IGF-I and IGF binding protein-1 (IGFBP-1) transgenic mice. J Neurosci 1995; 15:7344–7356.

149. Delhanty PJD, Han VKM. The expression of insulin-like growth factor (IGF)-binding protein-2 and IGF-II genes in the tissues of the developing ovine fetus. Endocrinology 1993; 132:41–52.

150. Wood TL, Rogler L, Streck RD, Cerro J, Green B, Grewal A, Pintar JE. Targeted disruption of IGFBP-2 gene. Growth Regul 1993; 3:3–6.

151. Pintar JE, Wood TL, Streck RD, Havton L, Rogler L, Hsu MS. Expression of IGF-II, the IGF-II/mannose-6-phosphate receptor and IGFBP-2 during rat embryogenesis. Adv Exp Med Biol 1991; 293:325–333.

152. Wood TL, Streck RD, Pintar JE. Expression of the IGFBP-2 gene in post-implantation rat embryos. Development 1992; 114:59–66.

153. Crystal RA, Giduice LC. Insulin-like growth factor binding protein (IGFBP) profiles in human fetal cord sera: ontogeny during gestation and differences in newborns with intrauterine growth retardation (IUGR) and large-for-gestational-age (LGA) newborns. In: Spencer EM, ed. Modern Concepts of Insulin-Like Growth Factors. Elsevier; New York, 1991:395–408.

154. Chessex P, Reichman B, Verellen G, Putet G, Smith JM, Heim T, Swyer PR. Metabolic consequences of intrauterine growth retardation in very-low-birthweight infants. Pediatr Res 1984; 18:709–713.

155. Collins J, Leonard JV. Hyperinsulinism in asphyxiated and small for dates infants with hypoglycemia. Lancet 1984; 2:311–313.

156. Kliegman RM. Alterations of fasting glucose and fat metabolism in intrauterine growth-retarded newborn dogs. Am J Physiol 1989; 256:E380–E385.

157. Holtrop PC. The frequency of hypoglycemia in full-term large-and small-for-gestational-age newborns. Am J Perinatol 1993; 10:150–154.

158. Shelly HJ, Neligan GA. Neonatal hypoglycemia. Br Med Bull 1966; 22:34–39.

159. Williams PR, Fiser RH Jr, Sperling MA, Oh W. Effects of oral alanine feeding on blood glucose, plasma glucagon, and insulin concentrations in small for gestational age infants. N Eng J Med 1975; 292:612–614.

160. Hawdon JM, Weddell A, Aynsley-Green A, Platt MPW. Hormonal and metabolic response to hypoglycemia in small for gestational age infants. Arch Dis Child 1993; 68:269–273.

161. Hawdon JM, Platt MPW. Metabolic adaptation in small for gestational age infants. Arch Dis Child 1993; 68:262–268.

162. King RA, Smith RM, Dahlenberg GW. Long-term postnatal development of insulin secretion in early premature neonates. Early Hum Dev 1986; 13:285–294.

163. Cowett RM, Oh W, Pollak A, Schwartz R, Stonestreet BS. Glucose disposal of low-birthweight infants: steady-state hyperglycemia produced by constant intravenous glucose infusion. Pediatrics 63:389–396.

164. Hay WW Jr, Fetal and neonatal glucose homeostasis and their relation to the small-for-gestational-age infant. Sem Perinatol 1984; 8:101–116.

165. Bougneres PF, Castano L, Rocchiccioli F, Gia HP. Medium-chain fatty acids increase glucose production in normal and low-birthweight newborns. Am J Physiol 1989; 256:E692–E697.

166. Sabel K, Olegard R, Mellander M, Hildingsson K. Interrelation between fatty acid oxidation and control of gluconeogenic substrates in small-for-gestational-age (SGA) infants with hypoglycemia and with normoglycemia. Acta Paediatr Scand 1982; 71:53–61.

167. Sinclair J. Heat production and thermoregulation in the small-for-date infant. Pediatr Clin North Am 1970; 17:147–158.

168. Chessex P, Reichman B, Verellen G, et al. Metabolic consequences of intra-uterine growth retardation in very-low-birthweight infants. Pediatr Res 1984; 18:709–713.

169. Cauderay M, Schutz Y, Micheli JL, Calame A, Jequier E. Energy–nitrogen balances and protein turnover in small- and appropriate-for-gestational-age low-birthweight infants. Eur J Clin Nutr 1988; 42:125–136.

170. Pencharz PB, Masson M, Desgranges F, Papageorgiou A. Total-body protein turnover in human premature neonates: effects of birthweight, intrauterine nutritional status and diet. Clin Sci 1981; 61:207–215.

171. Sinclair JC, Silverman WA. Relative hypermetabolism in undergrown human neonates. Lancet, 1966; ii:49.

172. Holliday M, Potter D, Jarrah A, et al. Relation of metabolic rate to body weight and organ size: a review. J Physiol 1967; 199:685–703.

173. van Goudoever JB, Sulkers EJ, Halliday D, et al. Whole-body protein turnover in preterm appropriate-for-gestational-age and small-for-gestational-age in-fants: comparison of [15N]glycine and [1-13C]leucine administered simulta-neously. Pediatr Res 1995; 37:381–388.

174. Kandil H, Darwish O, Hammad S, Zagloul N, Halliday D, Millward J. Nitrogen balance and protein turnover during the growth failure in newly born low-birthweight infants. Am J Clin Nutr 1991; 53:1411–1417.

175. Ehrenkranz RA, Younes N, Lemons JA, Fanaroff AA, Donovan EF, Wright LL, Katsikiotis V, Tyson JE, Oh W, Shankaran S, Bauer CR, Korones SB, Stoll BJ, Stevenson DK, Papile LA. Longitudinal growth of hospitalized very-low-birthweight infants. Pediatrics 1999; 104:280–289.

176. Morley R, Lucas A. Influence of early diet on outcome in preterm infants. Acta Paediatr Suppl 1994; 405:123–126.

177. Pauls J, Bauer K, Versmold H. Postnatal body weight curves for infants below

1000 g birthweight receiving early enteral and parenteral nutrition. Eur J Pediatr 1998; 157:416–421.

178. Carlson SJ, Ziegler EE. Nutrient intakes and growth of very-low-birthweight infants. J Perinatol 1998; 18:252–258.

179. Lucas A, Gore SM, Cole TJ, Bamford MF, Dossetor JF, Barr I, Dicarlo L, Cork S, Lucas PJ. A multicenter trial on feeding low-birthweight infants: effects of diet on early growth. Arch Dis child 1984; 59:722–730.

180. Clark R, Wagner CL, Merritt RJ, Bloom BT, Neu J, Young TE, Clark DA. Nutrition in the neonatal intensive care unit: how do we reduce the incidence of extrauterine growth restriction? J Perinatol 2003; 23:337–344.

181. Desai M, Crowther NJ, Lucas A, Hales CN. Organ-selective growth in the offspring of protein-restricted mothers. Br J Nutr 1996; 76:591–603.

182. Morgane PJ, Austin-LaFrance R, Bronzino J, Tonkiss J, Diaz-Cintra S, Cintra L, Kemper T, Galler JR. Prenatal malnutrition and development of the brain. Neurosci Biobehav Rev 1993; 17:91–128.

183. Winick M, Rosso P. The effect of severe early malnutrition on cellular growth of human brain. Pediatr Res 1969; 3:181–184.

184. Lucas A, Morley R, Cole TJ. Randomized trial of early diet in preterm babies and later intelligence quotient. BMJ 1998; 317:1481–1487.

185. Hediger M, Overpeck M, Maurer K, Kuczmarski R, McGlynn A, Davis W. Growth of infants and young children born small or large for gestational age: findings from the Third National Health and Nutrition Examination Survey. Arch Ped Adol Med 1998; 152:1225–1231.

186. Hales CN. Metabolic consequences of intrauterine growth retardation. Acta Paediatr Scand Suppl 1997; 423:184–187.

187. Yau K, Chang M. Growth and body composition of preterm, small-for-gestational-age infants at a postmenstrual age of 37–40 weeks. Early Hum Dev 1993; 33:117–131.

188. Hediger M, Overpeck M, Kuczmarski R, McGlynn A, Maurer K, Davis W. Muscularity and fatness of infants and young children born small- or large-for-gestational-age. Pediatrics 1998; 1025:e60.

189. Lucas A, Morely RM, Cole TJ, Gore SM. A randomized multicenter study of human milk versus formula and later development in preterm infants. Arch Dis Child 1994; 70:F141.

190. Lucas A, Morley R, Cole TJ, Lister G, Leeson-Payne C. Breast milk and subsequent intelligence quotient in children born preterm. Lancet 1992; 339: 261–264.

191. Brooke OG, Kinsey JM. High-energy feeding in small-for-gestation infants. Arch Dis Child 1985; 60:42–46.

192. Lucas A, Fewtrell MS, Davies PS, Bishop NJ, Clough H, Cole TJ. Breastfeeding and catch-up growth in infants born small for gestational age. Acta Paediatr Scand 1997; 86:556–564.

193. Karlberg J, Albertsson-Wikland K, Baber FM, Low LC, Yeung CY. Born small for gestational age: consequences for growth. Acta Paediatr Scand Suppl 1996; 417:8–13.

194. Albertsson-Wikland K, Karlberg J. Postnatal growth of children born small for gestational age. Acta Paediatr Scand Suppl 1997; 423:193–195.
195. Oken E, Gillman MW. Fetal origins of obesity. Obes Res 2003; 11:496–506.
196. Cianfarani S, Germane D, Brfanca F. Low birthweight and adult insulin resistance: the "catch-up growth" hypothesis. Arch Dis Child Fetal Neonatal Ed 1999; 81:F71–F73.
197. Singhal A, Fewtrell M, Cole TJ, Lucas A. Low nutrient intake and early growth for later insulin resistance in adolescents born preterm. Lancet 2003; 361:1089–1097.
198. Barker DJP. The fetal and infant origins of adult disease. BMJ 1993; 301:1111.
199. Snoeck A, Remacle C, Reusens B, Hoet JJ. Effect of a low-protein diet during pregnancy on the fetal rat endocrine pancreas. Biol Neonate 1990; 57:107–118.
200. Dahri S, Snoeck A, Reusens B, Remacle C, Hoet JJ. Islet function in offspring of mothers on a low protein diet during pregnancy. Diabetes 1991; 40:115–121.
201. Dahri S, Cherif H, Reusens B, Remacle C, Hoet JJ. Effect of an isolcaloric low-protein diet during gestation in rat on in vitro insulin secretion by islets of the offspring. Diabetologia 1994; 37:A80.
202. Rasschaert J, Reusens B, Dahri S, Sener A, Remacle C, Hoet JJ, Malaisse WJ. Impaired activity of rat pancreatic islet mitochondrial glycerophosphate dehydrogenase in protein malnutrition. Endocrinology 1995; 136:2631–2634.
203. Smart J. Undernutrition, learning and memory: review of experimental studies. In: Taylor TG, Jenkins NK, eds. Proceedings of XII International Congress of Nutrition. London: John Libbey, 1986:74–78.
204. Hay WW Jr, Catz CS, Grave GD, Yaffe SJ. Workshop summary: fetal growth: its regulation and disorders. Pediatrics 1997; 99:585–591.
205. Anderson S, Hay WW Jr. The small-for-gestational-age infant. In: Avery GB, Fletcher MA, MacDonald MG, eds. Neonatology: Pathophysiology and Management of the Newborn. 5th ed. Philadelphia: Lippincott-Raven, 1999: 411–444.
206. Lubchenco LO, Hansman C, Boyd E. Pediatrics 1966; 37:403–408.
207. Creasy RK, Resnik R. Intrauterine growth retardation. In: Creasy RK, Resnik R, eds. Maternal–Fetal Medicine. 2d ed. Philadelphia: Saunders, 1989.
208. Shelley HJ, Neligan GA. Br Med Bull 1966; 22:36.

6
Nutritional Influences on Infant Development

William C. Heird
Baylor College of Medicine, Houston, Texas, U.S.A.

Robert G. Voigt
Mayo Clinic, Rochester, Minnesota, U.S.A.

I. INTRODUCTION

The human brain increases in size from about 400 g at term to 1400–1500 g at maturity, and the bulk of this growth occurs between birth and 2 years of age. This period of rapid brain growth, the "brain growth spurt," begins about midgestation and does not slow perceptibly until about 18 months of age. Some further growth occurs after 2 years of age, but this is minor compared with the growth prior to 2 years of age; quantitatively, the increase in weight from 2 years of age to adulthood is about the same as that during the last half of pregnancy.

The major period of neuroblast multiplication occurs prior to the "brain growth spurt," with the adult complement of neurons being established in most brain regions by midgestation. However, a number of other processes, probably as important as or perhaps more important than the final number of neurons, are occurring during the "brain growth spurt." These include glial multiplication, dendritic growth, establishment of synaptic connectivity, and myelination. It has been estimated that the human brain has about 100 billion neurons at birth and that each of these develops approximately 15,000 synapses by 3 years of age. Some established synapses eventually disappear, but those that are used frequently are preserved.

Considering this remarkable activity of the human brain between about midgestation and 3 years of age and the fuel obviously required to support it, it seems quite likely that inadequate intake of either a single nutrient (e.g., iron, zinc, an indispensable amino acid or fatty acid) or all nutrients (e.g., protein and energy) might interfere with the orderly processes of the "brain growth spurt." Indeed, specific as well as global developmental delays have been attributed to an inadequate intake of a single nutrient or global malnutrition during this potentially vulnerable period of brain growth and development (1–5).

On the other hand, not all studies of nutrient inadequacy during early development have documented neurodevelopmental delays. This may be because the specific nutritional intervention was not applied during the most vulnerable period of overall brain development or during the most vulnerable period for inadequacy of a specific nutrient. It also could be due to the fact, as many maintain, that the brain is spared the most serious consequences of nutrient inadequacy. This clearly is true to some extent. But an equally probable reason is the lack of sensitivity of the test instruments available to assess neurodevelopmental outcomes during infancy and early childhood. The remainder of this chapter deals with aspects of this latter problem.

II. BIOLOGICAL INFLUENCES ON COGNITIVE DEVELOPMENT

Cognitive development is dependent upon complex interactions between genetic factors and multiple environmental factors, only one of which is nutrition. It is virtually impossible to control for all these environmental factors when attempting to determine the effect of a specific nutritional factor on cognitive development. Moreover, the primary outcome variable of most studies of the impact of a specific nutritional factor has been general intelligence, or IQ, the stability of which over time is questionable. This is particularly problematical if the IQ difference attributed to the nutritional factor is small. Even more problematical is the tendency to equate scores on tests of early childhood development to subsequent cognitive function. This is because the correlation between scores during childhood and later measures of IQ is weak to nonexistent until after the age of 2 years.

Genes appear to set the upper and lower limits on potential intellectual outcome, but environmental factors determine where within this range ultimate intellectual function falls (6). Numerous twin and adoption studies have shown that general intelligence is among the most heritable behavioral traits. These studies suggest that heritability of general intelligence increases from about 20% in infancy to 40% in childhood, 50% in adolescence, and

60% in adulthood (7). Thus, any study examining the effect of nutrition on intelligence must control for this significant genetic effect.

On the other hand, the twin and adoption studies indicate that 40% of the variation in ultimate adult IQ is unrelated to genetics. This allows a substantial role for environmental factors to influence IQ; however, nutrition is only one of these factors. Thus, considering the many prenatal, perinatal, and postnatal biologically based environmental factors that can affect intelligence, it is understandably difficult to quantitate the independent effect of specific nutritional factors on ultimate intellectual outcome. Prenatal factors include maternal nutritional status (8), maternal smoking (9), as well as maternal use of alcohol (10) and other drug abuse (11). Perinatal factors (12) and complications of prematurity (13) also exert significant effects on ultimate cognitive development. Postnatal factors that can influence a child's cognitive status include acute or chronic illness, medications (14), toxins (15), and sleep (16). Thus, to determine the specific effect of any nutritional factor on cognitive development, it is necessary to control for all these biologically based environmental factors.

III. PSYCHOSOCIAL INFLUENCES ON COGNITIVE DEVELOPMENT

Even more important than these biologically based environmental factors is the vast number of potential psychosocial factors that can influence cognitive development. One of the most important of these is the quality of the home caregiving environment. A nurturing, emotionally responsive, and developmentally stimulating home environment promotes a secure attachment between the infant and its caregivers and is critical to promoting optimal cognitive development. A neglectful or abusive home environment, on the other hand, has a detrimental effect on ultimate IQ. The quality of the home caregiving environment, in turn, is influenced by maternal and paternal age, maternal and paternal education level (17), parental psychopathology (particularly depression) (18), or substance abuse and family size/birth order (19). Family structure (divorce, single parents, stepfamilies, foster care, adoption) also may influence the quality of the caregiving environment (20). Adoption into a favorable environment can produce as much as a 10- to 12-point increase in IQ, whereas adoption into an unfavorable environment can result in a 10- to 12-point loss (21).

Socioeconomic status is also a critical determinant of developmental outcome. Poverty, for example, is often associated with overcrowding, homelessness, and exposure to violence, all of which have detrimental effects on cognitive development (22). Culture and ethnicity also influence scores on

IQ tests. Differences in IQ scores among different cultural, ethnic, and racial groups, for example, may reflect the importance placed on specific types of knowledge by the various groups as well as the differences among groups in familial and social interactions (6). Community factors affecting IQ include the quality of daycare, school, and recreational environments, neighborhood stability, and level of social support available for families (23).

IV. CONTROLLING FOR OTHER ENVIRONMENTAL INFLUENCES IN NUTRITIONAL STUDIES

It is extremely difficult to control for all these multiple environmental influences on cognitive development in studies focusing on the effect of a specific environmental factor (e.g., nutrition). However, failure to control for these factors may lead to inappropriate conclusions regarding the influence of specific nutritional factors on development. For example, iron deficiency is commonly thought to be associated with adverse cognitive, motor, and behavioral sequelae. However, in one study, controlling for maternal education and quality of the home caregiving environment removed the statistical significance of iron deficiency on the developmental outcome measures (2). Breast-feeding vs. formula feeding also is commonly thought to confer cognitive advantages as late as young adulthood. Indeed, a recent meta-analysis of 20 previous studies showed a 3-point advantage in IQ scores for breast-fed versus formula-fed infants (24). On the other hand, Jain et al, reviewing the evidence that breast-feeding promotes intelligence (25), noted that 69% of the 40 studies published from 1929 to 2001 concluded that breast-feeding promoted intelligence but that only nine of these controlled adequately for both socioeconomic status and level of developmental stimulation received by the child. Of these nine studies, four concluded that breast-feeding promoted intelligence and five concluded that it did not. Further, only two of these nine studies met the authors' preestablished methodological standards for an epidemiological study; one of these concluded that the effect of breast-feeding on intelligence was significant and the other did not.

V. DIFFICULTIES IN ASSESSING "INTELLIGENCE"

Studies evaluating the effects of nutritional factors on developmental outcome also are hampered by the methods available to assess intelligence. One problem is that results obtained from standardized tests of infant development during the first 2 years of life, including the Bayley Scales (26), which are considered the gold standard of early developmental assessment instruments, do not reliably predict IQ in later childhood or adulthood. Correlations between these early developmental measures and later IQ range only from about 0.1 to 0.2 at 1 year of age to no more than 0.40 at 2 years of age. In contrast, parental IQ, education level, and socioeconomic status all predict IQ in later childhood or adulthood with a correlation of approximately 0.50. Thus, these factors are considerably better at predicting adult IQ before 2 years of age (27) than is actually testing the child.

The correlation between early cognitive measures and adult IQ improves to 0.60 at 3 years of age, and the correlation between IQ scores at 6 years of age and adulthood is 0.8 (27). After 6 years of age, the stability of IQ is thought to be very high (6,27). However, while the IQ scores of most children do not change dramatically after 6 years of age, those of some children do. In a study examining 17 intelligence assessments between 2 1/2 and 17 years of age, as much as a 30-point difference between the highest and lowest IQ scores was noted in a third of the population, and the mean difference was 28.5 points (28). Thus, while IQ is considered one of the most stable behavioral measurements, substantial change is possible in a large number of individuals. Contributing to the variability in IQ scores is the standard error of the available measurements and the difficulty in testing children. For example, the standard error of WISC-III scores is about 3 IQ points (29). The overall state of the child also is important. Being hungry, fussy, tired, anxious, oppositional, unmotivated, or otherwise uncooperative during testing can alter performance immensely. The skills and qualifications of psychometric examiners can also be extremely variable. Thus, IQ and other developmental test scores appear to be moving targets, making correlations between a specific nutritional factor and any single IQ or other developmental measurement intrinsically suspect.

Historically, IQ has been considered one of the best predictors of school performance. However, there may be better predictors of more important long-term functional outcomes. In a review of 400 studies examining individuals with many different occupations, IQ correlated with job performance, with an r of 0.53, indicating that factors other than IQ accounted for 72% of the difference in job performance (30). One of the reasons is that IQ scores do not tap many important individual characteristics (i.e., motivation, work ethio, creativity, social skills, leadership abilities) that may play a greater role in long-term performance.

Recently the concept of emotional intelligence, or EQ, has been promoted as a better measure of long-term competence. This is conceptualized as an array of emotional and social abilities, competencies, and skills that enable individuals to cope with daily demands and to be more effective in their personal and social lives (31). Future studies of the effects of nutrition on developmental outcome should include efforts to measure differences in these skills in addition to or instead of IQ.

The very small differences that have been reported in studies investigating the effects of nutritional factors on IQ, the lack of correlation between infant tests of developmental function and future IQ, the plethora of genetic and environmental factors that contribute to differences in IQ, the difficulty of controlling for nutritional differences, and the potential instability of IQ across time in a significant number of individuals have led many to conclude that other experimental measures of developmental function are more appropriate measures of the effect of nutritional interventions. Instruments used to assess developmental functions of infants primarily assess sensorimotor development rather than information processing and, hence, are relatively insensitive for detecting deficits in specific cognitive abilities. This likely explains the lack of correlation between these measures and later IQ scores until about 2 years of age, when the available developmental tests first include tasks involving more mature information processing.

VI. ALTERNATIVES TO IQ FOR USE IN NUTRITIONAL STUDIES

In contrast, measures of infant information processing, such as tests of visual recognition memory, visual attention, processing speed, and electrophysiologic and imaging techniques such as event-related potentials and magnetic resonance imaging assess selected aspects of infant cognition rather than overall cognitive performance. These measures are thought to assess specific abilities that contribute to the formation of mature thinking (32). They also represent more subtle and sophisticated measures that can assess finergrained differences in brain development at the structural and functional levels (33). Thus, these techniques may be better measures for identifying the more subtle role that specific interventions, including dietary interventions, exert on long-term developmental outcomes. In fact, tests of visual recognition memory performed before 12 months of age have a median predictive correlation with later IQ (up to 11 years of age) (34) of 0.45 (35), far superior to global measures of infant development such as the Bayley Scales.

A. Measures of Infant Information Processing

Tests of visual recognition memory (e.g., the Fagan Test of Infant Intelligence) (36) have not been normed on a representative sample of infants. Thus, they cannot be used to identify individuals with processing deficits relative to the general population. However, these tests have been shown to discriminate between at-risk and control infants in studies of prematurity (37), cocaine- (38), PCB- (39), and alcohol-exposed (40) infants, infants with Down syndrome (41), and infants with different nutritional intakes (42).

Tests of visual recognition memory assess an infant's ability to detect and respond to something new in the environment. They have been shown to correlate with future IQ as well as with language and reading abilities. They also correlate with more discrete cognitive functions, such as delayed memory and processing speed (32). Tests of visual attention assess look duration and the number of shifts in looking at novel versus familiar stimuli. Shorter looking time during habituation to a familiar stimulus and more shifting of looks to novel stimuli are predictive of a higher IQ up to 12 years of age (43). Finally, tests of processing speed assess either reaction time or the time an infant needs to encode visual information. Infants are presented with a series of paired visual stimuli, with one remaining the same from trial to trial, and testing continues until the infant shows a consistent preference for the novel stimulus. This procedure, therefore, provides an index of the speed with which new visual stimuli are encoded. Infants with slower processing speeds have been shown to have lower IQ scores at age 4 years, and reaction times during infancy have been shown to correlate with reaction times at 4 years of age ($r = 0.51$) (44).

B. Event-Related Potentials

Event-related potentials (ERPs) are similar to auditory brainstem-evoked responses (ABERs) and visual evoked potentials (VEPs) but focus, instead, on cognitive rather than sensory processes (33,45,46). ERPs are extracted by averaging the electroencephalogram across multiple presentations of stimuli that are similar in physical properties but differ in cognitive attributes such as familiarity. Examples of such stimuli include a mother's face versus a stranger's face or a mother's voice versus a stranger's voice. The ERP waveform is the portion of the electroencephalogram that reflects cognitive processing. Since these can assess an infant's auditory, visual, and tactile recognition memory near the time of birth, they often circumvent the confounding effects of later environmental factors. ERPs performed at 38–42 weeks postmenstrual age in a group of infants of diabetic mothers and controls have been shown to correlate reasonably well with Bayley MDI scores at 1 year of age ($r = 0.47$) (45). ERPs measuring speech sound discrimination in newborn infants have been shown to predict verbal IQ scores at 5 years of age (47).

C. Magnetic Resonance Imaging

Magnetic resonance imaging (MRI) is just beginning to be used in developmental research (33). These high-resolution structural images allow quantitative volumetric measurements of specific brain structures that may be affected by injury, disease state, or, perhaps, nutritional factors (48). Other MRI scanning techniques include functional MRI scanning, which maps brain areas that are most active during specific cognitive tasks (49), and diffusion tensor imaging (DTI), which assesses axonal myelination and efficiency of neural communications in specific brain regions (50). Either or both of these MRI techniques can be used to study subtle effects of nutritional factors on specific cognitive processes. Finally, magnetic resonance spectroscopy can assess the concentration of biologic compounds, including metabolites related to membrane biochemistry (51). This technique may have particular relevance for studying changes in membrane phospholipids subsequent to dietary interventions.

VII. NUTRITIONAL EFFECTS ON SPECIFIC NEUROPSYCHOLOGICAL PROCESSES

Animal studies have shown that the hippocampus and cerebellum are most vulnerable to effects of malnutrition (52). Permanent alterations are often seen in these structures, whereas other brain areas tend to recover. If this is also true in humans, lack of nutrients would not be expected to affect global IQ but, rather, to affect only the cognitive processes mediated by these structures, e.g., working and long-term declarative memory (hippocampus) and/or motor coordination and procedural learning, such as reading and writing (cerebellum) (52,53).

Neuropharmacological studies have shown long-lasting, although not permanent, changes in neurotransmitter activity and receptor function in malnourished animals. This suggests that attentional and executive functions (planning, impulse inhibition) and emotional reactivity and/or motivation (frustration tolerance, adaptation to stress, anxiety), rather than global cognition, may be specifically affected by malnutrition (52). In fact, provided the testing situations do not evoke stress (53), malnourished animals perform as well as controls on a variety of complex learning and memory tasks.

Experimental measures of infant information processing, event-related potentials, and MRI scanning techniques hold promise as alternatives to global IQ measurements in studies investigating nutritional influences on cognitive development. These measures, in theory, should more reliably detect the very subtle differences in cognitive functioning, e.g., differences in attention, memory, motor control, and executive as well as emotional functioning, that are more likely to be associated with nutritional interventions than are global IQ scores. Many of these measurements can also be obtained at very young ages, avoiding the confounding effects of many of the multiple environmental factors that influence global IQ scores. These measures not only have better predictive validity for global IQ scores than standard infant developmental measures but, more important, also appear to tap basic cognitive processes that show measurable continuity throughout development and, hence, are predictive of the same related abilities in later childhood.

REFERENCES

1. Baer MT, Poulsen MK, Howard-Teplansky RB, Harris AB. Effects of nutrition on development and behavior. In: Carey WB, Crocker AC, Levine MD, eds. Developmental-Behavioral Pediatrics. 3rd ed. Philadelphia: Saunders, 1999: 294–311.
2. Lozoff B, Wolf AW, Jimenez E. Iron-deficiency anemia and infant development: effects of extended oral iron therapy. J Pediatr 1996; 129:382–389.
3. Golub MS, Keen CL, Gershwin ME, Hendricks PG. Developmental zinc deficiency and behavior. J Nutr 1995; 125:2263S–2271S.
4. McCullough AL, Kirksey A, Wachs TD, McCabe GP, Bassily NS, Bishry Z, Galal OM, Harrison GG, Jerome NW. Vitamin B6 status of Egyptian mothers: relation to infant behavior and maternal–infant interactions. Am J Clin Nutr 1990; 51:1067–1074.
5. Grantham-McGregor S. A review of studies of the effect of severe malnutrition on mental development. J Nutr 1995; 125:2233S–2238S.
6. Sattler JM. Issues related to the measurement and change of intelligence. Assessment of Children: Cognitive Applications. 4th ed. San Diego: Jerome M. Sattler, 2001:160–182.
7. McClearn GE, Johansson B, Berg S, Pedersen NL, Ahern F, Petrill SA, Plomin R. Substantial genetic influence on cognitive abilities in twins 80 or more years old. Science 1997; 276:1560–1563.
8. Dobbing J. Maternal nutrition in pregnancy and later achievement of offspring: a personal interpretation. Early Hum Dev 1985; 12:1–8.
9. Cornelius MD, Ryan CM, Day NL, Goldschmidt L, Willford JA. Prenatal tobacco effects on neuropsychological outcomes among preadolescents. J Dev Behav Pediatr 2001; 22:217–225.
10. Jacobson JL, Jacobson SW. Drinking moderately and pregnancy: effects on child development. Alcohol Res Health 1999; 23:25–30.
11. Mayes LC. Developing brain and in utero cocaine exposure: effects on neural ontogeny. Dev Psychopathol 1999; 11:685–714.

12. Robertson CM, Finer NN. Educational readiness of survivors of neonatal encephalopathy associated with birth asphyxia at term. J Dev Behav Pediatr 1988; 9:298–306.
13. Bhutta AT, Cleves MA, Casey PH, Craddock MM, Anand KJ. Cognitive and behavioral outcomes of school-aged children who were born preterm: a meta-analysis. JAMA 2002; 288:728–737.
14. American Academy of Pediatrics Committee on Drugs. Behavioral and cognitive effects of anticonvulsant therapy. Pediatrics 1995; 96:538–540.
15. Canfield RL, Henderson CR, Cory-Slechta DA, Cox C, Jusko TA, Lanphear BP. Intellectual impairment in children with blood lead concentrations below 10 micrograms per deciliter. NEJM 2003; 348:1517–1526.
16. Blunden S, Lushington K, Kennedy D, Martin J, Dawson D. Behavior and neurocognitive performance in children aged 5–10 years who snore compared to controls. J Clin Exp Neuropsychology 2000; 22:554–568.
17. Bradley RH, Corwyn RF, McAdoo HP, Coll CG. The home environments of children in the United States part I: variations by age, gender, ethnicity, and poverty status. Child Dev 2001; 72:1844–1867.
18. Petterson SM, Albers AB. Effects of poverty and maternal depression on early child development. Child Dev 2001; 72:1794–1813.
19. Zajonc RB. Family configuration and intelligence. Science 1976; 192:227–236.
20. Clarke-Stewart KA, Vandell DL, McCartney K, Owen MT, Booth C. Effects of parental separation and divorce on very young children. J Fam Psychol 2000; 14:304–326.
21. Locurto C. The malleability of IQ as judged from adoption studies. Intelligence 1990; 14:275–292.
22. Duncan G, Brooks-Dunn J, Klebanov P. Economic deprivation and early childhood development. Child Dev 1994; 65:296–318.
23. Brooks-Gunn J, Han WJ, Waldfogel J. Maternal employment and child cognitive outcomes in the first three years of life: the NICHD study of early child care. Child Dev 2002; 73:1052–1072.
24. Anderson JW, Johnstone BM, Remley DT. Breast-feeding and cognitive development: a meta-analysis. Am J Clin Nutr 1999; 70:525–535.
25. Jain A, Concato J, Leventhal JM. How good is the evidence linking breastfeeding and intelligence? Pediatrics 2002; 109:1044–1053.
26. Bayley N. The Bayley Scales of Infant Development. San Antonio: Psychological Corp, 1993.
27. McCall RB, Mash CW. Long-chain polyunsaturated fatty acids and the measurement and prediction of intelligence (IQ). In: Dobbing J, ed. Developing Brain and Behavior: The Role of Lipids in Infant Formula. San Diego: Academic Press, 1997:295–338.
28. McCall RB. Developmental changes in mental performance: the effect of the birth of a sibling. Child Dev 1984; 55:1317–1321.
29. Wechsler D. Wechsler Intelligence Scale for Children. 3rd ed. San Antonio: Psychological Corporation, 1991.
30. Hunter JE, Hunter RF. Validity and utility of alternative predictors of job performance. Psychol Bull 1984; 96:72–98.

31. McMullen B. Emotional intelligence. Br Med J 2003; 326:S19.
32. Rose SA, Feldman JF, Jankowski JJ. The building blocks of cognition. J Pediatr 2003; 143:S54–S61.
33. Thomas KM. Assessing brain development using neurophysiologic and behavioral measures. J Pediatr 2003; 143:S46–S53.
34. Rose SA, Feldman JF. Prediction of IQ and specific cognitive abilities at 11 years from infancy measures. Dev Psychol 1990; 26:759–769.
35. McCall RB, Carriger MS. A meta-analysis of infant habituation and recognition memory performance as predictors of later IQ. Child Dev 1993; 64:57–79.
36. Fagan J, Detterman DK. The Fagan test of infant intelligence: a technical summary. J Appl Dev Psychol 1992; 13:173–193.
37. Rose SA, Feldman JF, Jankowski JJ. Attention and recognition memory in the first year of life: a longitudinal study of preterms and fullterms. Dev Psychol 2001; 37:135–151.
38. Jacobson SW, Jacobson JL, Sokol RJ, Martier SS, Chiodo LM. New evidence for neurobehavioral effects of in utero cocaine exposure. J Pediatr 1996; 129:581–590.
39. Jacobson SW, Fein GG, Jacobson JL, Schwartz PM, Dowler JK. The effect of intrauterine PCB exposure on visual recognition memory. Child Dev 1985; 56:853–860.
40. Jacobson SW, Jacobson JL, Sokol RJ, Martier SS, Ager JW. Prenatal alcohol exposure and infant information processing ability. Child Dev 1993; 64:1706–1721.
41. Miranda SB, Fantz RL. Recognition memory in Down's syndrome and normal infants. Child Dev 1974; 48:651–660.
42. Carlson SE, Werkman SH. A randomized trial of visual attention of preterm infants fed docosahexaenoic acid until two months. Lipids 1996; 3:113–119.
43. Sigman M, Cohen SE, Beckwith L, Asarnow R, Parmelee AH. Continuity in cognitive abilities from infancy to 12 years of age. Cognit Dev 1991; 6:47–57.
44. Dougherty TM, Haith MM. Infant expectations and reaction time as predictors of childhood speed of processing and IQ. Dev Psychol 1997; 33:146–155.
45. DeRegnier RA, Nelson CA, Thomas KM, Wewerka S, Georgieff MK. Neurophysiologic evaluation of auditory recognition memory in healthy newborn infants and infants of diabetic mothers. J Pediatr 2000; 137:777–784.
46. Nelson CA, Wewerka SS, Borscheid AJ, DeRegnier RA, Georgieff MK. Electrophysiologic evidence of impaired cross-modal recognition memory in 8-month-old infants of diabetic mothers. J Pediatr 2003; 142:575–582.
47. Molfese DL, Molfese VJ. Discrimination of language skills at five years of age using event-related potentials recorded at birth. Dev Neuropsychol 1997; 13:135–156.
48. DeBellis MD, Casey BJ, Dahl R, Birmaher B, Williamson D, Thomas KM, Axelson DA, Frustaci K, Boring AM, Hall J, Ryan ND. A pilot study of amygdala volumes in pediatric generalized anxiety disorder. Biol Psychiatry 2000; 48:51–57.
49. Casey BJ, Cohen JD, Jezzard P, Turner R, Noll DC, Trainor RJ, Giedd J,

Kaysen D, Hertz-Pannier L, Rapoport JL. Activation of prefrontal cortex during a nonspatial working memory task with functional MRI. Neuroimage 1995; 2:221–229.

50. Hoon AH, Lawrie WT, Melhem ER, Reinhardt EM, Van Zijl PC, Solaiyappan M, Jiang H, Johnston MV, Mori S. Diffusion tensor imaging of periventricular leukomalacia shows affected sensory cortex white matter pathways. Neurology 2002; 59:752–756.

51. Yeo RA, Hill DE, Campbell RA, Vigil J, Petropoulos H, Hart B, Zamora L, Brooks WM. Proton magnetic resonance spectroscopy investigation of the right frontal lobe in children with attention-deficit/hyperactivity disorder. J Am Acad Child Adol Psychiatry 2003; 42:303–310.

52. Levitsky DA, Strupp BJ. Malnutrition and the brain: changing concepts, changing concerns. J Nutr 1995; 125:2212S–2220S.

53. Strupp BJ, Levitsky DA. Enduring effects of early malnutrition: a theoretical reappraisal. J Nutr 1995; 125:2221S–2232S.

7

Feeding the Preterm Infant

David H. Adamkin
University of Louisville and Kosair Children's Hospital, Louisville, Kentucky, U.S.A.

I. INTRODUCTION

The goal of nutritional management of very-low-birth weight (VLBW), <1500 g, infants that has been supported by the American Academy of Pediatrics Committee on Nutrition (1–3) is the achievement of postnatal growth at a rate that approximates the intrauterine growth of a normal fetus at the same postconceptional age. Yet in reality the growth of these infants' lags considerably after birth (4). These infants, especially those under 1000-g birth weight (VVLBW), do not even regain birth weight until 2–3 weeks of age. The growth of most VLBW infants proceeds at a slower rate than in utero, often by a large margin (4,5). While many of the smallest VLBW infants are also born small for gestational age (SGA), both appropriate-for-gestational-age (AGA) VLBW and SGA infants develop *extrauterine growth retardation* (EUGR). Figure 1, from the NICHD Neonatal Research Network, demonstrates the differences between normal intrauterine growth (4) and the observed rates of postnatal growth in the NICHD study. For each gestational age category the postnatal study growth curve was shifted to the right of the reference curve (4). Therefore, this "growth deficiency" is common in VVLBW infants. Nutrient intakes received by VLBW infants are lower than the uptakes by the fetus, and this intake deficit persists throughout much of the infants' stay in the hospital and even beyond (5). While nonnutritional factors are involved in the slow growth of VLBW infants, (6) nutrient intakes are low and critical in explaining the poor growth. There is considerable evidence that these early growth deficits have long-lasting effects, including short stature and poor neurodevelopmental out-

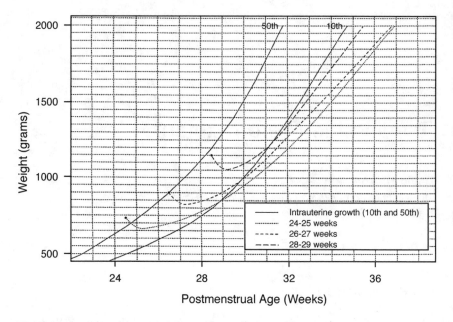

Figure 1 Mean body weight versus gestational age in weeks for all study infants who had gestational ages at birth of between 24 and 29 weeks. (From Ref. 4.)

comes (7). The most convincing data concerning the neurodevelopmental consequences of inadequate early nutrition are those of Lucas et al. (8,9). They demonstrated that premature infants fed a preterm formula and hence a higher intake of protein (and other nutrients) over the first month of life had higher neurodevelopmental indices at both 18 months and 7–8 years of age (9) than infants fed a term formula with a lower content of protein (and other nutrients) during this period (9).

Nutritional management of VLBW infants is marked by a lack of uniformity of practice from NICU to NICU as well as within a practice. This heterogeneity of practice regarding nutritional management persists from the first hours of life to hospital discharge and beyond. Diversity of practice thrives where there is uncertainty. Because undernutrition is, by definition, unphysiologic and undesirable, it makes sense that any measure that diminishes it is inherently good, providing safety is not compromised.

As elusive as the goal is that nutrition should support "postnatal growth" approximating in utero growth of the normal fetus (1–3), the fetal model is still unquestionably sound and there is no alternative model or gold standard. Similarly, estimates of required intakes to achieve fetal growth are available (10–14). Following is a summary of nutrients needed for achievement of fetal growth and discussion regarding nutritional strategies to promote postnatal growth.

II. NUTRIENTS NEEDED FOR ACHIEVEMENT OF FETAL GROWTH

The nutrient deposition (accretion) associated with postnatal growth that approximates the in utero growth of a normal fetus can be determined from data on the chemical composition of the human fetus. Many investigators have provided useful data describing the chemical composition of the human fetus (11,12,15). Gestational age is not accurately available for the majority of such analyzed fetuses. However, the body content of most components (except lipid) is available. The "Ziegler" reference fetus uses the limited available set of fetal data for which gestational age could be accurately assessed (16). From this he is able to construct calculated daily accretion of components. Recently Ziegler (17) compiled fetal accretion data, pulling together the work from Forbes (11) and Sparks (15), and the reference fetus (10,18) and also included contemporary fetal growth data (19). Table 1 (17) is a synthesis of the different models, showing estimates of nutrient intakes derived from this factorial approach. Nutrient intakes must not only meet needs for accretion but also replace ongoing losses. Accretion includes the amounts actually laid down in new tissues plus the cost of accretion. For example, for energy, cost includes the energy required for synthesis of new body tissue and for growth in general. An estimate of the energy cost of growth is 10 kcal/kg/day when protein is near that required for growth.

Protein losses via the skin and urine are estimated in the model and are referenced in Table 1. Energy losses comprise resting energy expenditure (REE) plus an allowance for miscellaneous expenditure, e.g., occasional cold exposure and physical activity; resting energy expenditures are assumed to be 45–50 kcal/kg/d, and miscellaneous expenditures are assumed to be 15–20 kcal/kg/d (Table 1) (17).

The sum of accretion plus losses provides an estimate of required nutrient intakes via the parenteral route. Correction for the efficiency of absorption (assumed 88% for protein and 85% for energy) provides the required intakes enterally.

Protein and energy are the key nutrients for growth. Both must be provided in appropriate proportion for optimal utilization of each. If there is protein but not enough energy provided, protein cannot be fully utilized for growth. Conversely, if not enough protein is provided, energy will be in relative excess and will be deposited as fat (23).

Table 1 Estimated Nutrient Intakes Needed to Achieve Fetal Weight Gain

	Body weight (g)				
	500–700	700–900	900–1200	1200–1500	1500–180
Fetal weight gain[a] (g/d)	13	16	20	24	26
(g/kg/d)	21	20	19	18	16
Protein (g) ($N \times 6.25$)					
Inevitable loss[b]	1.0	1.0	1.0	1.0	1.0
Growth (accretion)[c]	2.5	2.5	2.5	2.4	2.2
Required intake					
Parenteral[d]	3.5	3.5	3.5	3.4	3.2
Enteral[e]	4.0	4.0	4.0	3.9	3.6
Energy (kcal)					
Loss	60	60	65	70	70
Resting expenditure	45	45	50	50	50
Misc. expenditure	15	15	15	20	20
Growth (accretion)[f]	29	32	36	38	39
Required intake					
Parenteral[d]	89	92	101	108	109
Enteral[g]	105	108	119	127	128
Protein/Energy (g/100 kcal)					
Parenteral	3.9	4.1	3.5	3.1	2.9
Enteral	3.8	3.7	3.4	3.1	2.8

Because nutrient needs are closely related to body weight and weight gain, the nutrient needs apply to a postnatal ages. All values are per kilogram per day.
[a] Based on data of Kramer et al. (Ref. 19).
[b] Urinary nitrogen loss of 133 mg/kg/d (Refs. 20,21) and dermal loss of 27 mg/kg/d (Ref. 2).
[c] Includes correction of 90% efficiency of conversion from dietary to body protein.
[d] Sum of loss and accretion.
[e] Same as parenteral, but assuming 88% absorption of dietary protein.
[f] Energy accretion plus 10 kcal/kg/d cost of growth.
[g] Assuming 85% absorption of dietary energy.
Source: Ref. 17.

    Information regarding energy requirements in VVLBW infants has been sparse, largely because of practical and technical limitations in studying these infants. A new, noninvasive method to assess energy expenditure (doubly labeled water method), allows total energy expenditure to be determined over 5–7 days without altering clinical care of these infants (24). This methodology has been validated in premature infants (24–27).

    There is preliminary evidence in VVLBW infants with minimal respiratory disease but on mechanical ventilation suggesting high rates of energy expenditure in early postnatal life (85 cal/kg/d) (28). Those VVLBW infants still on ventilators at 3 and 5 weeks postnatal age still had high rates of energy expenditure of 86–94 kcal/kg/d, respectively (29). Therefore, based on these measured energy expenditures, ~ 130 kcal/kg/d of energy intake would be necessary to achieve the target energy balance (energy intake minus energy expenditures) of ~ 25–30 kcal/kg/d, as noted in the reference fetus. These studies suggest that the energy needs of this group of infants are very likely to exceed those of the healthy growing preterm infant population.

The protein requirement of VVLBW infants can be estimated in ways other than chemical composition. They are the rate of catabolism of the essential amino acid phenylalanine (determined by stable isotopic techniques) and the phenylalanine content of body protein (30). Assuming a rate of obligate protein loss of 1.1–1.5 g/kg/d (31,32), an efficiency of protein retention of 80–90% (30), and a protein accretion goal of 2 g/kg/d (10), protein requirements of 3.5–4 g/kg/d would be necessary.

It is apparent that protein and energy requirements are not being met in VVLBW infants. These intakes are difficult to achieve in the first 2 weeks of life in these infants; nevertheless, aggressive parenteral and enteral nutritional strategies can produce substantial improvements.

III. STRATEGIES TO PROMOTE GROWTH

Aggressive nutrition theoretically means that the transfer from fetal to extrauterine life should proceed with minimal, if any, interruption of growth and development. Therefore, for this to occur the transfer of nutrients to the fetus/infant should not be interrupted. Birth, when it occurs, particularly in these VVLBW infants, involves some temporary interruption of the transfer of nutrients. Reduction of this interruption to a reasonable minimum is the first goal of aggressive nutrition.

IV. PARENTERAL NUTRITION

Because immaturity of the gastrointestinal tract in these VLBW infants precludes substantive nutritional support from enteral nutrition, nearly all of those infants are supported with parenteral nutrition (PN). From a nutritional point of view, the liberal use of PN has been a huge success, particularly in the VVLBW infant.

Until recently, the initiation of PN has been delayed by a number of days. Reasons for this delay have not been clear but probably have been related to VLBW infants' ability to catabolize amino acids and, in general, concerns about "tolerance" in the first days of life in critically ill infants.

Amino acids are administered aggressively from the first hours of life to avoid the period of early neonatal malnutrition.

An understanding of fetal nutrition (Table 1) may be helpful in designing postnatal strategies in VVLBW infants. Extending those data to clinical application, we know that at 70% of gestation, there is little fetal lipid uptake. Fetal energy metabolism is not dependent on fat until early in the third trimester, and then it increases only gradually toward term. Glucose is delivered to the fetus from the mother at low fetal insulin concentrations, generally at a rate that matches fetal energy expenditure. The human placenta actively transports amino acids to the fetus, and animal studies indicate that fetal amino acid uptake greatly exceeds protein accretion requirements. Approximately 50% of the amino acids taken up by the fetus are oxidized and serve as a significant energy source. Urea production is a byproduct of amino acid oxidation. Relatively high rates of fetal urea production are seen in human and animal fetuses as compared with the term neonate and adult, suggesting high protein turnover and oxidation rates in the fetus. Therefore, a rise in blood urea nitrogen, which is often observed after the start of PN, is not an adverse effect or sign of toxicity. Rather, an increase in urea nitrogen is a normal accompaniment of an increase in the intake of amino acids or protein.

Several controlled studies have demonstrated the efficacy and safety of amino acids initiated within the first 24 hours of life (33–37). There were no recognizable metabolic derangements, including hyperammonemia, metabolic acidosis, or abnormal aminograms.

A strong argument for the early aggressive use of amino acids is the prevention of "metabolic shock." Concentrations of some key amino acids begin to decline in the VLBW infant from the time the cord is cut. This metabolic shock may trigger the starvation response, of which endogenous glucose production is a prominent feature. Irrepressible glucose production may be the cause of the so-called glucose intolerance that often limits the amount of energy that can be administered to the VLBW infant. It makes sense to smooth the metabolic transition from fetal to extrauterine life. Withholding PN for days, or even for hours, means sending the infant unnecessarily into a metabolic emergency. Thus, the need for parenteral nutrition may never be more acute than right after birth. It is noteworthy that Rivera et al. (21) made the surreptitious observation that glucose tolerance was substantially improved in the group receiving early amino acids. Early amino acids may stimulate insulin secretion, consistent with the notion that forestalling the starvation response improves glucose tolerance.

V. DOSE OF AMINO ACIDS

Figure 2 shows protein loss that occurs in mechanically ventilated, 26-weeks-gestation, 900-g-birth-weight infants at 2 days of age who were receiving glucose alone (31). Also shown are clinically stable 32-weeks-gestation premature infants and normal-term infants (36,37). It is clear that there is a significant effect of gestation on protein metabolism as the rate of protein loss in VVLBW infants is twofold higher than in normal-term infants.

The impact of this rate of protein loss is shown in Figure 3. A 26-weeks-gestation, 1000-g-birth-weight infant begins with body protein stores of ~88 g; without any protein intake, the infant loses over 1.5% of body protein per day (38). Contrast this with the normal fetus, who would be accumulating body protein at over 2% per day. It is obvious that significant body protein deficits can accumulate rapidly in VVLBW infants if early aggressive amino acid administration is not offered.

The studies of early PN used doses between 1.0 and 1.5 g/kg/d, an amount that will replace ongoing losses. This should be initiated within 24 hours of birth. Ultimate amino acid intake should be 3.0 g/kg/d; however, one can consider intakes of 3.5 g/kg/d for infants weighing less than 1200 g in situations where enteral feeds are extremely delayed or withheld for prolonged periods. A desirable protein-to-energy ratio is 25 kcal/kg for every gram of protein/kg or 2–3 mg/kg/min of glucose per gram of protein intake.

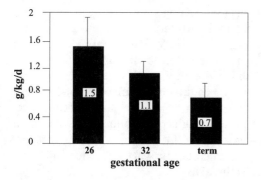

Figure 2 Protein losses measured in three groups of infants receiving glucose alone at 2–3 days of age. Protein losses are calculated from measured rates of phenylalanine catabolism (31,36,37). (From Ref. 38.)

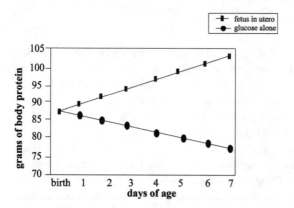

Figure 3 Change in body protein stores in a theoretical 26-weeks-gestation, 1000-g premature infant receiving glucose alone as compared with a fetus in utero. (From Ref. 38.)

VI. GLUCOSE

Carbohydrates are the main energy substrate for the fetus and the preterm infant receiving parenteral nutrition. At least at the outset, lipids play a minor role in supplying energy, although they play an important role at all times in providing essential fatty acids. Clearly, the infant must eventually transition to enteral feedings. These feedings provide about half the energy from fat. However, while on PN, carbohydrate remains the dominant energy substrate.

Glucose intolerance is common in VLBW infants and in some may also occur with nonoliguric hyperkalemia (39). Endogenous glucose production is elevated in VLBW infants as compared with term infants and adults (40). Also, high glucose production rates are found in VLBW infants who received only glucose as compared to those receiving glucose plus amino acids and/or lipids (41). Clinical experience with glucose intolerance suggests that glucose alone does not always suppress glucose production in VLBW infants. It is not clear what circumstances or metabolic conditions lead to glucose intolerance. It appears likely, however, that persistent glucose production is the main cause, fueled by ongoing proteolysis that is not suppressed by physiologic concentrations of insulin. There is uncertainty whether abnormally low peripheral glucose utilization is also involved.

The glucose infusion rate should maintain euglycemia. Depending on the degree of immaturity (<26 weeks), 5% glucose or 10% glucose may be used. Another objective becomes the achievement of higher energy intakes. Glucose intolerance, defined as the inability to maintain euglycemia at glucose administration rates greater than 6 mg/kg/min, is a frequent problem in VLBW infants, especially those weighing less than 1000 g. It can limit delivery of energy to the infant to a fraction of the resting energy expenditure, meaning that the infant remains in negative energy balance. Even with glucose intolerance of a lesser severity, the limitation it places on energy delivery is nutritionally deleterious.

Several strategies are used to manage this early hyperglycemia in VVLBW infants: (1) decreasing glucose administration until hyperglycemia resolves (unless the hyperglycemia is so severe that this strategy would require infusion of a hypotonic solution); (2) administering intravenous amino acids, which decrease glucose concentrations in VVLBW infants, presumably by enhancing endogenous insulin secretion; (3) initiation of exogenous insulin therapy at rates to control hyperglycemia (42–45); and (4) using insulin to control hyperglycemia and to increase nutritional uptake (46). The first three strategies prevent adequate early nutrition, and the safety of the last has been questioned in this population because of the possible development of lactic acidemia (47).

Several studies have shown that insulin used as a nutritional adjuvant successfully lowers glucose concentrations and increases weight gain in preterm infants without significant risk of causing hypoglycemia (44,46). However, little is known about its effects on the quality of weight gain and counterregulatory hormone concentrations. A 1998 study examined the effect of insulin using a hyperinsulinemic-euglycemic clamp in VVLBW infants receiving only glucose. These infants were normoglycemic prior to the initiation of insulin. They demonstrated a significant elevation in plasma lactate concentrations and the development of significant metabolic acidosis (47).

In our experience, the administration of amino acids early after birth appears to prevent the need for intravenous insulin, perhaps through stimulation of insulin by amino acids (arginine and leucine, for example) (48). Additionally, with this improved tolerance, appropriate energy for growth may also be achieved more readily.

VII. LIPIDS

There are two roles for lipid as a part of a PN regimen. The first function is to serve as a source of linoleic acid. When used in small amounts it can prevent or treat essential fatty acid deficiency (EFAD). The second function is its use as a energy source. Larger quantities serve as a partial replacement for glucose as a major source of calories.

The preterm neonate is especially susceptible to the development of EFAD because tissue stores of linoleic acid are small and requirements for essential fatty acids are large as a result of rapid growth. The human fetus depends entirely on placental transfer of essential fatty acids. A VLBW infant with limited nonprotein calorie reserve must mobilize fatty acids for energy when receiving intravenous nutrition devoid of lipid. Our own studies in these infants confirm other studies that show EFAD can develop in the VLBW infant during the first week of life on lipid-free regimens (49,50).

The importance of long-chain polyunsaturated fatty acids (LC-PUFAs) for the development of the brain and the retina has been recognized (51). Infants are not capable of forming sufficient quantities of LC-PUFAs from the respective precursor fatty acids (linoleic and alpha-linolenic acids) and thus depend on an exogenous source of LC-PUFAs. Intravenous lipid emulsions contain small amounts of these fatty acids as part of the egg phospholipid used as a stabilizer.

Clinically, it should be noted that infusion of 20% rather than 10% lipid emulsions results in lower plasma concentrations of phospholipid, cholesterol, and triglycerides (52). The mechanism for these differences are the lower phospholipid/triglyceride ratio of the 20% versus 10% emulsion. Phospholipids inhibit lipoprotein lipase (53); this difference may explain the lower triglyceride concentration.

The "routine" use of intravenous lipid emulsions has not been universally accepted in critically ill, ventilated VLBW infants because of potential complications that worry the practitioner. Hazards most pertinent to the ventilated VLBW infant include adverse effect on gas exchange and displacement of bilirubin from albumin. Both Brans et al. (54) and Adamkin et al. (55) found no difference in oxygenation between infants randomly assigned to various lipid doses (including controls without lipids) when using lower rates and longer infusion times of intravenous lipids. The displacement of bilirubin from binding sites on serum albumin may occur even with adequate metabolism of infused lipid, e.g., the increasing concentrations of free fatty acids (FFA) may compete with bilirubin for binding to albumin (ALB), a possible but preventable occurrence (56). In vitro, displacement of ALB-bound bilirubin by FFA depends on the relative concentrations of all three compounds (57,58). An in vivo study has shown no free bilirubin generated if the molar FFA/ALB ratio is less than 6 (59). Our data with lipid initiation at 0.5 g/kg/day of lipid in VLBW infants on assisted ventilation with respiratory distress syndrome showed a mean FFA/ALB ratio of less than 1; no individual patient value exceeded a ratio of 3 when daily doses were increased to 2.5 g/kg/day (in increments of 0.5 g/kg/day) over an 18-hour infusion time (60). Other investigators found no adverse effect on bilirubin binding when lipid emulsion was infused at a dose of 2 g/kg/day over either 15 or 24 hours (61).

Therefore, there is no credible evidence of adverse effects when intravenous lipid emulsions are used properly as we understand it today. Proper use includes slow infusion rates (≤ 0.15 g/kg/h), slow increases in dosage, and avoidance of unduly high doses, e.g., >3.0 g/kg/d). Gilbertson et al. (62) demonstrated that slow administration of intravenous lipids beginning on day 1 at a dose of 1.0 g/kg/d and increasing in stepwise fashion to 3.0 g/kg/d by day 4 is well tolerated without noticeable adverse effects. Also, there were no differences in plasma levels of triglycerides and nonesterified fatty acids as compared with infants who did not receive intravenous lipids (62).

We initiate intravenous lipids the second day of life, following initiation of amino acids shortly after delivery. Starting dose is 0.5 g/kg/d or 1.0 g/kg/d. Plasma triglycerides are monitored after each increase in dose, and levels are maintained at less than 200 mg/dL. A 20% lipid emulsion is used exclusively. Infusion rate is 0.15 or less g/kg/h. Therefore, a dose of 3.0 g/kg/d would be infused over 24 hours.

VIII. INITIATION AND ADVANCEMENT OF ENTERAL FEEDINGS

The timing of the initial feedings for the preterm infant has been debated for nearly a century (63) and remains controversial. As suitable PN solutions designed for neonates became available, many physicians chose to use parenteral nutrition alone in the sick, ventilated, preterm infant because of concerns about necrotizing enterocolitis (NEC). Total parenteral nutrition was thought to be a logical continuation of the transplacental nutrition the infants would have received in utero. However, this view discounts any role that swallowed amniotic fluid may play in nutrition and in the development of the gastrointestinal tract. In fact, by the end of third trimester, the amniotic fluid provides the fetus with the same enteral volume intake and approximately 25% of the enteral protein intake as that of a term, breast-fed infant (64). Parenteral nutrition does little to support the function of the gastrointestinal tract. Studies in animals deprived of enteral substrate despite being maintained in an anabolic state with TPN, showed that intraluminal nutrition was necessary for normal gastrointestinal structure and functional integrity (65,66). Enteral feedings have both direct trophic effects and indirect effects secondary to the release of intestinal hormones. Lucas et al. (67) demonstrated significant rises in plasma concentrations of enteroglucagon, gastrin, and gastric-inhibiting polypeptide in preterm infants after milk feeds of as little as 12 mL/kg/day. Similar surges in these trophic hormones were not seen in intravenously nourished infants.

Clearly, one of the important benefits of using PN is that it allows feedings to be advanced slowly, which probably increases the safety of enteral feedings. However, how neonatologists feed VLBW neonates has traditionally been based on local practices and not subjected to rigorous scientific investigation (68) because of the prevailing fear of NEC.

In addition, regardless of feeding strategy, the advancement of feedings is based on evidence of intolerance based on increased pregavage residuals or greenish aspirates. According to Ziegler, gastric residuals are very frequent in the early neonatal period and are virtually always benign, e.g., not associated with NEC (69).

A 2002 study (70) demonstrated that in VVLBW infants, excessive gastric residual volume (GRV) either determined by percent of the previous feed or an absolute volume (>2 mL or >3mL) did not necessarily effect feeding success, as determined by the volume of total feeding on day 14. Similarly the color of the GRV (green, milky, clear) did not predict feeding intolerance (70). Nonetheless, the volume of feeding on day 14 did correlate with a higher proportion of episodes of zero GRVs and with predominantly milky gastric residuals. Thus, isolated findings related to gastric emptying alone should not be the sole criteria in initiating or advancing feeds. Stooling pattern, abdominal distension, and the nature of the stools should also be considered (71).

The etiology of NEC remains unclear. Because NEC occurs rarely in infants who are not being fed, feedings have come to be seen as the cause of NEC. The association between feedings and NEC is likely to be explained by the fact that feedings act as vehicles for the introduction of bacterial or viral pathogens or toxins. They are more likely to survive the gastric barrier because of low acidity, against which the immature gut is poorly able to defend itself. Efforts aimed at minimizing the risk of NEC have focused on the time of introduction of feedings, on feeding volumes, and on the rate of feeding volume increments. One by one, the strategies that had been developed with the aim of reducing the risk of NEC were shown to be ineffective and unnecessary. Yet these strategies still linger today and distract neonatologists from concentrating on the real challenge, which is the continued growth faltering that VLBW infants so often show.

One of the main strategies intended to reduce the risk of NEC involved the withholding of feeding for prolonged periods of time (72). Although it was never shown that the prolonged withholding of feedings actually prevented NEC, some form of the strategy was widely adopted in the 1970s and 1980s. The withholding of feedings eventually came under scrutiny and was compared in a number of controlled trials with early introduction of feedings (73). A systematic review of the results of published trials (73) concluded that early introduction of feedings shorten the time to full feeds as well as the length of hospitalization and does not lead to an increase in the incidence of NEC. A controlled study involving 100 VLBW infants (74) confirmed these findings and found, in addition, a significant reduction of serious infections when feedings were introduced early. Thus, delayed introduction of feedings is now known to have no beneficial effects, e.g., reduction in incidence of NEC, and to have substantial negative effects.

Another strategy aimed at preventing NEC has been to keep the rate of feeding increments low. The strategy was based on the findings of Anderson and Kliegman (75), who in their retrospective analysis of 19 cases of NEC found that, in infants who went on to develop NEC, feedings were advanced more rapidly than in control infants without NEC. Based on these findings, they recommended that feedings not be advanced by more than 20 mL/kg each day (75). This recommendation has found wide acceptance, although its validity has not been confirmed. In the only prospective randomized trial, Rayyis et al. (76) compared increments of 15 mL/kg/d with increments of 35 mL/kg/d. They found, as was to be expected, that with fast advancement, full intakes were achieved sooner and weight gain set in earlier. But there was no difference in the incidence of NEC. Whether it protects against NEC or not, limiting feeding increments in VLBW infants to 20 mL/kg/d is an acceptable and not unduly onerous practice. It still permits achievement of full feedings in the reasonable period of about 8 days.

With the earlier introduction of enteral feedings, particularly in VLBW infants who are ventilator dependent and require invasive monitoring, the issue of safety of initiating enteral feedings while an umbilical artery catheter (UAC) is still in place must be considered (77). The presence of a UAC has been associated with an increased risk for NEC (78), and it is a common nursery policy to delay feedings until catheters are removed. However, few data from controlled studies support this policy. Davey et al. (79) examined feeding tolerance in 47 infants weighing less than 2000 g at birth who had respiratory distress and UACs. Infants were assigned randomly to begin feedings as soon as they met the predefined criterion of stability or to delay feeding until their UACs were removed for 24 hours. Infants who were fed with catheters in place started feeding significantly sooner and required half the number of days of parenteral nutrition. The incidence of NEC was comparable for infants fed with catheters in place and those whose catheters were removed before initiation of feedings (79). In addition, multiple large epidemiological surveys (80–83) have not shown a cause-and-effect relation between low-lying umbilical artery catheters and NEC.

The decision when to start these early enteral or trophic feeds may be influenced by what milk is available to feed the infant. Lucas and Cole (84), in a multicenter feeding trial involving almost 1000 preterm infants with birth weights less than 1850 g, demonstrated that the incidence of confirmed NEC was six times greater in formula-fed infants than in those receiving human milk. In addition, NEC was rare for infants greater than 30 weeks' gestation who were fed human milk, but this was not the case for formula-fed babies. A delay of feeding in the formula-fed group was associated with a reduced risk of NEC, whereas the use of early human milk feedings had no correlation with the occurrence of NEC. Therefore, strategizing when to initiate feeds for individual patients should take into account individual risk and the milk available for the patient.

Feedings should be started within the first days of life. A frequently encountered problem is that breast milk takes at least 2 days to come in and often does not come in for 3, 4, or 5 days. During that time, only small amounts of colostrum are available, which is very valuable and must be fed. Gastric residuals should not be allowed to interfere with feeding. Initial feeding volumes should be kept low (1–2 mL/feed), and frequency of feeding to every 3 hours. Feeding volumes should be increased slowly. Increments should be about 20 mL/kg/d when a decision is made to advance feedings.

For extremely-low-birth-weight (<750 g) infants on life support and invasive monitoring, one may introduce trophic feedings with 1 mL/feed every 8 hours for a period of a few days and then proceed as described earlier above. Each nursery should establish criteria of stability to be reached before such feeds are initiated. These may include normal blood pressure and pH, $paO_2 > 55$, 12 hours or more from last surfactant or indomethacin dose, normal gastrointestinal exam, heme-negative stools, and under two desaturation episodes per hour to less than 80%.

IX. FEEDING THE GROWING VLBW INFANT

Preoccupation with preventing NEC has contributed to the chronic undernourishment of stable, growing VLBW infants (Fig. 1). Inadequate nutrient intakes have the potential for adversely effecting neurocognitive development (9). Probably, protein and energy are limiting factors, and both need to be provided in greater amounts than are now used.

Currently, fortified breast milk provides around 3.1–3.25 g of protein/ 100 kcal, assuming that the breast milk has a protein content of about 1.5 g/100 kcal. But protein content of breast milk drops with the duration of lactation and fortified breast milk; therefore, it is likely to provide less protein than 3.1–3.25 g/100 kcal. Formulas provide between 2.7 and 3.0 g/100 kcal. Thus, feedings are typically providing less protein (relative to energy) than is required (Table 1), at least until the infant reaches a weight of 1500 g. This suggests that inadequate protein intake is at least partially responsible for the poor growth of VLBW infants. Supplementation with additional protein and increasing the amount of commercial fortifier beyond the standard amount are options if growth is unsatisfactory and/or if low blood urea concentration (<4 mg/dL) suggests that protein intake is low, e.g., is growth-limiting.

There is a strong suspicion that most infants also need considerably more calories than indicated in Table 1 for achievement of growth that matches fetal growth. Yet the notion is widely held that infants need 120 kcal/kg/d regardless of size or age. Moreover, it is common practice to adjust the feeding volume of growing infants only after there has been a demonstrated need, e.g., a decrease in weight gain. The net effect is that energy intakes are generally lower than average needs for adequate growth.

Energy requirements are uncertain and very variable. The unmet challenge is to determine the energy requirement of each individual VLBW infant and then to meet it. Hopefully technologies in the future will allow for such individualization of energy requirements. Until then, feeding volumes must be adjusted daily to meet requirements that sustain growth of greater than 15 g/kg/d. This means providing nutrients to support not only the intrauterine rate of growth but also "catch-up" growth (that require to correct deficits incurred prior to regaining birth weight) after birth weight is regained and the infant is more stable.

Embleton et al. (6), compared actual energy intake vs. using an energy requirement of 120 kcal/kg/d, and documented an energy deficit of (406 ± 92 kcal)/kg/d over the first week of life and a deficit of (813 ± 542 kcal)/kg/d over the first 5 weeks of life in infants born prior to 30 weeks' gestation. Interestingly, an additional 24 kcal/kg/d, which would be provided with 180 mL/kg/d of preterm formula vs. 150 mL/kg/d, would provide an additional 840 kcal/kg over a 35-day period. This meets the energy deficit documented in the study (6).

Therefore, preterm formulas should be fed at 180 mL/kg/d during convalescence to meet protein requirements and enhance growth. If feeding volumes are restricted, as they often are because of pulmonary disease, feedings should be concentrated to 90 or 100 kcal/dL so as to enable adequate energy intakes to be delivered. Still, volumes must be adequate to provide adequate protein as well. Fortification of breast milk should be initiated well before a full feeding volume is reached (100 mL/kg/d). Remember that the composition of expressed breast milk is quite variable and that with standard fortification regimes, either energy or protein intake can be less than is assumed (85). If there is evidence that protein intake is inadequate (e.g., low serum urea concentration BUN <4), supplementation with additional protein may be indicated.

When fluid restriction is indicated, milk concentration, formula, and/or modular additives may be considered. There is a wide practice of milk manipulation for premature infants, but documentation is lacking on the nutrient adequacy, tolerance, or safety of theses concoctions (86). There are seven "formula recipes" for 27- and 30-kcal/oz milks to meet the nutrient needs of infants requiring fluid restrictions, which can be found in the third

Table 2 Comparison of Nutrient Values for Various Preterm Formulas

Formula	Protein (g/100 cal)	Calcium (mg/100 cal)	Phosphorus (mg/100 cal)	Iron (mg/100 cal)
SHMF + MBM[a]	3.0	142	80	0.5
EHMF + MBM	3.1	115	58	1.2
EPF	3.0	165	83	1.8
SSC	2.7	180	90	1.5
EPF 30 with MCT oil and Polycose	2.4	132	66	1.4
SSC 30 with MCT oil and Polycose	2.2	144	72	1.2
BPD-B 30	2.6	144	89	1.2
BPD-F 30	2.4	148	75	1.0

[a] Abbreviations: SHMF (Similac Human Milk Fortifier); EHMF (Enfamil Human Milk Fortifier); EPF (Enfamil Premature Formula); SSC (Similac Special Care); BPD-B 30 (breast milk based, B) 30 mL; 19 mL human milk, 1 packet HMF, 10 mL liquid concentrate (40 cal/oz) term formula; BPD-F 30 (formula based, F) 30 mL; 20 mL Similac Natural Care Liquid Fortifier, 10 mL liquid concentrate (40 cal/oz) term-formula

edition of Nutritional Care for High-Risk Newborns (Precept Press, Chicago, 2000). At the University of Louisville, concoctions have been developed and used. They are known as BPD (bronchopulmonary dysplasia) formulas, since they are used exclusively in these infants. Table 2 provides a comparison for those formula vs. preterm formulas, fortified human milk, and preterm formula in which only medium-chain triglycerides (MCT oil) and polycose are added. Clearly, more liberal volumes of intake with concentrated feeds will be necessary to increase both energy and protein to attain adequate protein in these fluid-restricted infants (~130 mL/kg/d). Attainment of adequate protein intakes will remain difficult in a few, and supplemental protein may be necessary. Currently such protein use is the only way of selectively increasing protein intake of VLBW infants fed breast milk or formula.

X. POSTNATAL GROWTH IN THE NICU

The plotting of growth facilitates the assessment of trends in growth. There are two types of charts for the premature infant. They are the intrauterine and postnatal charts.

The intrauterine charts represent the growth of the fetus that is the goal for premature infants to achieve. The charts do not allow for the initial weight loss seen in the newborn, so the infant's weight at 1 week will be below the birth percentile. There is a wide range in the years, geographical location related to altitude, and ethnicity among the various intrauterine growth curves available (87,88). These differences may alter birth growth parameters. It is also likely that birth weight, length, and head circumference measurements of normal undelivered fetuses at the same gestational age are underestimated to some degree by the reference curves.

In 1996 Alexander et al. (87) described fetal growth data from 20 to 44 weeks' gestation for the United States from data collected on more than 3.8 million single live births. These babies were born to U.S. resident mothers, and the data are contained in the 1991 U.S. Live Birth File created by the National Center for Health Statistics.

The postnatal charts reflect the initial weight loss that occurs with infants during the first week of life. Many studies demonstrate rate of weight gain similar to the fetus at 15 g/kg/d after the VVLBW infant returns to birth weight at 2–3 weeks of age (4,89,90). Table 3 reviews available postnatal growth curves (4,89–92).

The most recent chart from the National Institute of Child Health and Human Development Neonatal Research Network center offers the following advantages: (1) sample size is large, (2) sample reflects care of modern-day newborn intensive care units, (3) sample size is from 12 newborn intensive care units (NICUs) throughout the United States, and (4) weight, length, head circumference, and midarm circumference data were obtained (4). This should be considered a "growth observation study." These grids are *not* intended to be considered as "optimal" growth but rather to focus attention on postnatal growth and factors affecting it. As shown (Figure 1), although the birth weights of the study infants are similar to the birth weights of the infants show on the reference intrauterine curve, most of the infants born between 24 and 29 weeks of gestation would not have achieved the median birth weight of the reference fetus of the same postmenstrual age, and many would be less than the 10th percentile at hospital discharge. Infants who experience major morbidities, such as chronic lung disease and late-onset sepsis, also tend to gain weight more slowly (4). Unless growth at a rate that exceeds the intrauterine growth rate can be achieved, most VLBW infants fail to demonstrate catch-up growth and at hospital discharge have not reached the 50th percentile body weight, length, and head circumference of the reference fetus at the same postmenstrual age. Following discharge from the NICU, these infants are at risk for growth failure and their growth must be followed closely.

XI. SUMMARY

The aggressive approach to nutrition of the VLBW infant described in this chapter aims at minimizing the interruption of nutrient uptake that occurs

Table 3 Comparison of Postnatal Growth Charts

Measurements chart	Birth year(s)	Infant sample size	Birthweight (g)	Geographic location	Days of life followed	Obtained
Dancis J, O'Connell JR, Holt LE (Ref. 91)	1948	100	1000–2500	New York, New York	50	Weight
Shaffer SG, Quimir CL, Anderson JV, et al. (Ref. 89)	1984–1985	385	<2500	Kansas City, Kansas	40	Weight
Wright K, Dawson JP, Fallis D, et al. (Ref. 90)	1987–1991	205	501–1500	Knoxville, Tennessee	105	Weight, length, head circumference
Adamkin DH, Klingbeil R, Radmacher PG (Ref. 92)	1988–1990	99	<1200	Louisville, Kentucky	50	Weight
Ehrenkranz RA, Younes N, Lemons J, et al. (Ref. 4)	1995–1994	1660	501–1500	12 Sites, United States	120	Weight, length, head circumference, midarm circumference

with premature birth. A 1998 article using these practices has shown favorable results. Pauls and coworkers (93) constructed postnatal body weight gain curves for the first 30 days of life from retrospective data collected on 136 survivors with birth weight less than 1000 g who were born between 1991 and 1997 and who received early parenteral and enteral nutrition. All infants received a parenteral glucose and amino acid (1 g/kg/d) solution on day 1 and a lipid emulsion (0.5 g/kg/d) on day 2; both were increased by 0.5 g/kg/d to 3 g/kg/d as tolerated. Minimal enteral feedings were initiated with human milk, if available, or a preterm formula during the first day of life and advanced as tolerated; full enteral nutrition was achieved at a median of 20 days. Birth weight was regained at a mean of 11 ± 3.7 days, and subsequent weight gain was 15.7 ± 7.2 g/kg/d. These postnatal growth curves reflect growth of VVLBW infants who received early parenteral and enteral nutritional support. These curves do show improved growth versus the other postnatal curves (Table 3). This is also our experience in comparing most recent growth performance with previous data (92,94). Therefore, these curves are the most current reflecting aggressive strategies.

Our first nutritional goal in these patients is to achieve positive energy balance as soon after birth as possible. A nutrient regimen providing intakes of 2.0, 5.0, and 0.5 to 1.0 g/kg/day of parenteral amino acid, glucose, and lipid emulsion, respectively, is tolerated by most low-birth-weight infants (63). This regimen supports positive nitrogen retention and prevents the development of classic essential fatty acid deficiency. These intakes provide less total energy than needed for achieving positive energy balance, and additional energy is added as extra glucose and/or lipid parenterally. Next comes the integration of trophic feedings to prime the gut in order to prepare the immature intestine for its intended function.

Total parenteral nutrition used for these VLBW infants should include a pediatric amino acid solution designed to normalize plasma amino acid pattern, improve nitrogen retention and growth, and attenuate TPN-associated complications (95). These solutions provide essential amino acids, including taurine and tyrosine (96), and semiessential amino acids such as cysteine, as well as the nonessential amino acids, glutamic acid, and aspartic acids, not found in standard crystalline amino acid solutions. This allows for lower amounts of glycine to balance the solutions, avoiding significantly elevated plasma glycine concentrations, which have been seen in VLBW infants infused with the standard solutions (96). Twenty percent lipid emulsions are preferred in premature infants because they result in lower triglycerides and other plasma lipids (52). Balanced parenteral nutrition, including both fat and carbohydrate (as nonnitrogen calories), is the ideal regimen, especially for VLBW infants with RDS. Such a regimen decreases the respiratory quotient and prevents excessive fluid administration.

Concerning enteral nutrition, there is no evidence to support the use of dilute formula in the management of VLBW infants. It is our practice to use intermittent bolus gavage feeding as the standard. However, continuous nasogastric feeding is used if feeding intolerance persists despite manipulation of the amount and frequency of feedings agreed upon. Specific guideline definition and management of feeding intolerance are necessary for each NICU. As far as determining the best type of feeding, studies comparing premature human milk and premature infant formula have focused on short-term outcomes and lack long-term follow-up. Breast milk is almost universally accepted as the best feeding substrate for these infants (97). Human milk fortification, especially with sodium, calcium, phosphorous, and protein, will be necessary to maintain adequate growth, nutrient retention, and biochemical homeostasis (97,98).

We must continue to seek and evaluate ways to improve the growth of VLBW infants. In 1948, Dancis said that the "chief variable in determining the weight curve of such infants is the feeding policy" (91). Marked changes in perinatal medicine and in the understanding of the nutritional requirements of VLBW infants have occurred since the Dancis growth curves. Figure 4

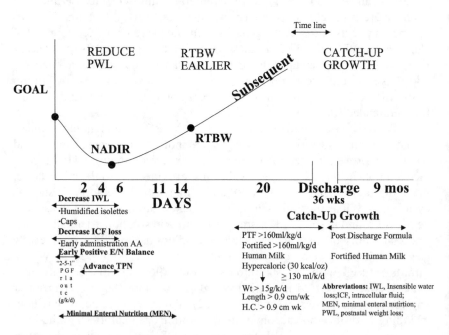

Figure 4 Aggressive nutrition: prevention of EUGR.

demonstrates a "time line" of many of the strategies and goals presented in this chapter to provide aggressive nutrition and prevent EUGR. Advances and technologies will continue to improve our care and understanding of these unique patients and their nutritional needs. The rewards will be, not only improved longitudinal growth, but also better neurodevelopmental outcome.

REFERENCES

1. American Academy of Pediatrics, Committee on Nutrition. Nutritional needs of low-birth-weight infants. Pediatrics 1977; 60:519–530.
2. American Academy of Pediatrics, Committee on Nutrition. Nutritional needs of low-birth-weight infants. Pediatrics 1985; 75:976–986.
3. American Academy of Pediatrics, Committee on Nutrition. Nutritional needs of low-birth-weight infants. In: Pediatric Nutrition Handbook. 4th ed. Elk Grove Village, IL: American Academy of Pediatrics, 1998:55–87.
4. Ehrenkranz RA, Younes N, Lemons J, et al. Longitudinal growth of hospitalized very-low-birth-weight infants. Pediatrics 1999; 104:280–289.
5. Carlson SJ, Ziegler EE. Nutrient intakes and growth of very-low-birth-weight infants. J Perinatol 1998; 18:252–258.
6. Embleton NE, Pang N, Cooke RJ. Postnatal malnutrition and growth retardation: an inevitable consequence of current recommendations in preterm infants? Pediatrics 2001; 107:270–273.
7. Hay WW Jr, Lucas A, Heird WC, Ziegler H, Levin E, Grave GD, Catz CS, Yaffee SJ. Workshop summary: nutrition of the extremely-low-birth-weight infant. Pediatrics 1999; 104:1360–1368.
8. Lucas A, Morley R, Cole TJ, Gore SM, Lucas PJ, Crowle P, Pearse R, Boon AJ, Powell R. Early diet in preterm babies and developmental status at 18 months. Lancet 1990; 335:1477–1481.
9. Lucas A, Morley R, Cole TJ. Randomised trial of early diet in preterm babies and later intelligence quotient. BMJ 1998; 317:1481–1487.
10. Ziegler EE, Biga RL, Fomon SJ. Nutritional requirements of the premature infant. In: Suskind RM ed. Textbook of Pediatric Nutrition. New York: Raven Press, 1981:29–39.
11. Forbes GB. Human Body Composition. New York: Springer-Verlag, 1987: 101–124.
12. Forbes G. Nutritional adequacy of human breast milk for premature born infants. In: Lebenthal E, ed. Gastroenterology and Nutrition in Infancy. New York: Raven Press, 1989:27–34.
13. Ziegler EE. Protein in premature feeding. Nutrition 1994; 10:69–71.
14. Thureen PJ, Hay WW Jr. Intravenous nutrition and postnatal growth of the micropreemie. Clin Perinatol 2000; 27:197–219.

15. Sparks JW. Human intrauterine growth and nutrient accretion. Semin Perinatol 1984; 8:74–93.

16. Ziegler EE, O'Donnell AM, Nelson SE, et al. Body composition of the reference fetus. Growth 1976; 40:329–341.

17. Ziegler EE, Thureen PJ, Carlson SJ. Aggressive nutrition of the very-low-birth-weight infant. Clin Perinatol 2002; 29:225–244.

18. Ziegler EE. Protein requirements of preterm infants. In: Fomon SJ, Heird WC, eds. Energy and Protein Needs During Infancy. New York: Academic Press, 1986:69–85.

19. Kramer MS, Platt RW, Wen SW, et al. A new and improved population-based Canadian reference for birth weight for gestational age. Pediatrics 2001; 108: 1–7.

20. Saini J, Macmahon P, Morgan JB, et al. Early parenteral feeding of amino acids. Arch Dis Child 1989; 64:1362–1366.

21. Rivera JA, Bell EF, Bier DM. Effect of intravenous amino acids on protein metabolism of preterm infants during the first three days of life. Pediatr Res 1993; 33:106–111.

22. Snyderman SE, Boyer A, Kogut MD, et al. The protein requirement of the premature infant. I. The effect of protein intake on the retention of nitrogen. J Pediatr 1963; 74:872–880.

23. Reichman B, Chessex P, Putet G, et al. Diet, fat accretion, and growth in premature infants. N Engl J Med 1981; 305:1495–1500.

24. Schoeller DA, van Santen E. Measurement of energy expenditure in humans by doubly labeled water method. J Appl Physiol 1982; 53:955–959.

25. Jensen CL, Butte NF, Wong WW, et al. Determining energy expenditure in preterm infants: comparison of $^2H_2^{18}O$ method and indirect calorimetry. Am J Physiol 1992; 263:R685–R692.

26. Roberts S, Coward W, Schlingenseipen KH, et al. Comparison of the doubly labeled water ($^2H_2^{18}O$) method with indirect calorimetry and a nutrient-balance study for simultaneous determination of energy expenditure, water intake, and metabolizable energy intake in preterm infants. Am J Clin Nutr 1986; 44:315–322.

27. Jones PJH, Winthrop AL, Schoeller DA, et al. Validation of doubly labeled water for assessing energy expenditure in infants. Pediatr Res 1987; 21:242–246.

28. Carr BJ, Denne SC, Leitch CA. Total energy expenditure in extremely premature and term infants in early postnatal life. Pediatr Res 2000; 47:284.

29. Leitch CA, Ahlrichs JA, Karn CA, et al. Energy expenditure and energy intake during dexamethasone therapy for chronic lung disease. Pediatr Res 1999; 46:109–113.

30. Thompson GN, Pacy PJ, Merritt H, et al. Rapid measurement of whole-body and forearm protein turnover using a $^2H_5$ phenylalanine model. Am J Physiol 1989; 256:E631–E639.

31. Denne SC, Karn CA, Ahlrichs JA, et al. Proteolysis and phenylalanine hydroxylation in response to parenteral nutrition in extremely premature and normal newborns. J Clin Invest 1996; 97:746–754.

32. Kashyap S, Heird WC. Protein requirements of low-birth-weight, very-low-birth-weight, and small-for-gestation-age infants. New York: Vevey/Raven Press, 1994.

33. Bauer K, Bovermann G, Roithmaier A, et al. Body composition, nutrition, and fluid balance during the first two weeks of life in preterm neonates weighting less than 1500 grams. J Pediatr 1991; 118:615–620.

34. van Lingen RA, van Goudoever JB, Luijendijk IHT, et al. Effects of early amino acid administration during total parenteral nutrition on protein metabolism in preterm infants. Clin Sci 1992; 82:199–203.

35. Murdock N, Crighton A, Nelson LM, et al. Low-birth-weight infants and total parenteral nutrition immediately after birth. II. Randomized study of biochemical tolerance of intravenous glucose, amino acids, and lipid. Arch Dis Child 1995; 73:F8–F12.

36. Poindexter BB, Karn CA, Ahlrichs JA, et al. Amino acids suppress proteolysis independent of insulin throughout the neonatal period. Am J Physiol 1997; 272:R592–R599.

37. Clark SE, Karn CA, Ahlrichs JA, et al. Acute changes in leucine and phenylalanine kinetics produced by parenteral nutrition in premature infants. Pediatr Res 1997; 41:568–574.

38. Denne SC. Protein and energy requirements in preterm infants. Semin Nonatal 2001; 6:377–382.

39. Stefano JL, Norman ME, Morales MC, et al. Decreased erythrocyte Na-K^{+}-ATPase activity associated with cellular potassium loss in extremely-low-birth-weight infants with nonoliguric hyperkalemia. J Pediatr 1993; 122:276–284.

40. Keshen T, Miller R, Jahoor F, et al. Glucose production and gluconeogenesis are negatively related to body weight in mechanically ventilated, very-low-birth-weight neonates. Pediatr Res 1997; 41:132–138.

41. Kalhan SC, Parimi P, Van Beek R, et al. Estimation of gluconeogenesis in newborn infants. Am J Physiol Endocrinol Metab 2001; 281:E991–E997.

42. Goldman SL, Hirata T. Attenuated response to insulin in very-low-birth-weight infants. Pediat Res 1980; 14:50–53.

43. Vaucher YE, Walson PD, Morrow G III. Continuous insulin infusion in hyperglycemic, very-low-birth-weight infants. J Pediatr Gastroenterol Nutr 1982; 1:211–217.

44. Ostertag SG, Jovanovic L, Lewis B, et al. Insulin pump therapy in the very-low-birth-weight infant. Pediatrics 78:625–630.

45. Binder ND, Raschko PK, Benda GI, et al. Insulin infusion with parenteral nutrition in extremely-low-birth-weight infants with hyperglycemia. J Pediatr 1989; 114:273–280.

46. Collins JW Jr, Hoppe M, Brown K. A controlled trial of insulin infusion and parenteral nutrition in extremely-low-birth-weight infants with glucose intolerance. J Pediatr 1991; 118:921–927.

47. Poindexter BB, Karn CA, Denne SC. Exogenous insulin reduces proteolysis and protein synthesis in extremely-low-birth-weight infants. J Pediatr 1998; 132:948–953.

48. Michelli JL, Schutz Y, Jund S, Calame A. Early postnatal amino acid administration ELBW PT infants. Sem Neonatal Nutr Metab, 1994; 2.
49. Friedman Z, Danon A, Stahlman MT, et al. Rapid onset of essential fatty acid deficiency in the newborn. Pediatrics 1976; 58:640.
50. Adamkin DH. Use of intravenous fat emulsions, Part 1. Perinatology–Neonatology May/June, 1986; 10(3):16–23.
51. Uauy R, Mena P. Lipids and neurodevelopment. Nutr Rev 2001; 59:S34–S48.
52. Haumont D, Deckelbaum RJ, Richelle M, et al. Plasma lipid and plasma lipoprotein concentrations in low-birth-weight infants given parenteral nutrition with 20% compared to 10% intralipid. J Pediatr 1989; 115:787–793.
53. Fielding CJ. Human lipoprotein lipase inhibition of activity by cholesterol. Biochem Biophys Acta 1970; 218:221–226.
54. Brans YW, Dutton EB, Drew DS, et al. Fat emulsion tolerance in very-low-birth-weight neonates: effect on diffusion of oxygen in the lungs and on blood pH. Pediatrics 1986; 78:79–84.
55. Adamkin DH, Gelke KN, Wilkerson SA. Clinical and laboratory observations: influence of intravenous fat therapy on tracheal effluent phospholipids and oxygenation in severe respiratory distress syndrome. J Pediatr 1985; 106:122–124.
56. Thiessen H, Jacobsen J, Brodersen R. Displacement of albumin-bound bilirubin by fatty acids. Acta Pediatr Scand 1972; 61:285.
57. Jacobsen J. Binding of bilirubin to human serum albumin. FEBS Lett 1969; 5:112.
58. Starinsky R, Shafrir E. Displacement of albumin-bound bilirubin by free fatty acids: implications for neonatal hyperbilirubinemia. Clin Chim Acta 1970; 29:311.
59. Andrew G, Chan G, Schiff D. Lipid metabolism in the neonate: II. The effect of intralipid on bilirubin binding in vitro and in vivo. J Pediatr 1976; 88:279.
60. Adamkin DH, Radmacher PG, Klingbeil RK. Use of intravenous lipid and hyperbilirubinemia. J Pediatr Gastroenterol Nutr 1992; 14:135.
61. Spear ML, Stahl GE, Hamosh M, et al. Effect of heparin dose and infusion rate on lipid clearance and bilirubin binding in premature infants receiving intravenous fat emulsions. J Pediatr 1988; 112:94.
62. Gilbertson N, Kovar IZ, Cox DJ, et al. Introduction of intravenous lipid administration on the first day of life in the very-low-birth-weight neonate. J Pediatr 1991; 119:615–623.
63. Heird WC, Jensen CL, Gomez MR. Practical aspects of achieving positive energy balance in low-birth-weight infants. J Pediatr 1992; 120:120–128.
64. Lucas A. Minimal enteral feeding. Seminars in Neonatal Nutrition and Metabolism 1993; 1:22.
65. Dworkin LD, Levine GM, Farber NJ, et al. Small intestinal mass of the rat is partially determined by indiscrete effects intraluminal nutrition. Gastroenterology 1976; 71:626–630.
66. Levine GM, Deren JJ, Steiger E, et al. Role of oral intake in maintenance of gut mass and disaccharide activity. Gastroenterology 1974; 67:975–982.

67. Lucas A, Bloom SR, Aynsley-Green A. Gut hormones and "minimal enteral feeding." Acta Pediatr Scan 1986; 75:719–723.

68. Kliegman RM. Experimental validation of neonatal feeding practices. Pediatrics 1999; 103:492–493.

69. Ziegler EE. Trophic feeds. In: Ziegler EE, Lucas A, Moro GE, eds. Nutrition of the Very-Low-Birth-Weight Infant. Philadelphia: Lippincott Williams & Wilkins, 1999:233–244.

70. Mihatsch WA, von Schoenaich P, Fahnenstich H, et al. The significance of gastric residuals in the early enteral feeding advancement of extremely-low-birth-weight infants. Pediatrics 2002; 109:457–459.

71. Kliegman RM. Studies of feeding intolerance in very-low-birth-weight infants: definition and significance [commentary]. Pediatrics 2002; 109(3).

72. Brown EG, Sweet AY. Preventing necrotizing enterocolitis in neonates. JAMA 1978; 240, 2452–2454.

73. Tyson JE, Kennedy K, Minimal enteral nutrition in parenterally fed neonates, 1997. Available at: http://www.nichd.nih.gov/cochraneneonatal/tyson/tyson/htm.

74. McClure RJ, Newell SJ. Randomized control study of clinical outcome following trophic feeding. Arch Dis Child Fetal Neonatal Ed 2000; 82:F29–F33.

75. Anderson DM, Kliegman RM. The relationship of neonatal alimentation practices to the occurrence of endemic necrotizing enterocolitis. Am J Perinatol 1991; 8:62–67.

76. Rayyis SF, Ambalavanan N, Wright L, et al. Randomized trial of "slow" versus "fast" feed advancements on the incidence of necrotizing enterocolitis in very-low-birth-weight infants. J Pediatr 1999; 134:293–297.

77. Caeton AJ, Goetzman BW. Risk business, umbilical arterial catheterization. Am J Dis Child 1985; 139:120.

78. Kliegman RM, Fanaroff AA. Neonatal necrotizing enterocolitis: a nine-year experience. Am J Dis Child 1981; 135:603–607.

79. Davey AM, Wagner CL, Phelps DL, et al. Do premature infants with umbilical artery catheters tolerate oral feeds? Pediatr Res 1993; 31:199A.

80. Frantz ID, L'Heureux P, Engel RR. Necrotizing enterocolitis. J Pediatr 1975; 86:259.

81. Kerner JA. The use of umbilical catheters for parenteral nutrition. In: Kerner JA, ed. Manual of Pediatric Parenteral Nutrition. New York: Wiley, 1993:303.

82. Lehmiller DJ, Kanto WP. Relationships of mesenteric thromboembolism, oral feeding, and necrotizing enterocolitis. J Pediatr 1978; 92:96.

83. Wesstrom G, Finnstrom O, Stenport G. Umbilical artery catheterization in newborns: I. Thrombosis in relation to catheter type and position. Acta Pediatr Scand 1979; 68:575.

84. Lucas A, Cole TJ. Breast milk and neonatal necrotizing enterocolitis. Lancet 1990; 336:1519–1523.

85. Ziegler EE. Breast-milk fortification. Acta Paediat 2001; 90:1–4.

86. Nein-Folino NL, Loughead IL, Loughead MK. Enhanced-calorie formulas: considerations and options. Neonatal Netw 2001; 20(1):7–15.

87. Alexander GR, Himes JH, Kaufman RB, et al. A United States national reference for fetal growth. Obstet Gynecol 1996; 87:163–168.
88. Yip R. Altitude and birth weight. J Pediatr 1987; 111:869–876.
89. Shaffer SG, Quimiro CL, Anderson JV, et al. Postnatal weight changes in low-birth-weight infants. Pediatrics 1987; 79(5):702–705.
90. Wright K, Dawson JP, Fallis D, et al. New postnatal growth grids for very-low-birth-weight infants. Pediatrics 1993; 91(5):922–926.
91. Dancis J, O'Connell JR, Holt LE. A grid for recording the weight of premature infants. J Pediatr 1948; 33:570–572.
92. Adamkin DH, Klingbeil RK, Radmacher PG. Forty years after Dancis: the very-very-low-birth-weight-infant grids. J Perinatol 1994; 14(3):187–189.
93. Pauls J, Bauer K, Versmold H. Postnatal body weight curves for infants below 1000-g birth weight receiving early enteral and parenteral nutrition. Eur J Pediatr 1998; 157:416–421.
94. Rafail S, Radmacher P, Adamkin D. Early postnatal weight loss and return to birth weight in VVLBW (<1001 g) and ELBW (<751 g) during three eras in the NICU. J Invest Med 2001; 786.
95. Adamkin DH, Anderson AH. Preliminary comparison of TPN-associated cholestasis (TPN-AC) in neonates receiving aminosyn vs. aminosyn-pediatric formulation (PF). Pediatr Res 1987; 21, 422A.
96. Adamkin DH, Benawra RS, Desai NS, Marchildon MB, McClead RE, McCulloch KM. Clinical comparison of two neonatal intravenous amino acid formulations in preterm infants. J Perinatol 1991; 11(4):375–382.
97. Atkinson SA. Human milk feeding of the micropreemie. Clin Perinatol 2000; 27:235–247.
98. Schanler RJ. The role of human milk fortification for premature infants. Clin Perinatol 1998; 25:645–657.

8
Post-Hospital-Discharge Nutrition for the Premature Infant

Anjali P. Parish and Jatinder Bhatia
Medical College of Georgia, Augusta, Georgia, U.S.A.

I. INTRODUCTION

As perinatal medicine advances, the survival of premature infants at younger gestational ages is improving, and their special needs are becoming more complex. The responsibility for their long-term care has fallen on the primary care physician as well. These infants have ongoing issues with nutrition and growth, chronic lung disease, retinopathy of prematurity, gastroesophageal reflux, apnea, and immunizations. However, assessment of growth and development still remains the cornerstone of their well-child visits, and they depend on optimal nutrition for good outcomes. The focus of this chapter is the nutritional goals of the premature infant and ways to achieve them. Our ability to provide in-hospital nutrition, while still not optimal, has vastly improved; care of the preterm infant, especially the very low birthweight infant, after hospital discharge still lags behind.

II. EXPECTED WEIGHT GAIN

Every office visit should begin with measurement of weight, occipitofrontal head circumference, and crown–heel length. These are key parameters for assessing growth based on corrected gestational age (CGA) and not chronological age. For example, an infant born at 28 weeks' gestation when 2 months old chronologically would actually be at 36 weeks' CGA. Suggested gains for healthy term infants in anthropometric measures are weight gain of 16–40 g per day and length gain of 0.6–1.0 cm per week in the first 3 months of life (1). Premature infants fed standard-term formulas had average gains in weight and head circumference of 13.0 g/kg/d and 1.21 mm/d, respectively, while those fed preterm formula gained 16.6 g/kg/d in weight and 1.53 mm/d in head circumference, respectively (2). In general, 110–130 kcal per kilogram per day should allow for the observed average growth for most premature infants. Infants with a confounding health problem, such as chronic lung disease or being small for gestational age, may require higher-energy and/or protein intakes.

Several methods exist to determine energy expenditure and estimate needs. The more commonly employed are direct calorimetry, indirect calorimetry, and the doubly labeled water technique (3). Although necessary for research, none of these methods is practical for everyday office use. One study showed premature infants increased their volume of intake when fed 67-kcal/dL formula to match the caloric intake of their counterparts being fed 81-kcal/dL formula (4). Since most premature infants may not be able to ingest more than 150–180 mL/kg/d, determining the infant's energy needs will help determine which caloric density formula he/she should receive. Currently, the best measure of energy intake versus expenditure is adequate growth along appropriate growth curves.

III. EXTRAUTERINE GROWTH RESTRICTION AND CATCH-UP GROWTH

Despite aggressive use of total parenteral nutrition in the NICU, most premature infants still suffer from extrauterine growth restriction at the time of hospital discharge. Multiple issues contribute to growth delays, including repeated infections, use of steroids, delayed commencement of parenteral nutrition, intolerance to parenteral glucose and/or lipids, delayed advancement to full enteral feedings, and inappropriate feedings once enteral feeds are started, i.e., unfortified human milk or term-infant formula. A multicenter NICHD study found that the average weight of an initial 28- to 29-week infant was 715 g less than expected by 32 weeks' CGA. Furthermore, the younger the gestational age at birth, the greater the weight deficit by 32 weeks, and growth curves for all groups of infants originally less than 29 weeks were below the 10th percentile for in utero growth (5,6). Since the optimal growth trajectory of a premature infant is not known (in utero growth curves provide an in utero standard), simply maintaining the premature infant along his own growth curve may still prove to be inadequate, because it does not take catch-up growth into account. *Catch-up growth* refers to the difference in weight/HC/length between a fetus in utero and his prematurely born counterpart at the same postconception age. In many instances, premature infants are 2 standard deviations and more below the growth of what they should have been if they had not been born early (7). Partial catch-up growth can be achieved by manipulating the dietary intake of premature infants; however, the best way to achieve this goal has yet to be determined (8). The growth deficits are associated with changes in body composition, with premature infants having a higher percentage of body fat and lower lean body mass (9). In larger infants, Bhatia and Rassin (10) demonstrated differences in triceps and subscapular skinfold thicknesses between infants fed "ex utero" and infants who were studied at similar body weights, but within the first few days of life, "in utero." Body length was significantly greater in the "in utero" group, but there were no differences in total body water or midarm circumferences. These data suggest that feeding of a standard premature-infant formula during the initial hospitalization supported a similar rate of weight gain and body water content as the transplacentally nourished infant but resulted in dissimilar deposition of fat. Embelton et al. (11) have attributed the failure in catch-up to the practice of calculating feeds on the baby's current weight rather than on the expected weight. They demonstrated substantial energy and protein deficits over the period of study. Moreover, these deficits were associated with a decreasing weight z-score that reached a nadir of approximately -1 by 2 weeks (in infants over 31 weeks) and recovered slightly by discharge; in infants under 31 weeks, the weight z-score nadir was lower, occurring at approximately 3 weeks, and improved very slightly by discharge. Similar findings were recently reported by Ernst et al. (12). For now, the currently available premature-infant formulas, with their higher energy and nutrient content, or appropriately fortified human milk are superior to term formulas in assisting with catch-up growth.

IV. ADVANTAGES OF PRETERM AND TRANSITION FORMULAS

Once an infant's energy needs are established, the best way to deliver these calories must be determined. Simply increasing the carbohydrate content of the formula will increase the calories, but this method may not result in very desirable growth. Studies have established the importance of supplementing the premature infant with more protein and fat per kilogram of body weight per day than the term infant to achieve adequate growth (8). The increase in growth among premature infants fed specialized preterm formula may not be due simply to increase in body fat stores (13). Premature infants fed specialized preterm formula from discharge to 12 months' CGA took in less volume and equal calories per day but more protein than those fed term formulas; these infants had better weight gain and head growth. Furthermore, these growth advantages appear to be more in males than in females, for reasons not well understood (14).

The leading cause of osteopenia in the premature infant is calcium and phosphorus deficiency (7). Fetuses accumulate their largest quantities of calcium and phosphorus in the last trimester of pregnancy (7). Calcium and phosphorus needs for the premature infant approach 200 mg/kg/d of calcium and 100 mg/kg/d of phosphorus (3). Premature infants fed fortified preterm formula until 6 months' corrected gestational age were, on average, longer than those fed standard term formula (67.1 cm vs. 64.9 cm) At 8 weeks postdischarge, low-birthweight infants fed a premature-infant formula with higher levels of calcium and phosphorus had higher bone mineral contents than those fed standard-term formula or unsupplemented human milk. Most commercially available preterm-infant formulas will supply adequate calcium and phosphorus if the infant takes at least 150 mL/kg/d; term formulas or unfortified human milk will not. Metabolic bone disease is a well-recognized complication of prematurity, especially in infants provided prolonged parenteral nutrition or unfortified human milk. The preterm infant at 40 weeks postconceptional age (PCA) has a bone mineral content approximately half of that of a term counterpart (15). Expremature infants studied at 8 years of age still demonstrated a significant reduction in bone mineral mass and reduced bone mineral density in the hips (16). It should be noted that the lower-bone-mineral-mass effect largely disappears when corrected for differences in height and weight.

Of particular interest is the neurodevelopmental outcome for the otherwise-healthy preterm infant. A preliminary study demonstrated that premature infants (at 18 months' postterm age) fed specialized preterm formula had higher developmental and social quotient scores than those fed standard-term formula. Furthermore, they had a lower incidence of moderate developmental impairment. Unpublished data from this same study suggest that this effect of diet on developmental performance persists at 7.5–8 years of age (7). These infants were fed preterm formula for only 4 weeks postnatally. In longer feeding trials, feeding of preterm formulas after hospital discharge did not improve developmental outcome at 18 months' corrected age (17).

If a mother does not desire to breast-feed, an appropriate commercial formula must be selected for her premature infant. In general, currently available soy formulas are inappropriate for premature infants prior to 6 months CGA. These formulas have a caloric density of 67 kcal/dL. Levels of calcium/phosphorus are not high enough to prevent metabolic bone disease, and the absence of lactose impairs calcium absorption. They also lack adequate protein and fat content necessary for the premature infant. If true milk protein allergy exists, elemental formulas that can be concentrated to higher caloric content may be a better option for these infants.

Always of concern to parents as well as physicians is how well the infants tolerate these formulas. One study comparing preterm to term formula asked mothers to keep log books on number of spit-ups/vomits, colic episodes per 2 weeks, frequency of stools, and perceptual size/consistency of stools. Data showed no difference between the diet groups for any of these factors (18). Parental reassurance, rediscussing the benefits of preterm formulas, and confirming appropriate growth for size and age are the best ways to prevent formula change before needed.

V. DHA AND THE PREMATURE INFANT

Preterm infants provided human milk are reported to have advanced neuro-developmental outcome as compared to formula-fed infants, measured by electroretinograms, visual evoked potentials, and psychometric tests (19–22). The better performance, although possibly multifactorial, has been related to dietary docosahexanoic (DHA) and arachdonic (AA) acids, since plasma and erythrocyte phospholipids contents of AA and DHA are higher in breast-fed infants than in infants fed formulas lacking these fatty acids (23,24), and inadequate long-chain fatty acids in the diet may be related to performance on tests of cognitive function (25,26). The inability to synthesize enough DHA and AA from their precursors and the lack of preformed DHA may be the cause of the lower content of these fatty acids in formula-fed infants. The recent addition of these fatty acids to formulas in the United States has led to renewed interest and debate about the effects of long-chain fatty acids and later neurodevelopmental outcome, and has been reviewed elsewhere (27). In a large prospective, randomized controlled trial, preterm infants were assigned to one of three formula-feeding groups with or without long-chain fatty acids: control, AA + DHA from a fish/fungal source, or AA + DHA from egg-derived triglyceride. Subsequently, they were fed human milk or a preterm formula with or without added AA (0.42%) and DHA (0.26%) to term-corrected age and then human milk or a transitional formula with or without similar amounts of AA and DHA to 12 months' corrected age. Visual acuity measured by visual evoked potentials, and not by acuity cards, was better in both the AA + DHA-supplemented infants than control and were closer to that of human milk-fed term infants at 6 months of age. Scores on the Fagan test of novelty preference were greater in AA + DHA (egg) than AA + DHA (fish/fungal) and control at 6 months but not later. There were no differences in the Bailey Mental Developmental Index at 12 months of age. However, in infants less than 1250 g, there was an almost 9-point difference between AA + DHA (fish/fungal) and control infants, suggesting the benefit of the added fatty acids. Vocabulary comprehension was also greater at 14 months in both supplemented groups as compared to control when Spanish-speaking infants and twins were excluded from the analyses. There were no demonstrable growth benefits or adverse effects (28). In contrast, Innis et al. (29) demonstrated that preterm infants fed DHA (0.14%) and AA (0.27%) from single-cell triglycerides gained weight significantly faster during preterm formula feeding than control infants and had weight:length ratios similar to those of term breast-fed infants at 48 and 57 weeks' postmenstrual age (PMA). No effects on visual acuity could be demonstrated. In a similar study, preterm infants were fed formulas with DHA + AA or control formulas without DHA and AA from two different sources until 92 weeks' postmenstrual age (30). Infants were evaluated at 118 weeks with the Bayley Scales of Infant Development II (BSID). Infants fed the formula containing single-cell source of the fatty acids had greater achieved weights at 66–118 weeks' PMA than control and were comparable to term human milk-fed infants at 118 weeks' PMA. These infants also had greater length at 79 and 92 weeks' PMA than control and fish/single-source formula-fed infants and were comparable to human milk-fed infants by 79 weeks' PMA. Term infants had higher BSID scores than the preterm infants; however, both groups of supplemented infants had significantly higher scores than control. These studies, therefore, demonstrate the effects of short- and long-term feeding of the supplemented formulas on growth and development. In neither study were there documented adverse effects on growth. These studies differ from the short-term feeding study by Fewtrell et al. (31), where there were no significant differences in developmental scores between the supplemented and unsupplemented infants. Of concern is that the supplemented infants were shorter than control infants at 18 months. The duration of the feeding trial was short (mean 33 days, SD 17 days). The difference between the results could be due to a combination of level of supplementation, source of the fatty acids, and duration of feeding. Nonetheless, one needs to be vigilant for any adverse effect of a similar nature.

The meta-analysis of data from randomized studies in preterm infants demonstrates an advantage in supplemented vs. unsupplemented infants on both behaviorally and electrophysiologically based measures of visual function (32). There appears to be a visual benefit through the first year of age, and the benefit is probably not clinically significant. However, long-term follow-up studies should be able to demonstrate whether this advantage early in life confers an advantage later in life.

The available sources of DHA include fish oil, egg phospholipid, and triacylglycerol and algal oils, whereas AA can be obtained from fungal oils, egg phospholipid, and triacylglycerol. The FDA has accepted the single-cell sources of DHA and AA as "generally regarded as safe," and these are the only sources approved for addition to infant formula. Several regulatory bodies have recommended that these fatty acids be added to formulas for both preterm and term infants, and currently available formulas in the United States contain both fatty acids, albeit at different concentrations. The American Academy of Pediatrics has not endorsed the use of these supplemented formulas. The Life Science Research Office (LSRO) recently provided recommendations for minimum and maximum levels of linoleic acid, alpha-linolenic acid, and the ratio of the two precursors; however, the Expert Panel only recommended a maximum concentration of AA to be 0.6% of total fatty acids, DHA to be 0.35%, and EPA to be 30% of the concentration of DHA. The final ratio of AA to DHA in any preterm formula was recommended to be between 1.5 and 2.0 (33). Nonetheless, the formulas in the United States and abroad are now supplemented with these fatty acids, and postmarketing surveillance does not appear to raise any safety concerns. Long-term data, if they confirm the initial findings, should allay the concerns about these fatty acids and their inclusion in infant formulas. Maternal supplementation during pregnancy and lactation appears to have a favorable outcome for later development to at least 4 years of age (34). Other studies are now being reported where the beneficial effects extended to reducing blood pressure in later childhood in a cohort of infants fed these fatty acids in their formula (35).

VI. HUMAN MILK AND THE PREMATURE INFANT

Much attention has been given to the adequacy of human milk as the sole dietary source for the premature infant. Most centers will fortify human milk while premature infants are in the hospital. The debate is whether this supplementation should continue after discharge, and how. A multicenter trial in Great Britain showed infants fed preterm formula regained birth-weight more quickly than those exclusively fed human milk (36). Human milk-fed infants who received preterm formula supplementation also gained weight more quickly than exclusively human milk-fed infants, but not at the same rate as formula-fed babies (36). Furthermore, fortified human milk has been shown to improve mineral balance in preterm infants, bringing them closer to the reference fetus range as well as meeting the nutrient needs that exceed the content of human milk (37–39).

Human milk, however, contains undefined properties that aid the premature infant. Most notably, it seems to have a neurodevelopmental stimulatory effect. Early research found that preterm babies who were exclusively provided human milk had an average IQ score 10% higher than those fed preterm formula, even after adjustment for social and educational factors. By supplementing human milk, growth can be enhanced while providing the many advantages of mother's milk to the premature infant.

Human milk remains best for most babies; supplemented human milk may be even better for the premature baby. Unfortunately, most mothers do not continue to breast-feed beyond the first few weeks of life. A study from Case Western Reserve showed that of 84 mothers who originally wanted to breast-feed their premature infants, 30 (34%) provided milk until 40 weeks' CGA and only 14 (16%) were breast-feeding by 4 months' CGA. Furthermore, only 12 had achieved actual nursing by 4 months' CGA (40).

VII. RECOMMENDATIONS FOR WEANING

In general, it is recommended not to decrease an infant's energy intake until the growth velocity has recovered along the infant's natural curve. Smaller premature infants at birth remain significantly smaller than larger premature infants by 3 years CGA (41). Once the infant is stable for 1–2 months, the caloric density can be decreased by 2 kcal/oz every 1–2 months until back on term formula.

Transitional formulas or human milk fortifiers should be provided as full diet or supplementation to human milk until at least 4–6 months CGA regardless of adequate growth, because they contain significantly more calcium and phosphorus than term formulas. This becomes problematic when full breast-feeding is established and fortification is still felt to be needed. Some practitioners use devices to aid a breast-feeding mother; others find it easier to use a formula as a partial supplement. Very low birthweight infants fed supplemented human milk in the NICU but switched to human milk only at discharge showed progressive mineral deficiency until 25 postnatal weeks when compared to commercial formula-fed babies of the same weight and age (42). These deficits persisted at 52 postnatal weeks, even after other foods and commercial formula had been introduced in the same babies. The younger the gestational age at birth, the longer the need may be for transitional formulas in order to recover from mineral deficits.

VIII. IRON SUPPLEMENTATION

The growing fetus accumulates iron at a rate of 1.6–2.0 mg/kg/d in the third trimester, to reach a total body iron content of 75 mg/kg at term (3,43). When born prematurely, an infant loses this period of iron accumulation, resulting in lower iron stores; and the more ill the infant, the more blood lost through laboratory sampling and procedures, further depleting body iron content.

Though the use of r-erythropoeitin may decrease early anemia of prematurity (44), and the need for blood transfusions (45,46), many infants become anemic by discharge. Minimum daily iron intake should equal 4–6 mg/kg/d. Current commercial formulas provide 2.0 mg/kg/d if the infant consumes at least 150 cc/kg/d; therefore, iron supplementation is necessary for all premature infants.

IX. SUMMARY

Extrauterine growth will never replace a good intrauterine growth environment. As medicine advances and even younger infants are deemed viable, extrauterine growth restriction will become an increasing problem. Today's understanding of the nutritional needs of premature infants is improving but still minimal at best. As knowledge improves, physicians will need to adapt their practices to accommodate the changes. Frequent reformulation of commercial formula should be expected and welcomed. Most importantly, the premature infant will remain a very different patient from the term infant, and the two cannot be fed in the same way.

The goals for the premature infant should be to achieve maximal gain in all parameters without adverse metabolic consequences and to achieve better neurodevelopmental outcome (43). Although the premature infant will lag behind its term counterpart in neurodevelopmental outcome, recent studies with DHA/ARA-supplemented formulas demonstrated that preterm infants can catch up with the term breast-fed counterpart and have improved neurodevelopmental outcome as compared to nonsupplemented infant but remain lower than term breast-fed infants. Continued research into long-term outcomes associated with feeding strategies is required as this cohort of infants continues to be smaller at birth and at hospital discharge.

REFERENCES

1. Guo SM, Roche AF, Fomon SJ, Nelson SE, Chumlea WC, Rogers RR, Baumgartner RN, Ziegler EE, Siervogel RM. Reference data on gains in weight and length during the first two years of life. J Pediatr 1991; 119(3):355–362.
2. Lucas A, Morley R, Cole TJ, Gore SM, Lucas PJ, Crowle P, Pearse R, Boon AJ, Powell R. Early diet in preterm babies and developmental status at 18 months. Lancet 1990; 335:1477–1481.
3. Report of the 108th Ross Conference on Pediatric Research. Human Milk for Very-Low-Birth-Weight Infants, 1999.
4. Cooke RJ, Griffin J, McCormick K, Wells JCK, Smith JS, Robinson SJ,

Leighton M. Feeding preterm infants after hospital discharge: effect of dietary manipulation on nutrient intake and growth. Pediatr Res 1998; 43(3): 355–360.

5. Erenkranz RA, Younes N, Lemons JA, et al. Longitudinal growth of hospitalized very-low-birth-weight infants. Pediatrics 1999; 104:280–289.

6. Alexander GR, Himes JH, Kaufman RB, et al. A United States national reference for fetal growth. Obstet Gynecol 1996; 87:163–168.

7. Report of the 106th Ross Conference on Pediatric Research. Posthospital Nutrition in the Preterm Infant, 1996

8. Kashyap S, Schulze KF, Ramakrishnan R, Dell RB, Heird WC. Evaluation of a mathematical model for predicting the relationship between protein and energy intakes of low-birth-weight infants and the rate and composition of weight gain. Pediatr Res 1994; 35(6):704–712.

9. Cooke RJ, Rawlings DJ, McCormick K, et al. Body composition of preterm infant during infancy. Arch Dis Child Fetal Neonatal Ed 1999; 80:F188–F191.

10. Bhatia J, Rassin DK. Growth and total body water in premature infants fed "in-utero" or "ex-utero." Acta Paediatr Scand 1988; 77:326–331.

11. Embleton NE, Pang N, Cooke RJ. Postnatal Malnutrition and growth retardation: An inevitable consequence of current recommendations in premature infants? Pediatrics 2001; 107:270–273.

12. Ernst KD, Radmacher PG, Rafail ST, Adamkin DH. Postnatal malnutrition of extremely-low-birth-weight infants with catch-up growth postdischarge. J Perinatol 2003; 23(6):477–482.

13. Lucas A, Bishop NJ, King FJ, Cole TJ. Randomized trial of nutrition for preterm infants after discharge. Arch Dis Child 1992; 67(3):324–327.

14. Cooke RJ, Griffin J, McCormick K, Wells JCK, Smith JS, Robinson SJ, Leighton M. Feeding preterm infants after hospital discharge: effect of dietary manipulation on nutrient intake and growth. Pediatr Res 1998; 43(3):355–360.

15. Horsman A, Ryan SW, Congdon PJ, Truscott JG, Simpson M. Bone mineral content and body size 65–100 weeks' post-conception in preterm and full term infants. Arch Dis Child 1989; 64:1579–1586.

16. Bowden LS, Jones CJ, Ryan SW. Bone mineralization in ex-preterm infants aged 8 years. Eur J Pediatr 1999; 158:658–661.

17. Cooke RJ, Emblleton ND, Griffin IJ, et al. Feeding preterm infants after hospital discharge: growth and development at 18 months of age. Pediatr Res 2001; 49:719–722.

18. Lucas A, Bishop NJ, King FJ, Cole TJ. Randomized trial of nutrition for preterm infants after discharge. Arch Dis Child 1992; 67(3):324–327.

19. Uauy RD, Birch DG, Birch EE, Tyson JE, Hoffman DR. Effect of dietary omega-3 fatty acids on retinal function of very-low-birth-weight neonates. Pediatr Res 1990; 28:485–492.

20. Birch DG, Birch EE, Hoffman DR, Uauy RD. Retinal development in very-low-birth-weight infants fed diets differing in omega-3 fatty acids. Invest Ophthalmol Vis Sci 1992; 33:2365–2376.

21. Birch EE, Birch DG, Hoffman DR, Uauy RD. Dietary essential fatty acid supply and visual acuity development. Invest Ophthalmol Vis Sci 1992; 32:3242–3253.

22. Lucas A, Morley R, Cole TJ, Lister G, Leeson-Payne C. Breast milk and subsequent intelligence quotient in children born preterm. Lancet 1992; 339: 261–264.

23. Carlson SE, Rhodes PG, Ferguson MG. Docosahexanoic acids status of preterm infants at birth and following feeding of human milk or formula. Am J Clin Nutr 1986; 44:798–804.

24. Innis SM, Akrabawi SS, Diersen-Scgade DA, et al. Visual acuity and blood lipids in term infants fed human milk or formulae. Lipids 1997; 32:63–72.

25. Lucas A, Morley R, Cole TJ, et al. Early diet in preterm babies and developmental status at 18 months. Lancet 1990; 335:1477–1481.

26. Lucas A, Morley R, Cole TJ. Randomized trial of early diet in preterm babies and later intelligence quotient. BMJ 1998; 317:1481–1487.

27. Jensen CL, Heird WC. Lipids with an emphasis on long-chain polyunsaturated fatty acids. Clin Perinatol 2002; 29:261–281.

28. O'Connor DL, Hall R, Adamkin D, Auestad N, Castillo M, et al. Growth and development in preterm infants fed long-chain polyunsaturated fatty acids: a prospective, randomized controlled trial. Pediatrics 2001; 108(2):359–371.

29. Innis SM, Adamkin DH, Hall RT, Kahlan SC, Lair C, Lim M, et al. Docosahexaenoic acid and arachadonic acid enhance growth with no adverse effects in preterm infants fed formula. J Pediatr 2002; 140:547–554.

30. Clandinin M, VanAerde J, ANtonson D, Lim M, Stevens D, Merkel K, Harris J, Hansen J. Formulas with docosahexaenoic acid (DHA) and arachadonic acid (ARA) promote better growth and developmental scores in very-low-birth-weight infants (VLBW). Ped Res 2002; 51(4):1092.

31. Fewtrell MS, Morley R, Abbott RA, Singhal A, Isaacs EB, Stephenson T, MacFadyen U, Lucas A. Double-blind, randomized trial of long-chain polyunsaturated fatty acid supplementation in formula fed to preterm infants. Pediatrics 2002; 110(1):73–82.

32. San Jiovanni JP, Parra-Cabrera S, Colditz GA. Meta-analysis of dietary essential fatty acids and long-chain polyunsaturated fatty acids as they relate to visual function in healthy preterm infants. Pediatrics 2000; 105:1292–1298.

33. Klein CJ. Nutrient requirements for preterm infant formulas. J Nutr 2002; 132:1395S–1577S.

34. Helland IB, Smith LS, Saarem K, Saugstad OD, Drevon CA. Maternal supplementation with very-long-chain n-3 fatty acids during pregnancy and lactation augments children's IQ at 4 years of age. Pediatrics 2003; 111(1): e39–e44.

35. Forsyth JS, Willatts P, Agostoni C, Bissenden J, Casaer P, Boehm G. Long-chain polyunsaturated fatty acid supplementation in infant formula and blood pressure in later childhood: follow-up of a randomized controlled trial. BMJ 2003; 326:1–5.

36. Lucas A, Gore SM, Cole TJ, Bamford MF, Dossetor JF, Barr I, Dicarlo L, Cork S, Lucas PJ. Multicenter trial on feeding low-birth-weight infants: effects of diet on early growth. Arch Dis Child 1984; 59:722–730.

37. Schanler RJ, Garza C. Improved mineral balance in very-low-birth-weight infants fed fortified human milk. J Pediatr 1988; 112(3):452–456.

38. Schanler RJ, Hurst NM, Lau C. The use of human milk and breast-feeding in premature infants. Clin Perinatol 1999; 26:379–398.
39. Lucas A. Enteral nutrition. In: Tsang RC, Lucas A, Uauy R, Zlotkin S, eds. Nutritional Needs of the Preterm Infant: Scientific Basis and Practical Guidelines. Baltimore: Williams and Wilkins, 1993:209–223.
40. Furman L, Minich N, Hack M. Correlates of lactation in mothers of very-low-birth-weight infants. Pediatrics 2002; 109(4):e57.
41. Casey PH. Growth status and growth rates of a varied sample of low-birth-weight, preterm infants: a longitudinal cohort from birth to three years of age. J Pediatr 1991; 119:599–605.
42. Abrams SA, Schanler RJ, Tsang RC, Garza C. Bone mineralization in former very-low-birth-weight infants fed either human milk or commercial formula: one-year follow-up observation. J Pediatr 1989; 114:1041–1044.
43. Bhatia J, Bucher C, Bunyapen C. Feeding the premature infant. In: Berdanier CD, ed. Handbook of Nutrition and Food. Boca Raton, FL: CRC Press, 2002:203–218.
44. Bechensteen AG, et al. Erythropoietin, protein, and iron supplementation and the prevention of anaemia of prematurity. Arch Dis Child 1993; 69:19–23.
45. Ohls RK, Harcum J, Schibler KR, Christensen RD. The effect of erythropoietin on the transfusion requirements of preterm infants weighing 750 g or less: a randomized, double-blind, placebo-controlled study. J Pediatr 1997; 131:661–665.
46. Ohl RK, Ehrenkranz RA, Wright LL, Lemons JA, Korones SB, Stoll BJ, Stark AR, Shankaran S, Donovan EF, Close NC, Das A. Effects of erythropoietin therapy on transfusion requirements of preterm infants below 1250 grams birth weight: a multicenter, randomized, controlled trial. Pediatrics 2001; 108(4):934–942.

9

Breast-Feeding the Term Infant

Krystal Revai and David K. Rassin
The University of Texas Medical Branch, Galveston, Texas, U.S.A.

I. INTRODUCTION

It may seem unnecessary to present another essay extolling the virtues of breast-feeding for the healthy term infant. But as recently as 1993, the eminent pediatric nutritionist Sam Fomon stated that "Human milk is a superb food for the human infant, *but it is not ideal*" (1). Despite such doubts, the evidence has continued to mount that human milk *is* the ideal food for the human infant, resulting in an extremely strong endorsement of breast-feeding by the American Academy of Pediatrics (2).

There is little doubt that in the developing world, breast-feeding results in healthier infants by protecting them from exposure to poor-quality water and inadequate formula availability due to cost. Proving similar benefits in the industrialized world has been more difficult, but the cumulative total of the evidence is convincing and reflects an interesting progression in the appreciation of those benefits. This progression has reflected, first, mortality and then morbidity, progressing to psychological, social, and, most recently, improved cognitive outcomes.

The recommendations of various professional groups are discussed next, followed by the evolution of outcomes related to infant feeding, a discussion of who breast-feeds and why, possible mechanisms that may explain the relationship of outcomes to the form of infant feeding, a description of mothers who breast-feed, and, finally, factors that may interfere in a mother's ability to successfully breast-feed.

II. RECOMMENDATIONS FOR INFANT FEEDING

A variety of national and international organizations have recommended that breast-feeding be the preferred form of feeding for all healthy term infants (2–5). The Surgeon General of the United States has issued two reports defining specific goals for breast-feeding (75% of mothers at hospital discharge and 25% at 6 months of age) (6,7). Similar numbers have been proposed as part of the health goals for the United States, first in Healthy People 2000 (8) and then in the succeeding report, Healthy People 2010 (9).

The most recent recommendations regarding breast-feeding in the United States have gone beyond the usual statement that it is the preferred form of feeding to include a list of tasks for the pediatrician (2). The basic recommendation is that human milk is the preferred form of feeding for *all* infants, that nursing should begin as soon as possible, and that nursing should continue for 12 months (exclusively for 6). In addition, it is recommended that pediatricians strongly promote breast-feeding and educate themselves about the physiology and management of lactation. Promotion is to include supporting hospital policies that enable lactation, educating obstetricians about the importance of breast-feeding, and improving societal acceptance and encouragement of breast-feeding.

In addition to the recommendation sponsored by the American Academy of Pediatrics (2), the Healthy People 2010 (9) report has set national health care goals for the United States that address breast-feeding. These goals are that 75% of women will breast-feed during the early postpartum period, 50% at 6 months, and 25% at a year. These numbers are considerably higher than current breast-feeding rates (discussed later) and, in particular, are higher than the rates in the indigent or most vulnerable population.

III. EVOLUTION OF OUTCOMES RELATED TO INFANT FEEDING

As early as 1741 there was documentation of the advantage of human-milk-feeding over other feeds for infants. In a comparison of wet nursing versus "dry nursing" or pap (wheat and water) in a population of foundlings, it was noted that the mortality rate was 19% in the former and 53% in the latter group (10). In a more recent investigation, published in 1951, it was noted that in a United States urban population, there was an advantage of breast-feeding over bottle-feeding with respect to both morbidity and mortality (11).

Probably one of the more important investigations in this area was that of Cunningham (12,13), carried out in a private hospital in New York State in the 1970s. He documented increased morbidity, as measured by hospital admissions, in formula-fed as opposed to breast-fed infants. The results of this study were published at a time when the benefits of breast-feeding were beginning to be appreciated more broadly in response to especially low rates of breast-feeding in the United States.

The Cunningham (12,13) studies were followed by numerous investigations into specific diseases related to infections that might be impacted by breast-feeding. These include otitis media (14), gastroenteritis (15), respiratory infections (16), necrotizing enterocolitis (17), and neonatal sepsis (18). In addition, there are hints that breast-feeding may be somewhat protective with respect to atopic disease and asthma (19). The role of human milk in these diseases has been extensively reviewed (20).

In addition to the protective effect of breast-feeding in diseases related directly to infection and immune function, there have been reports that there is a reduced incidence of other disease and health-related processes in breast-fed infants. These processes include diabetes (21), obesity (22), sudden infant death syndrome (23), and increased cholesterol and ischemic heart disease (24). While the mechanisms by which breast-feeding may convey such benefits to the infant are unclear, the preponderance of evidence is that benefits do exist with respect to health outcomes. Indeed, there also may be physiologic benefits to the mother (in addition to economic—formula is expensive— and psychological—better mother–infant bonding) reflected in a lower rate of breast cancer in women who have lactated (25).

The most interesting outcome of interest in recent years has been the increased benefit to cognitive outcome that appears to be conveyed by human milk. A study by Rodgers in 1978 (26) that looked at cognitive performance in children and found advantages to breast-feeding stimulated numerous investigations in this area. While the confounding variables are complex, especially the fact that well-educated higher-social class mothers are more likely to breast-feed, the consistency of the results of these many studies would suggest that the positive effects of breast-feeding on cognition are real.

Of the various studies that we have critically reviewed (27), three have fulfilled fairly vigorous criteria (28–30) regarding the nature of the experimental design and the cognitive tests used. All three of these studies found positive effects of breast-feeding on cognition, although the strength of the effect varied and the methodology of one such study (28) raised the question of whether or not the effect was due to parenting rather than actual human milk components. An additional study that did not satisfy our criteria did tend to support this latter hypothesis (31). In this study, controlling for parenting appeared to abolish the breast-feeding effect in a middle-class Caucasian population (31). It may be that the advantages of breast-feeding are most apparent in populations that are at risk due to social stresses or poor public health conditions.

This latter consideration may be supported by the finding that human milk appears to offer a strong cognitive advantage to preterm infants (32,33). In this series of longitudinal investigations, a relatively short exposure to human milk appears to confer a long-term, fairly large advantage (8 plus I.Q. points).

Lastly, regarding the long-term effects of breast-feeding on cognition, it is of interest to note that in an adult (mean age 27.2 years) Danish sample of men, this form of feeding appeared to have conferred a significant advantage (34).

Thus, the overall benefits of breast-feeding to the term infant seem both profound and long-lasting. Obviously, some infants will not be able to successfully breast-feed. But this very small group should not be used as an excuse for not providing the vast majority of infants with the optimal form of feeding.

IV. MECHANISMS THAT TRANSLATE TO OUTCOMES

Presumably most of the differences in mortality observed between breast-fed and formula-fed infants reflect issues such as clean water availability and cost of adequate amounts of formula. These issues continue to be a major cause of infant mortality in the developing world today. Less obvious are the mechanisms by which breast-feeding results in improved health and cognitive outcomes. While various mechanisms have been proposed to account for these differences, there is no definitive explanation to date. The lack of a definitive mechanism probably reflects the numerous differences between human milk composition and infant formulas, even when the latter have been "adapted" by various additions. For example, the proteins in formulas are bovine or soy derived and differ in their amino acid composition from their human-derived counterparts. The lipids (which are usually of vegetable origin and so do not contain docosahexaenoic or arachidonic acids, unless they are added separately) exist in different triglyceride structures in human milk than in formulas. These differences reflect the fact that human milk is a wonderfully complex mixture that contains nutrients, cells, structures (such as micelles), and physical compartments that may protect immunologic constituents. In addition, mothers who breast-feed appear to have a different attitude toward their infants than do mothers who formula-feed (35,36). Those who breast-feed appear to place their infants at a higher priority than themselves, while those who formula-feed do the opposite, placing themselves first (35,36).

The appreciation of the role of human milk components in protecting the infant against infection was probably first stimulated by Gyorgy (37,38) in the 1960s and then given an additional impetus by the studies of Goldman (39,40). In the former investigations, the potential for human milk to antagonize infectious agents was documented; in the latter studies, actual cells from the immune system were identified in human milk. Since these investigations there has been an explosion of information regarding the anti-infective agents contained in human milk—these include proteins, lipids, carbohydrates, and cells. This catalogue of agents has been extensively reviewed (20). In addition, human milk may have more subtle immunologic effects on the infant, such as enhancing the response to vaccinations, that confer lifelong protection against infection (41).

Several questions still remain regarding how these agents might confer their benefits on the infant. For example, if all the immunologically protective proteins are subtracted from the total milk proteins, there might be insufficient nutritional protein to support the growth of the infant. Another question relates to how the proteins are protected after ingestion during their passage through the gut such that they may confer their protective effects. With respect to the former, it is clear that breast-fed infants grow well, so either human proteins are extremely efficient growth promoters or the protective proteins are also used for nutritional support.

With respect to the latter question, protection during passage through the gut, it would appear that a complex packaging of protective components exists in human milk. For example, the anti-inflammatory cytokine IL-10 appears to bind to a structure in human milk and is then released by the action of bile salts (42). Thus, the infant may ingest a packaged immunoprotective agent that is released by bile salts at the place in the gut appropriate for its action or absorption.

The protection of the infant against diseases such as obesity and diabetes has less clear mechanisms. It has been suggested that a lack of cholesterol in infant formulas may stimulate excessive synthesis in these infants later in life (43) and that bovine proteins may contribute to the induction of diabetes in formula-fed infants (44,45). But these relationships remain unproved.

The area that has garnered the most attention in recent years is the relationship between human milk constituents and cognition. We have suggested that the difference in amino acid composition between formulas and human milk may contribute to this effect (46). The amino acid milieu in which the term infant develops reflects the type of protein fed (47), and such differentiation is apparent by 48–72 hours of life (48). Amino acids may influence brain development via their roles as neurotransmitters and neurotransmitter precursors; this influence may have a large impact because the altered amino acid environment persists as long as the differing formulas are fed (47).

Others have supported the notion that the long-chain polyunsaturated fatty acids (LCPUFAs)—arachidonic acid and docosahexaenoic acid—are responsible for these differences in cognition (49–51). The LCPUFAs are components of brain cell membranes and may exert effects by altering the actual structure of these cells. However, their effects usually seem to be transient. All these proposed mechanisms reflect differences in human milk and formula composition, and despite efforts by those who manufacture formulas, these differences cannot be completely eradicated. Changing ratios of proteins derived from cows or adding algal-derived fatty acids (not necessarily bonded to triglycerides in the same way as they are in human milk) does not produce a product identical to human milk. Even attempts to improve immune function by adding nucleotides are only a partial improvement, for the manufacturers do not mimic the actual nucleic acids in human milk.

The ability to mimic human milk composition is hampered by the complex nature of this ideal food for the infant. A true copy probably won't be available until genetic engineering reaches a stage at which cows can be persuaded to produce human milk.

V. WHO BREAST-FEEDS?

Although tainted by obvious bias (it is ironic that the best data on breast-feeding incidence come from a formula-manufacturing company), Ross Laboratories has maintained the best national record of breast-feeding rates in the United States for the past few decades. However, we have criticized their data as underestimating rates in the indigent population (52). During this time, breast-feeding rates, both exclusive and partial, have risen and fallen in parallel. The current trends show a 69.5% exclusive breast-feeding rate in the hospital and 32.5% at 6 months. These rates surpass the highs of 61.9% and 27.1% for exclusive and partial breastfeeding, respectively, in the early 1980s (53).

The disparities in breast-feeding rates parallel other disparities in health care related to race and economic status that plague the United States today. In contradistinction to the perception that breast-feeding is for the poor or uneducated, it is educated women from the higher socioeconomic classes who breast-feed. The Pediatric Nutrition Surveillance Survey (PedNSS) tracks pediatric nutrition data collected from a number of programs, including: Women, Infants and Children (WIC); Early Periodic Screening, Diagnosis and Treatment (EPSDT); Title V of Maternal and Child Health (MCH); and Head Start. This surveillance of mostly low-income children documented an increase in the percentage of women breast-feeding. The prevalence of breast-feeding children increased from 35% in 1989 to 46% in 1997. Of these children in 1997, 46.2% of infants 6–8 months were ever breast-fed, and 20% were exclusively breast-fed until 6 months of age. Unfortunately, these data do not tell us how long the infants were breast-fed and when the introduction of formula began (54).

The group that has shown the largest gain in rate was that composed of teenage black women in the west south central part of the United States. These women were mostly unemployed, with no more than a high school education. The Ross and CDC studies are consistent in their findings that black women have the lowest breast-feeding rates and that this group had the largest percentage increase in breast-feeding rate both in the hospital and at 6 months of age (53,54).

Breast-feeding support needs to come from different levels within the health care community. From the perspective of the community, a culture of breast-feeding acceptance as the normative way of nourishing infants needs to be adopted. At the systems level, health care agencies need to back up noble goals with structural support. On the institutional level, hospitals, specifically newborn nurseries, should adopt baby-friendly and baby-centered care. Finally, at the patient level, health care practitioners treating women and children need to have basic skills with regard to management of breast-feeding.

VI. BREAST-FEEDING PROBLEMS AND TECHNIQUES

The keys to successful breast-feeding lie in education of both parents and health care providers. Mothers need to be encouraged and educated from the first prenatal visit to breast-feed their infants. WHO and UNICEF developed the Baby-Friendly Hospital Initiative in 1992 in an effort to increase breast-feeding rates around the world. The keys to this initiative lie in the "Ten Steps to Successful Breastfeeding" outlined in the initiative, which have become the basis for the Baby-Friendly Hospital Initiative—USA, The Texas Ten Steps Hospital Program, and others. The ten steps are as follows:

1. Have a written breast-feeding policy that is regularly communicated to all health care staff.
2. Train all staff in skills necessary to implement this policy.
3. Inform all pregnant women about the benefits and management of breast-feeding.
4. Help mothers initiate breast-feeding within 30–60 minutes of birth.
5. Show mothers how to breast-feed and how to sustain lactation, even if they should be separated from their infants.
6. Make sure babies are not fed anything other than breast milk unless medically indicated.

7. Practice rooming-in, which allows mothers and infants to remain together 24 hours a day.
8. Encourage breast-feeding on demand.
9. Give no artificial pacifiers to breast-feeding infants.
10. Establish breast-feeding support groups and refer mothers to them.

The list of baby-friendly hospitals in the United States and around the world continues to grow as more and more hospitals make the commitment to support breast-feeding women and infants (2,55,56).

Neonatal blood glucose monitoring is becoming more and more common in today's nurseries. This increase in glucose monitoring is largely due to the increasing prevalence of insulin resistance and frank gestational diabetes in the pregnant population (57). This increased incidence translates into more infants of diabetic mothers and more large-for-gestational-age babies. These groups of children routinely have glucose monitoring for some time after birth. The management of transient hypoglycemia in the newborn period has been to feed infants formula out of a bottle. Most of these children, however, can be treated successfully with breast-feeding. The initial step in preventing hypoglycemia in the newborn is to have the child nurse as soon as possible after birth, preferably in the first 30–60 minutes. Skin-to-skin contact with the mother helps the baby maintain body temperature while stimulating milk production. After the initial feed, the baby should be nursed regularly, either every 2–3 hours or when it begins to show early signs of hunger (crying is often a *late* sign of hunger). If the blood glucose does not improve or the baby becomes symptomatic, then an intravenous infusion of glucose is indicated, either a bolus of 2 cc/kg of D10W or a continuous infusion of a glucose-containing solution. As always, babies who continue to have hypoglycemia in the absence of any obvious risk factor should be assessed for other etiologies, such as sepsis, Beckwith–Wiedemann syndrome, inborn errors of metabolism, or midline CNS defects (58).

Many physicians, especially residents, take comfort in seeing the amount of formula consumed by the infant. They hear from mothers that they "have no milk" and only see a few drops of colostrum dripping from the mother's nipples and worry that this small amount will not be sufficient to adequately nourish the new baby. Short of weighing the infant before and after a feed, there is no easy way to quantify the amount of colostrum or milk that the infant ingests while nursing at the breast. We do, however, have some subjective and objective findings that can help.

The most important step in establishing successful lactation is their latch onto the mother. Babies need to be latched on properly in order to achieve good milk transfer at the breast. An inappropriate latch will lead to nipple irritation and pain. Babies that latch on well have lips that are flanged out asymmetrically around the areola. The mother should feel very little pain as the baby begins to suckle the breast (although she may feel uterine contractions during the first few days). Babies will frequently start out with a rapid, short burst of sucking followed by long, slow sucks interrupted by audible swallowing. Satisfied babies will frequently fall off the breast when finished and assume a relaxed, open-handed position. Mothers should feel milk transfer at the breast, and those who have some breast fullness should feel decreased fullness after a feed.

Objectively assess the hydration status of the baby to determine whether or not enough milk is being consumed. This assessment is done by counting wet diapers. A newborn baby should have one wet diaper for every 24 hours of age until the mother's milk is established, i.e., one in the first 24 hours, two in the second 24 hours, etc. During this time, urate crystals, frequently manifested as an orange/red discoloration in the diaper, can be seen. This finding is not a sign of dehydration in the initial newborn period but should no longer be observed after the mother's milk is established.

Jaundice is a common newborn problem. For breast-feeding babies, jaundice can be separated into two entities: breast-feeding jaundice and breast-milk jaundice. *Breast-feeding jaundice*, called by some *lack of breast-feeding jaundice* or *early jaundice*, is physiologic jaundice in the breast-fed baby. This situation may occasionally be worsened by inefficient breast-feeding and milk transfer. Babies with breast-feeding jaundice will usually have peak bilirubin concentrations between days 2 and 5 and often have infrequent stools and infrequent, inefficient feeds. This situation will often occur in primipara mothers who are inexperienced at breast-feeding a baby and whose milk does not become established for several days. The American Academy of Pediatrics (AAP) does not recommend cessation of breast-feeding or the introduction of dextrose water for these infants. The treatment of choice for infants with early jaundice is to assess breast-feeding timing and technique. Increasing the number of feeds and improving technique to maximize milk transfer at the breast will aid in meconium passage and decrease bilirubin concentration (59). Phototherapy should be initiated in accordance with AAP guidelines (59).

Breast milk jaundice, also referred to as *late jaundice*, is a process unique to breast-feeding babies. There are a few theories as to the pathophysiology behind the development of breast milk jaundice but no definite answers. The prevailing thought is that 5β-pregnane-$3\alpha,20\alpha$-diol inhibits the hepatic enzyme glucuronyl transferase and prevents bilirubin conjugation. Bilirubin will peak in the first to second week of life and rise to concentrations of 20 mg/dL or more. At lower concentrations, mothers can continue to breast-feed. If bilirubin concentrations approach 20 mg/dL, mothers should cease breast-feeding for 12–48 hours. Babies are supplemented during this time, and mothers should use an effective breast pump to express milk so as to maintain supply and prevent engorgement and mastitis. Bilirubin should drop within 12 hours and breast-feeding can be restarted. Bilirubin concentrations may increase slightly once breast milk is reintroduced; however, it usually will not reach a dangerous concentration. Bilirubin clearance should be documented. Babies may be clinically jaundiced for up to 3 months (60). If there are any lingering doubts in the clinician's mind, other causes or jaundice such as Crigler–Najjar syndrome, biliary atresia, or glucose-6 phosphate dehydrogenase deficiency should be ruled out.

Breast milk is the ideal nutrition for infants. The discussion presented in this chapter has focused on the long- and short-term advantages of breast milk for the child. An equally lengthy discussion could be initiated about advantages for the breast-feeding mother. Very few contraindications for breast-feeding exist. Why is it then that neither the lay nor health care communities rally around low breast-feeding rates in the same way that we have rallied around car seats, seat belt usage, or the back-to-sleep campaigns?

In a nationwide survey of graduates from pediatric residency program, graduates as recently as 1997 felt that they received insufficient training in breast-feeding management (61). A survey of pediatricians found that they do recommend breast-feeding to their patients but that only a slight majority make specific recommendations about the duration of exclusive breast-feeding, when to initiate breast-feeding, or the importance of rooming-in in the hospital. A small but significant majority of pediatricians felt that formula-feeding and breast-feeding were equally acceptable forms of infant feeding. Over 10% of pediatricians went as far as to suggest that mothers supplement with formula. Less than half of the pediatricians surveyed had attended a continuing medical education conference on breast-feeding (62). Pediatricians need to be aware of the techniques needed to support successful breast-feeding for mothers will usually turn to them for advice rather than to their obstetricians.

Physicians are often unaware of the subtle clues that can lead mothers to believe that there is no difference between breast milk and formula. Physician's will often acknowledge and accept a new mother's plan to combine breast- and bottle-feeding or to supplement with formula without any discussion about why she is supplementing or how this may impact the infant or her milk supply. Formula company paraphernalia that litters physician's offices, from gift bags to pens to calendars to samples left out on display, announce to families that it is OK to feed this to your baby. Finally, child health care providers routinely ask questions regarding development so that any developmental delays can be addressed early. Yet few, if any, routinely screen for problems that may lead to breast-feeding failure.

VII. CONCLUSION

Human milk is a species-specific infant nutrition. The availability of safe, nutritionally sound formula is a luxury in the United States and many industrialized countries with government-sponsored nutritional programs and a clean water supply. It is wonderful to have replacement nutrition for the relatively few infants who need formula secondary to a maternal or infant indication. However, in the United States and some other industrialized countries this replacement has become the standard. Given the overwhelming benefits of human milk, it is clear that health care professionals have an obligation to advocate and support breast-feeding for as many infants as possible.

REFERENCES

1. Fomon SJ. Nutrition of Normal Infants. St. Louis: Mosby, 1993; 1.
2. American Academy of Pediatrics, Workgroup on Breast-feeding. Breast-feeding and the use of human milk. Pediatr 1997; 100:1035–1039.
3. American College of Obstetricians and Gynecologists. Committee Statement: Breast-Feeding. Washington, DC: ACOG, 1985.
4. ESPGAN Committee on Nutrition. Guidelines on infant nutrition. I. Recommendations for the composition of an adapted formula. Acta Paediatr Scand 1977; 262(suppl):1–20.
5. Ambulatory Pediatric Association. The World Health Organization code of marketing of breastmilk substitutes. Pediatr 1981; 68:432–434.
6. Report of the Surgeon General's Workshop on Breast-Feeding and Human Lactation. Washington, DC: U.S. Department of Health and Human Services, Public Health Service, 1984.
7. Second Follow-up Report: The Surgeon General's Workshop on Breastfeeding and Human Lactation. Washington, DC: National Center for Education in Maternal and Child Care, 1991.
8. Healthy People 2000: National Health Promotion and Disease Prevention Objectives. Washington, DC: U.S. Department of Health and Human Services, Public Health Service, 1990:379–380.
9. Healthy People 2010: With Understanding and Improving Health and Objectives for Improving Health. 2 Vols. Washington, DC: Department of Health and Human Services, Government Printing Office, 2000, Section 16-46.
10. Fildes VA. Breasts, Bottles and Babies: A History of Infant Feeding. Edinburgh: Edinburgh University Press, 1986:279.
11. Robinson M. Infant morbidity and mortality: a study of 3266 infants. Lancet 1951; 1:788–794.
12. Cunningham AS. Morbidity in breast-fed and artificially fed infants. J Pediatr 1977; 90:726–729.

13. Cunningham AS. Morbidity in breast-fed and artificially fed infants. II. J Pediatr 1979; 95:685–689.
14. Saarinen UM. Prolonged breast-feeding as prophylaxis for recurrent otitis media. Acta Paediatr Scand 1982; 71:567–571.
15. Duffy LC, Byers TE, Riepenhoff-Taltz M, et al. The effects of infant feeding on rotavirus-induced gastroenteritis: a prospective study. Am J Public Health 1986; 76:259–263.
16. Cushing AH, Samet JM, Lambert WE, Skipper BJ, Hunt WC, Young SA, McLaren LC. Breast-feeding reduces the risk of respiratory illness in infants. Am J Epidemiol 1998; 147:863–870.
17. Pitt J. Necrotizing enterocolitis: a model for infection–immunity interaction. In: Ogra PL, ed. Neonatal Infections: Nutritional and Immunologic Interactions. Orlando, FL: Grune and Stratton, 1984:173–184.
18. Fallot ME, Boyd JL, Oski FA. Breast-feeding reduces incidence of hospital admissions for infection in infants. Pediatrics 1980; 65:1121–1124.
19. Kramer MS. Does breast-feeding help protect against atopic disease? Biology, methodology, and a golden jubilee of controversy. J Pediatr 1988; 112:181–190.
20. Rassin DK, Garofalo RP, Ogra PL. Human milk. In: Remington JS, Klein JO, eds. Infectious Diseases of the Fetus and Newborn Infant. 5th ed. Philadelphia: Saunders, 2000:169–203.
21. Pettitt DJ, Forman MR, Hanson RL, Knowler WC, Bennett PH. Breast-feeding and incidence of non-insulin-dependent diabetes mellitus in Pima Indians. Lancet 1997; 350:166–168.
22. Kramer MS. Do breast-feeding and delayed introduction of solid foods protect against subsequent obesity? J Pediatr 1981; 98:883–887.
23. Gunther M. The neonate's immunity gap, breast-feeding and cot death. Lancet 1975; 1:441.
24. Fall CHD, Barker DJP, Osmond C, Winter PD, Clark PMS, Hales CN. Relation of infant feeding to adult serum cholesterol concentration and death from ischaemic heart disease. Brit Med J 1992; 304:801–805.
25. Katsouyani K, Lipworth L, Trichopoulou A, Samoli E, Stuver S, Trichopoulous D. A case-control study of lactation and cancer of the breast. Br J Cancer 1996; 73:814–818.
26. Rodgers B. Feeding in infancy and later ability and attainment: a longitudinal study. Dev Med Child Neurol 1978; 20:421–426.
27. Rassin DK, Smith KE. Nutritional approaches to improve cognitive development during infancy: antioxidant compounds. Acta Paediatr 2003; 442(suppl):34–41.
28. Morrow-Tlucak M, Hande RH, Ernhart CB. Breastfeeding and cognitive development in the first 2 years of life. Soc Sci Med 1988; 26:635–639.
29. Rogan WJ, Gladen BC. Breast-feeding and cognitive development. Early Hum Dev 1993; 31:181–193.
30. Horwood LJ, Fergusson DM. Breast-feeding and later cognitive and academic outcomes. Pediatrics 1998; 101:e9.

31. Jacobson SW, Chiodo LM, Jacobson JL. Breast-feeding effects on intelligence quotient in 4- and 11-year-old children. Pediatrics 1999; 103:e71.
32. Lucas A, Morley R, Cole TJ, Gore SM. A randomized multicenter study of human milk versus formula and later development in preterm infants. Arch Dis Child 1994; 70:F141–F146.
33. Lucas A, Morely R, Cole TJ, Lister G, Leeson-Payne C. Breast milk and subsequent intelligence quotient in children born preterm. Lancet 1992; 339:261–264.
34. Mortensen EL, Michaelsen KF, Sanders SA, Reinisch JM. The association between duration of breast-feeding and adult intelligence. JAMA 2002; 287:2365–2371.
35. Baranowski T, Rassin DK, Richardson CJ, Brown JP, Bee DE. Attitudes toward breast-feeding. J Dev Behav Pediatr 1986; 7:367–372.
36. Baranowski T, Rassin DK, Richardson CJ, Bee DE, Palmer J. Expectancies of infant-feeding methods among mothers in three ethnic groups. Psychol Health 1990; 5:59–75.
37. Gyorgy P. A hitherto-unrecognized biochemical difference between human milk and cow's milk. Pediatrics 1953; 11:98–108.
38. Gyorgy P, Dhanamitta S, Steers E. Protective effects of human milk in experimental *Staphylococcus* infection. Science 1962; 137:338–340.
39. Smith CW, Goldman AS. The cells of human colostrum. I. In vitro studies of morphology and functions. Pediatr Res 1968; 2:103–109.
40. Smith CW, Goldman AS. Interactions of lymphocytes and macrophages from human colostrums: characteristics of the interacting lymphocyte. Res J Reticuloendothelial Soc 1970; 8:91–104.
41. Pickering L, Granoff DM, Erickson JR, et al. Modulation of the immune system by human milk and infant formula containing nucleotides. Pediatrics 1998; 101:242–249.
42. Garofalo R, Chheda S, Mei F, Palkowetz KH, Rudloff HE, Schmalstieg FC, Rassin DK, Goldman AS. Interleukin-10 in human milk. Pediatr Res 1995; 37:444–449.
43. Lourdes M, Cruz A, Wong WW, Mimouni F, Hachey DL, Setchell KDR, Klein PD, Tsang RC. Effects of infant nutrition on cholesterol synthesis. Pediatr Res 1994; 35:35–140.
44. Saukkonen T, Savilahti E, Madácsy L, Arató A, Körner A, Barkai L, Sarnesto A, Åkerblom HK. Increased frequency of IgM antibodies to cow's milk proteins in Hungarian children with newly diagnosed insulin-dependent diabetes mellitus. Eur J Pediatr 1996; 155:885–889.
45. Saukkonen T, Virtanen SM, Karppinen M, Reijonen H, Ilonen J, Räsänen L, Åkerblom HK, Savilahti E. Childhood Diabetes in Finland Study Group: significance of cow's milk protein antibodies as risk factor for childhood IDDM: interactions with dietary cow's milk intake and HLA-DQB1 genotype. Diabetologia 1998; 41:72–78.
46. Rassin DK. Essential and nonessential amino acids in neonatal nutrition. In: Räihä NCR, ed. Protein Metabolism During Infancy. New York: Raven Press, 1994:183–192.

47. Järvenpää A-L, Räihä NCR, Rassin DK, et al. Milk protein quantity and quality in the term infant. II. Effects on acidic and neutral amino acids. Pediatrics 1982; 70:221–230.

48. Cho F, Bhatia J, Rassin DK. Amino acid responses to dietary intake in the first 72 hours of life. Nutrition 1990; 6:449–455.

49. Scott DT, Janowsky JS, Robin E, Carroll MS, Taylor JA, Auestad N, Montalto MB. Formula supplementation with long-chain polyunsaturated fatty acids: are there developmental benefits? Pediatrics 1998; 102:1–3.

50. Birch EE, Garfield S, Hoffman DR, Uauy R, Birch DG. A randomized controlled trial of early dietary supply of long-chain polyunsaturated fatty acids and mental development in term infants. Develop Med Child Neuro 2000; 42:174–181.

51. Auestad N, Halter R, Hall RT, Blatter M, Bogle ML, Burks W, Erickson JR, Fitzgerald KM, Dobson V, Innis SM, Singer LT, Montalto MB, Jacobs JR, Qiu W, Bornstein MH. Growth and development in term infants fed long-chain polyunsaturated fatty acids: a double-masked, randomized, parallel, prospective, multivariate study. Pediatrics 2001; 108(2):372–381.

52. Rassin DK, Richardson CJ, Baranowski T, Nader PR, Guenther N, Bee DE, Brown JP. The incidence of breast-feeding in a lower-socioeconomic group of mothers in the United States: ethnic patterns. Pediatrics 1984; 73:132–137.

53. Ryan AS, Wenjun Z, Acosta A. Breast-feeding continues to increase into the new millennium. Pediatrics 2002; 110:1103–1109.

54. Centers for Disease Control and Prevention, US Department of Health and Human Services. Pediatric Nutrition Surveillance 1997. Full Report.

55. http://www.tdh.state.tx.us/lactate

56. http://www.cdc.gov/breastfeeding/compend-babyfriendlywho.htm

57. Kramer MS, Morin I, Yang H, Platt RW, Usher R, McNamara H, Joseph KS, Wen SW. Why are babies getting bigger? Temporal trends in fetal growth and its determinants. J Pediatr 2002; 141:538–542.

58. Academy of Breastfeeding Medicine Clinical Protocol Number 1—Guidelines for Glucose Monitoring and Treatment of Hypoglycemia in Term Breastfed Neonates. http://www.bfmed.org

59. Provisional Committee for Quality Improvement and Subcommittee on Hyperbilirubinemia. American Academy of Pediatrics Practice parameter: management of hyperbilirubinemia in the healthy term newborn. Pediatrics 1994; 94:558–565. (Published erratum appears in Pediatrics 95:458-61, 1995.)

60. Lawrence RA. Breastfeeding: A Guide for the Medical Profession. 5th ed. St. Louis: Mosby, 1998.

61. Walton DM, Edwards MC. A nationwide survey of pediatric residency training in newborn medicine: preparation for primary care practice. Pediatrics 2002; 110:1081–1087.

62. Schanler RJ, O'Conner KG, Lawrence RA. Pediatricians' practices and attitudes regarding breast-feeding promotion. Pediatrics 1999; 103:e35.

10
Introducing Solid Foods to Infants

Suzanne Domel Baxter
University of South Carolina, Columbia, South Carolina, U.S.A.

I. INTRODUCTION

There is a considerable body of literature available regarding how to introduce solid foods to infants. The purpose of this chapter is to review some of this information and identify consistencies as well as inconsistencies among various sources. The reader is asked to keep three caveats in mind when reading this chapter. First, this chapter regards introducing solid foods to normal, healthy infants. Second, this chapter regards introducing solid foods to infants in developed or industrialized countries, except for a section which regards infants in developing countries ("Complementary Feedings of Infants in Developing Countries" Section). Third, in many ways, introducing solid foods to infants is more of an art than a science. In other words, only some of the guidelines are explained or justified by scientific evidence.

II. GUIDELINES FOR INTRODUCING SOLID FOODS

A. Definition and Goal of Weaning

According to Webster's II *New College Dictionary* (1), wean is defined as "1. to withhold mother's milk from the young of a mammal and substitute other nourishment; 2. to cause to give up an interest or habit." The use of the term weaning in the context of infant feeding varies. Some use weaning to refer to weaning an infant from the breast or bottle to a cup (2–8), while others use the term to refer to the introduction of solid foods into an infant's diet (9,10). The process of introducing foods other than breast milk or formula into an infant's diet has been referred to as introducing solids (4,11), feeding solid

217

foods (2), supplemental feeding (6), and starting solids (12). Fomon uses the term beikost to refer to foods other than breast milk or formula that are fed to infants (13). Whatever term is used, the goal of weaning is to transition the infant from a liquid diet of breast milk or formula to a solid diet that includes a variety of foods and textures, meets the infant's nutrient needs, and encourages the development of feeding skills (9).

B. Periods of Infant Feeding

During the first year of life, the dietary intake of infants changes considerably as they transition from a totally liquid diet of breast milk or formula to a diet that includes a variety of solid and liquid foods. This transition can be described as occurring in three overlapping periods (14). Progression through the periods should be determined by an individual infant's developmental readiness and maturation of the intestinal tract and kidneys.

The first period is the nursing period. During this period, breast milk or formula is the only source of nutrients (14). Although the infant's digestive and mucosal barrier functions are maturing, the kidneys lack the maturity to handle large osmolar loads of protein and electrolytes. According to the American Academy of Pediatrics (AAP), the nursing period (i.e., when infants consume breast milk or formula exclusively) should last 4–6 months (14).

The second period is the transitional period. During this period, foods that are specially prepared (i.e., pureed, strained, mashed) are introduced to supplement breast milk or formula (14). By 4–5 months of age, the extrusion, or tongue thrust, reflex of early infancy has disappeared; until this is gone, it is difficult to give solid foods by spoon. At the beginning of this period, infants can sit with help; by the end of this period they can sit alone. During this period, infants develop the abilities and coordination necessary for recognizing a spoon, for chewing, and for swallowing solid foods, and they can appreciate the variety of colors and tastes provided by foods. By 5–6 months of age, infants can open their mouths and lean forward to indicate a desire for food; likewise, they can lean back and turn away to indicate disinterest or satiety. The ability to digest and absorb protein, carbohydrate, and fat is virtually mature. In most infants, renal concentrating ability allows for the excretion of osmolar loads without excessive water loss. At 4–6 months of age, recommendations for introducing solid foods are based on concepts of the infant's developmental processes along with social, cultural, economic, and psychological considerations. As solid foods are added, consumption of breast milk or formula decreases proportionally (14).

The third period is the modified adult period. During this period, most nutrients come from table foods (14). The infant's physiologic mechanisms have matured to near-adult proficiency when this period begins. The table foods that infants consume during this period require only minimal alteration, such as being cut into small pieces. Food preferences and taste ability are becoming established. The modified adult period generally begins after 10 months of age (14).

As weaning occurs during the first year of life, feeding is transitional in at least three different senses between the type of feeding characteristic of infants and the type of feeding (or eating) characteristic of adults (15). These three transitions are linked loosely in time. First, the infant changes from feeding on liquids (breast milk or formula) to feeding on the solid foods that progressively approximate an adult diet. Second, the infant's feeding behavior changes from sucking to chewing and biting. This is not simply due to changes in the diet from liquids to solid foods, because liquids are consumed by older children and adults as well, although not usually with the sucking behavior characteristic of infants. Third, the obligatory interaction between the infant and mother or caregiver that is characteristic in feeding infants is gradually replaced by independent feeding (15).

Feeding behavior during the weaning period is important theoretically and practically (15). Theoretically, the weaning period is the earliest period during which the mother or caregiver can influence the kind of feeding behavior that continues into adulthood. Insight into the weaning period is of practical importance because infants commonly develop feeding problems during the weaning period (15).

C. Recommendations Regarding When to Introduce Solid Foods

During the 20th century, the recommended age for introducing solid foods to infants fluctuated widely (16). Before 1920, solid foods were seldom recommended until 1 year of age (12,17). Between 1920 and 1950, the trend was for earlier and earlier introduction of solid foods (16); some even advocated feeding solid foods within the first few days of life (17). In the 1950s and 1960s, solid foods were commonly fed during the first and second months of life. But in the 1970s and 1980s, there was a trend toward a somewhat later introduction of solid foods (18). For example, in 1983, 52% of formula-fed infants were fed solid foods between 1 and 2 months of age and 67% were fed solid foods between 2 and 3 months of age; in 1988, the corresponding values were 36% and 53% (18). Although the percentages were lower in 1988 than in 1983, many infants were fed solid foods during the first 2 months of life. For additional information regarding the history of infant feeding and trends in infant feeding since 1950, refer to Fomon's book (19).

A review of information regarding weaning infants reveals several consistencies as well as inconsistencies. For example, although most sources indicate that solid foods are expected to supplement or complement breast milk or formula, instead of replace it (11,12,14,17,20–26), there are slight inconsistencies regarding the age range for when solid foods should be introduced (14). The AAP (5,14) and many others (2,4,6,9–11,20,24,27–32) recommend delaying the introduction of solid foods until 4–6 months of age; some sources cite the AAP recommendation (12,26). Other sources recommend introducing solid foods at 4 months of age (33,34), although the preference is to wait until 5 or 6 months of age (25) and introducing solid foods at 5–7 months of age (23).

Further review of information for weaning infants reveals that the rationale for when solid foods should be introduced varies somewhat, based on the source. Nutrient needs become greater than breast milk or formula can provide as the infant reaches 4–6 months of age, and supplemental foods become necessary for adequate satiety (9). An infant's age alone does not determine readiness for solid foods (4,9,14,23,27,35), nor does an infant's weight alone (2,4,27). Instead, the introduction of solid foods depends on the infant's developmental readiness (2,4–6,9,11,14,17,20,23–29,31), although other factors, such as growth (9,14,20), level of activity (14), and gastrointestinal maturation, may be included as well (11,26). One source states that an infant is ready for solid foods if the birth weight has doubled, s/he can hold his/her own head up, s/he can sit with help, s/he shows interest in the foods others are eating, and s/he nurses more than eight times a day or drinks more than 32 ounces of formula (32).

According to the Dietary Guidelines for Infants (35), the initial sign of an infant's readiness for supplemental foods is the weight cue, which is when infants (1) double their birth weight and (2) weigh at least 13 pounds; both weight criteria must be met due to variability in birth weight. Another sign of readiness for supplemental foods is frequent hunger, even after nursing 8–10 times a day or drinking 32 ounces of formula a day (35). Infants who have reached the weight criteria and are frequently hungry are ready for a developmental evaluation of eating readiness (35). Eating readiness cues include (1) the ability to sit with support, (2) the ability to hold up their head and support their weight with straight elbows when placed on their stomach, and (3) deliberate and frequent "mouthing" of their hands and toys (35). An infant who is ready for supplemental foods will quickly (i.e., within a week) learn to suck thin purees from a spoon and swallow them without gagging (35).

The disappearance of the extrusion, or tongue thrust, reflex is cited by numerous sources as a major developmental milestone for determining when an infant is ready for solid foods (2,4,5,9,14,17,20,23–28,30,31). The extrusion reflex causes an infant's tongue to protrude when solid foods or a spoon is put in the mouth (20); this makes it difficult to give solid foods by spoon. The reported age at which the extrusion reflex disappears varies from 3 or 4 months of age (17) to 4–5 months of age (14,20) to 4–6 months of age (4,9,11), according to the source.

Other developmental milestones as an indication of an infant's readiness for solid foods include the ability to sit with support and good neuromuscular control of the head and neck (2,4,6,14,25,27–29,31,32). In addition, by 5 or 6 months of age, an infant can indicate a desire for food by opening his/her mouth and/or leaning forward as well as disinterest or satiety by leaning back and/or turning away (4,9,11,14,17,20,21,24,27,28,33,34). Table 1 provides an overview of the sequence of development and feeding skills in normal, healthy full-term infants during the first year.

Although Fomon recommends that the introduction of solid foods be deferred until the infant reaches a stage of developmental readiness (33), he contends that limitations in the digestive capability of infants are insufficient to constitute a valid argument against feeding solid foods during the early months of life (13,33,34). As evidence, he points to the ability of infants during the 1950s and 1960s to tolerate solid foods during the early weeks of life (13). In addition, he states that it is doubtful that early introduction of solid foods is an important contributor to the development of allergic reactions, except for infants with a strong family history of food allergies (33,34). Instead, Fomon contends that the major objection to introducing solid foods prior to 4 months of age is based on the possibility that it may contribute to overfeeding and interfere with the establishment of sound eating habits (33,34). His rationale is this: If mothers or caregivers are to encourage infants to discontinue eating at the earliest sign of satiety, then infants must be able to communicate in some way with the people feeding them. By 4 months of age, most infants are able to sit with support, indicate desire for food by opening their mouths and leaning forward, and indicate disinterest or satiety by leaning back and turning away (36). Until an infant can express him- or herself in this way, feeding solid foods would seem to represent a type of forced feeding (9,11,13,28,33,34). It is important to note that although infants as young as 4 months of age are quite capable of taking control of the feeding interaction and demonstrating satiety as well as food preferences (36,37), mothers or caregivers must not ignore or override infants' behavioral signals.

In addition to representing a type of forced feeding, introducing solid foods too early can cause other problems. Before age 4–6 months, there is no nutritional need for solid foods (6,14,29,31). Infants require only breast milk or iron-fortified formula during the first 4–6 months of life (2,4,7,30–32). If solid foods are introduced too early, they may displace breast milk or formula, resulting in inadequate energy and nutrient intake (2,4,20). Feeding

Table 1 Sequence of Development and Feeding Skills in Normal, Healthy Full-Term Infants During the First Year

Infant's approximate age	Mouth patterns	Hand and body abilities	Feeding skills	Food textures to serve, and rationale

Birth–5 months	• Rooting reflex: When an infant's mouth, lips, cheeks, or chin are touched by an object, the infant's head and mouth turn toward the object and the infant opens his/her mouth. This reflex is seen from birth to about 4 months; it allows an infant to seek out and grasp a nipple.
	• Suck/swallow reflex: When lips and mouth area are touched, infant opens mouth and begins sucking movements; as liquid moves into the mouth, the tongue moves it to the back of the mouth for swallowing. This reflex is seen from birth to about 4 months; it facilitates feeding from the breast or bottle but not from a spoon or cup.
		• Poor control of head, neck, and trunk
		• Brings hand to mouth around 3 months
			• Swallows liquids, but pushes most solid objects from the mouth	Birth–3 months:
				  Serve liquids only.
				  Rationale: At this age, infants are only able to suck and swallow.

- Tongue thrust reflex: When lips are touched, infant's tongue extends out of mouth. This reflex is seen from birth to about 4–6 months; it allows for feeding from the breast or bottle but not from a spoon or cup.
- Gag reflex: When an object, such as a spoon or solid food, is placed at the back of the mouth, the object is quickly moved forward out of the mouth on the tongue. This reflex diminishes by 4 months but is retained to some extent in adults. This reflex is another reason to delay solid foods, and the use of a spoon, until 4–6 months.

4–6 months

- Draws in upper or lower lip when spoon is removed from mouth
- Up-and-down munching movement
- Can transfer food from front to back of tongue to swallow
- Tongue thrust reflex begins to disappear

- Sits with support
- Good head control
- Uses whole hand to grasp objects (palmer grasp)

- Takes in spoonful of pureed or strained food and swallows it without choking
- Drinks small amounts from cup, with spilling, when held by another person

4–7 months:
Add semisolid (strained) foods.
Rationale: At this age, infants can draw in upper or lower lip as spoon is removed from mouth, move tongue up and down, sit up with support, swallow semisolid

Table 1 Continued

Infant's approximate age	Mouth patterns	Hand and body abilities	Feeding skills	Food textures to serve, and rationale
	• Rooting reflex begins to disappear • Gag reflex diminishes • Opens mouth when sees spoon approaching			food without choking, open the mouth when seeing food, and drink from a cup, with spilling, with help.
5–9 months	• Begins to control the position of food in the mouth • Up-and-down munching movement • Positions food between jaws for chewing	• Begins to sit alone unsupported • Follows food with eyes • Begins to use thumb and index finger to pick up objects (pincher grasp)	• Begins to eat mashed food • Eats from a spoon easily • Drinks from a cup with some spilling • Begins to feed self with hands	See earlier and later entries.
8–11 months	• Moves food from side to side in mouth	• Sits alone easily	• Begins to eat ground or finely chopped	8–11 months: Add modified

Age				Rationale
	• Begins to curve lips around rim of cup	• Transfers objects from hand to mouth	food and small pieces of soft food	(mashed or diced) table foods and liquids in a cup.
	• Begins to chew in rotary pattern (diagonal movement of the jaw as food is moved to the side or center of the mouth)		• Begins to experiment with spoon but prefers to feed self with hands	Rationale: At this age, infants can move tongue from side to side, begin spoon-feeding themselves with help, begin to chew, begin to have some teeth, begin to hold food and use their fingers to feed themselves, and drink from a cup with less spilling, with help.
			• Drinks from a cup with less spilling	See earlier entries.
10–12 months	• Rotary chewing (diagonal movement of the jaw as food is moved to the side or center of the mouth)	• Begins to put spoon in mouth	• Eats chopped food and small pieces of soft, cooked table food	
		• Begins to hold cup	• Begins self-spoon-feeding with help	
		• Good eye–hand–mouth coordination		

Source: Adapted from Refs. 2 and 4.

solid foods too early may increase the risk of choking (2,4,11,28), the development of food allergies or intolerances (2,4,12,29,31), especially in susceptible infants (28), the risk of insulin-dependent diabetes mellitus in susceptible infants (28), diarrhea (28), and overeating and obesity (25).

Reasons for the early introduction of supplemental foods include the ready availability of convenient forms of solid foods, the desire of mothers to see their infants gain weight rapidly, and the belief that it will help infants sleep through the night (14). However, feeding solid foods before infants are ready will not help them sleep through the night (2,4,11,29,31) or make them eat fewer times throughout the day (2,4,31). Numerous studies indicate that early introduction of solid foods is common. For example, Skinner et al. (38) reported that among 98 mother/infant pairs of middle and upper socioeconomic status, the percentages of infants for whom solid foods were introduced prior to 4 months of age were 60% for cereal, 35% for juice, 34% for fruit, and 17% for vegetables. Mothers who introduced cereal the earliest were more likely to be formula-feeding, to feed cereal in the infant's bottle, to be primiparous, to be employed outside the home, and/or not to cite the physician as a source for guiding the introduction of solid foods (38). Nevling et al. (39) reported that among 60 adolescent and 60 adult mothers, the mean respective age in months that infants were introduced to solid foods was 2.1 and 3.1 for cereal, 3.2 and 3.6 for fruit, and 3.8 and 4.0 for vegetables; the authors concluded that the degree to which mothers follow current feeding guidelines when introducing solid foods is influenced by factors other than early motherhood. Bronner et al. (40) reported that among 217 African–American women who were participants in the Special Supplemental Nutrition Program for Women, Infants, and Children (WIC) and thus received nutrition education about infant feeding, 32% introduced nonmilk liquids or solid foods to their infants by 7–10 days postpartum; this escalated to 77% by 8 weeks of age and 93% by 16 weeks postpartum. Feeding cereal in a bottle was the most common practice at each of the time periods. Mothers breast-feeding exclusively (i.e., not adding nonmilk liquids or solid foods) were least likely, and mothers providing mixed feedings (i.e., breast milk and formula) were more likely than mothers feeding formula exclusively to introduce nonmilk liquids and solid foods (40). Heath et al. (41) reported that although current recommendations in New Zealand are to introduce solid foods at 4–6 months of age and to delay cow's milk until 12 months of age, among 74 white mothers, 45% introduced nonmilk foods to their infants before 4 months of age, and 69% gave unmodified cow's milk before 12 months of age.

Waiting too late to introduce solid foods may cause problems as well. According to the AAP, delaying the introduction of solid foods beyond 6 months may delay the timely appearance of other developmental milestones (14). However, another source indicates that the introduction of solid foods should not be delayed beyond 8 months of age (4). Other sources indicate that delaying the introduction of solid foods beyond the time when an infant is developmentally ready for them increases the risk that infants will not learn to eat solid foods properly (2,4,17,23,28), develop iron-deficiency anemia (2,28) especially if breast-fed (23), become malnourished (2,4,28), and not grow normally (2,28). The importance of introducing a variety of solid foods at specific intervals as the infant develops is evident in deprived environments, in which the introduction of solid foods is delayed or the eating pattern is unvaried and monotonous (42). Harris et al. (36) found that preference declined with infant age among 12 infants, aged 16–25 weeks and formerly breast-fed, who were tested for their preferences for salt in the first food fed to them. The authors commented that if food preferences begin to develop in the early months, delaying the introduction of solid foods may induce infants to accept only a limited range of foods (36).

D. One at a Time, Wait, and Watch

When solid foods are introduced, single-ingredient or plain foods should be selected (2,4,11,14,21,26,32,35); for example, rice cereal should be fed instead of a mixed-grain cereal. Combination foods or mixtures may be given to older infants after they have been introduced to each food item separately (2,12,14,26,29,30,32).

New foods should be introduced one at a time (2,4–7,11,12,17,21,23–25,27,29,30,35) and fed daily (12) for several days (9). Although waiting before another new food is introduced to allow for signs of food intolerances to be identified is recommended (2,4–6,11,12,14,17,20,23,24,27,29,30,35), inconsistencies exist in the recommended length of the waiting period. For example, before introducing the next new food, the waiting period ranges from "several" days (30,35) to at least 2 or 3 days (5,17,23,24), to 3–5 days (12), to 1 week (2,4,7,11,12,14,20,21,25,29) or more (6). Signs of intolerance or sensitivity may include rashes (2,4,5,17,20,23–25,27,30), hives (2,4,17), vomiting (2,4,5,17,20,27), diarrhea (2,4,5,17,20,23–25,27,30), irritability (2,4,20), wheezing (2,4,17,20,23,24), coughing (2,4), respiratory symptoms (4), congestion or stuffiness (2), ear infections (2,4), stomachache (2,4,23,24), cramps (17), headache (17), asthma (30), systemic reactions such as anaphylactic shock or failure to thrive (4), and runny nose (25). If an infant appears to have a reaction to a particular food, remove it from his/her diet for 1–3 months before trying it again; if the food provokes a reaction on a subsequent try, eliminate it again for several months (17). If an infant has had an allergic reaction to a particular food, consult a pediatrician (5) or health care provider (12) before trying it again.

Allowing time between the introduction of new foods also provides time for the infant to become accustomed to each new flavor and texture (2,4,17,20). The initial refusal of new flavors and textures is not uncommon;

parents and caregivers should be encouraged to offer another food and reintroduce the refused food several weeks later (2,4,20). It may take numerous tastes in numerous meals for an infant to become accustomed to the flavor of a new food and to accept it (6,23). The more a food is offered to an infant, the better chance s/he has of liking it (32). If foods that are rejected on the first introduction are never offered again, an infant is denied the opportunity to learn to like a variety of foods (23). However, if an infant rejects a food after repeated offerings, s/he probably really does not like that food (43).

E. Progression of Texture and Consistency

When solid foods are first introduced around 4–6 months of age, the texture or consistency of foods should be strained or pureed (2,4,20). This progresses to mashed foods around 6 months of age, ground or finely chopped food around 8 months of age, and chopped food around 10 months of age (2,4,20).

A small study by Lundy et al. (44) with 12 infants between 4 and 8 months of age who were just starting solid foods indicated that infants who experienced a variety of differently textured applesauces (e.g., pureed, lumpy, and diced) preferred greater texture complexity. The results highlight the importance of texture variations within the infant's feeding skill range and suggest that parents and caregivers need to provide variety and novelty in the food choices they offer to infants (44).

If infants are not introduced to chewable foods at the recommended age, they may be less likely to accept new textures later in life, which may limit the variety of their diet (45). In a study with 9360 infants in England, Northstone et al. (45) determined the development of feeding difficulties as perceived by the mother according to the age at which the infant was first introduced to lumpy solid foods. Results indicated a significant difference in the variety of foods given to infants at both 6 and 15 months according to the age at which they began to have lumps in their food, and feeding difficulties were more likely to occur when lumpy solid foods were first introduced to infants at or after 10 months of age. The authors concluded that solid foods containing chewable lumps should be introduced to infants between 6 and 9 months of age, because delayed introduction is associated with increased levels of feeding difficulty at 15 months (45). These results suggest a "critical window" for introducing "lumpy" solid foods to infants.

F. How Much and How Often

Start with 1–2 teaspoons of a new food once a day (2,4–6,17,21); be patient and allow the infant time to adapt to the new textures and flavors of solid foods (2,4). Because it is not uncommon for infants initially to refuse new flavors and textures, it is important to offer another food and to reintroduce the refused food several weeks later and then to keep offering a variety of flavors and textures as infants' tastes grow and change (20). Always begin with small amounts of foods, and offer seconds if necessary; infants will indicate hunger or satiety (20). Gradually increase until the infant will eat 2–4 tablespoons of each food at meals (4,17). An infant 4–6 months of age may eat one meal per day that includes solid foods; by 8 months of age, each day an infant may be eating three meals and two to three snacks that include solid foods (4). Table 2 provides a suggested feeding schedule, along with daily servings. Table 3 provides sample menus.

Infants are the best judges of how much food they need, so allow them to determine how much they will eat (4). Infants indicate their interest in consuming additional solid foods by opening their mouths and leaning forward (4). Feed until infants indicate they are full and satisfied by (1) pulling away from the spoon, (2) turning their heads away, (3) playing with the food, (4) sealing their lips, (5) pushing the food or spoon out of their mouths, or (6) throwing the food on the floor (2,4). Follow the infant's lead on how often and how fast to feed, food preferences, and amount of food (4). There is day-to-day variation in the quantity of food consumed, because an infant's appetite varies, which influences the amount of food eaten on a particular day (4).

III. FEEDING RELATIONSHIP

Fomon (33) identified 10 infant feeding recommendations appropriate for the 21st century along with the rationale for each recommendation. The 10 recommendations are listed in Table 4. This paragraph discusses the rationale for the 7th recommendation (i.e., actions of caregivers should be conducive to establishing habits of eating in moderation) as described by Fomon (33,34). During the early weeks of infancy, the goal of providing adequate intake of energy and essential nutrients should be combined with efforts to establish sound eating habits, including, perhaps most importantly, the habit of eating in moderation. In theory, establishing a habit of eating in moderation early in life may decrease the risk of obesity in adult life, and no harm is likely to result from efforts to achieve this goal. Thus, delaying a recommendation for moderation does not seem necessary. It appears that breast-fed infants have more control over the amount consumed at a feeding than formula-fed infants; thus, breast-feeding may in itself aid in establishing habits of eating in moderation. However, the same attitudes of the parents/caretakers are required with either mode of feeding (33,34). To establish habits of eating in

Table 2 Suggested Feeding Schedule, with Daily Servings[a]

	Birth to 4 months	4–6 months	6–8 months	8–10 months	10–12 months
Breast milk or infant formula	8–12 nursings or 4–6 formula feedings: 0–1 mo: 18–24 oz 1–2 mo: 22–28 oz 2–3 mo: 25–32 oz 3–4 mo: 28–32 oz	4–6 nursings or 4–6 formula feedings: 4–5 mo: 27–39 oz 5–6 mo: 27–45 oz	3–5 nursings or 3–5 formula feedings (24–32 oz)	3–4 nursings or 2–4 formula feedings (24–32 oz)	3–4 nursings or 2–4 formula feedings (24–32 oz)
Grain products	None	Iron-fortified infant cereal: begin with rice cereal; 2 or 3 daily servings (total of 4–8 tbsp after mixing)	Iron-fortified infant cereal: 2–3 tbsp 2 times daily (total of 4–6 tbsp after mixing) Crackers, zwieback, toast: 1 small serving (for relief when teething)	Iron-fortified infant cereal: 2–3 tbsp 2 times daily (total of 4–6 tbsp after mixing) Other grain products: 2–3 daily servings of soft breads in bite-sized pieces	Iron-fortified infant cereal: 2–3 tbsp 2 times daily (total of 4–6 tbsp after mixing) Other grain products: 2–3 daily servings
Vegetables	None	None	Plain, strained or pureed, cooked: 1–2 daily servings (total of 3–4 tbsp)	Finger foods: cooked, mashed, soft, bite-sized pieces: 2 daily servings (total of 6–8 tbsp)	Finger foods: cooked, soft, bite-sized pieces: 2 daily servings (total of 6–8 tbsp)

Fruits	None	None	Plain, strained or pureed, cooked: 1–2 daily servings (total of 3–4 tbsp)	Finger foods: cooked, mashed, soft, bite-sized pieces: 2 daily servings (total of 6–8 tbsp)	Finger foods: chopped soft, fresh or cooked: 2 daily servings (total of 6–8 tbsp)
Juices	None	None	100% juice, vitamin C–fortified, plain: 2–4 oz per day; only in a cup	100% juice, vitamin C–fortified, plain: 4 oz per day; only in a cup	100% juice, vitamin C–fortified, plain: 4 oz per day; only in a cup
Protein foods	None	None	Meats: plain, strained or pureed; 1–2 tbsp per day	Pureed or finely chopped, plain meat or poultry, or fish: egg yolk, yogurt, cheese, cottage cheese, mashed beans or peas: 4–6 tbsp per day	Strips of tender meat or poultry; ground meats, fish, egg yolk, yogurt, cheese strips, mashed beans or peas: 2 oz or 1/2 cup per day

[a] Serving sizes may vary for individual infants.
Source: Adapted from Refs. 4 and 20.

Table 3 Sample Menus

	4–6 months[a]	6–8 months[a]	8–10 months[a]	10–12 months[a]
Breakfast	Iron-fortified infant cereal (2 tbsp after mixing) Breast milk or iron-fortified formula (6 oz)	Iron-fortified infant cereal (3 tbsp after mixing) Vitamin C-fortified apple juice (1 oz, in a cup) Breast milk or iron-fortified formula (6 oz)	Iron-fortified infant cereal (3 tbsp after mixing) Orange juice (2 oz, in a cup) Breast milk or iron-fortified formula (6 oz)	Iron-fortified infant cereal (3 tbsp after mixing) Orange juice (2 oz, in a cup) Breast milk or iron-fortified formula (6 oz)
Midmorning snack	Breast milk or iron-fortified formula (6 oz)	Pears (2 tbsp, pureed) Breast milk or iron-fortified formula (6 oz)	Banana (3 tbsp, mashed) Breast milk or iron-fortified formula (6 oz)	Grapes (1/4 cup, cut into quarters) Breast milk or iron-fortified formula (6 oz)
Lunch	Iron-fortified infant cereal (2 tbsp after mixing) Breast milk or iron-fortified formula (6 oz)	Chicken (1 tbsp, pureed) Green peas (2 tbsp, pureed) Applesauce (2 tbsp, pureed) Water (2 oz)	Finely shredded chicken (2 tbsp) Macaroni (1/4 cup, mashed) Green peas (3 tbsp, mashed) Applesauce (3 tbsp) Water (2 oz)	Finely shredded chicken (1/4 cup) Macaroni (1/4 cup) Green beans (4 tbsp) Pear (4 tbsp, fresh, soft, diced) Water (2 oz)

Midafternoon snack	Breast milk or iron-fortified formula (6 oz)	Zwieback (1) Breast milk or iron-fortified formula (6 oz)	Cheerios (1/4 cup) Breast milk or iron-fortified formula (6 oz)	Cheerios (1/4 cup) Breast milk or iron-fortified formula (6 oz)
Dinner	Iron-fortified infant cereal (2 tbsp after mixing) Breast milk or iron-fortified formula (6 oz)	Beef (1 tbsp, pureed) Iron-fortified infant cereal (3 tbsp after mixing) Carrots (2 tbsp, pureed) Vitamin C-fortified white grape juice (1 oz, in a cup) Water (2 oz)	Ground beef (2 tbsp) Iron-fortified infant cereal (3 tbsp after mixing) Cooked carrots (3 tbsp, mashed) Vitamin C-fortified apple juice (2 oz, in a cup) Water (2 oz)	Ground beef (1/4 cup) Iron-fortified infant cereal (3 tbsp after mixing) Cooked carrots (4 tbsp) Vitamin C-fortified apple juice (2 oz, in a cup) Water (2 oz)
Evening snack	Breast milk or iron-fortified formula (6 oz)	Breast milk or iron-fortified formula (8 oz)	Graham cracker made without honey (1) Breast milk or iron-fortified formula (8 oz)	Graham cracker made without honey (1) Breast milk or iron-fortified formula (8 oz)

[a] Serving sizes may vary for individual infants.
Source: Adapted from Refs. 2 and 4.

Table 4 Infant Feeding Recommendations for the 21st Century (by Fomon)

---

1. Every mother should be encouraged to breast-feed her infant—but not coerced to do so.
2. Every infant should be given an injection of vitamin K as soon as feasible after birth.
3. While in the hospital, every woman who breast-feeds her infant should be given instructions about breast-feeding.
4. Follow-up approximately 48 hours after discharge from the hospital should be arranged for women who breast-feed.
5. Every breast-fed infant should receive a daily supplement of iron and vitamin D.
6. Formula-fed infants should receive iron-fortified formulas.
7. Actions of caregivers should be conducive to establishing habits of eating in moderation.
8. Introduction of beikost (i.e., foods other than breast milk or formula) should be deferred until the infant reaches the state of developmental readiness for such feeding.
9. Beikost items should be thoughtfully selected.
10. Cow's milk should not be fed before 1 year of age.

Source: Adapted from Ref. 33.

moderation, parents and caregivers should encourage infants to discontinue eating at the earliest sign of desire to stop (33,34). Every variation of forced feeding should be avoided. Although the effects of the frequency of feeding in infancy have not been studied, there is little basis for believing that it is nutritionally desirable to widely space an infant's feedings. Thus, it may not be in the infant's best interests to sleep through the night as early in life as possible or to adapt to a pattern of three feedings per day as early as possible. The effort to establish habits of eating in moderation applies first to breast-feeding and formula-feeding and later to the predominantly solid diet of children and adults (33,34).

Fomon's recommendation encourages parents/caregivers to respect and encourage their infant's internal indications of satiety. This is similar to Satter's division of responsibility regarding feeding, in which parents are responsible for the what, when, and where of feeding and infants are responsible for the how much and whether of eating (23,46). According to Satter, appropriate feeding is built on trust—trust in the infant's ability to eat and in his/her ability to grow in the way nature intended. When feeding infants, parents are responsible for controlling what food comes into the house, for preparing and presenting meals and snacks that are appropriate for the infant's age and developmental level, and for making meal- and snack times pleasant. Infants are responsible for how much they eat and whether they eat (23,46).

Several other sources regarding the introduction of solid foods to infants advocate a division of responsibility in feeding. Most sources specify that infants should not be forced to eat but should be trusted and allowed to decide whether they will eat and how much they will eat (2,4,6,7,12,17,20,21, 24,26,30,31,33–35,47). Studies indicate that infants are born with the ability to self-regulate their caloric intake by adjusting their formula intake when the caloric level of the formula changes (48) and when solid foods are added (49). Parents and caregivers who adjust their feeding approach to accommodate their infant's appetite also give their infant the opportunity to learn about self-regulation, social interactions, and communicating complex needs; this strengthens the infant's basic physical abilities, helps to ensure adequate nutrition, and establishes patterns of eating in moderation (35). If infants and children are encouraged to respect their internal cues of satiety, they can maintain the habit of eating when they are hungry and stopping when they are full, and perhaps they can avoid problems with eating that are related to obesity or eating disorders later in life (24).

IV. LEARNING TO EAT

As infants make the transition from consuming a liquid diet of only breast milk or formula to consuming a diet with a variety of solid foods, an enormous amount of learning about food and eating occurs (50). Some of this learning occurs because of exposure to new foods as well as the parents' decision to breast-feed or formula-feed (50). For example, in a study with 36 infants 4–6 months of age, Sullivan and Birch (51) found that after 10 opportunities to consume their first vegetable, intake was significantly increased as the number of opportunities increased, regardless of whether the vegetable was salted or unsalted; furthermore, breast-fed infants showed greater increases in intake of the vegetable after exposure and had an overall greater level of intake than formula-fed infants. The authors concluded that acceptance increases as infants become familiar with a new food through repeated opportunities to taste and consume that food; in addition to familiarity, acceptance of new foods may be facilitated by exposure to different flavors in breast milk (51). In a study with 17 breast-fed infants who had been fed their first solid food, cereal prepared with water only, for less than 1 month, Mennella and Beauchamp (52) found that consumption was greater when the cereal was prepared with their mothers' milk than when it was prepared with water; furthermore, the infants' willingness to accept the cereal prepared with their mothers' milk was correlated with their mothers' reported willingness to try novel foods and flavors. Mennella and Beauchamp (52) concluded that "the transition from a diet exclusively of human milk to a mixed diet may be facilitated by providing the infant with bridges of familiarity such that the infant experiences a commonality of flavors in the two feeding situations."

How many exposures to a new food are needed before an infant learns to like it? Some sources indicate that it may take 5–10 or as many as 15–20 exposures for an infant to learn to like a new food (6,23). However, in a study with 39 infants 4–7 months of age who had been introduced to only cereal on a regular basis, Birch et al. (53) found that after only one exposure to a novel target food (i.e., either bananas or peas), intake of the target, same (i.e., same food prepared by another manufacturer), and similar (i.e., other fruits for infants receiving a target fruit) foods nearly doubled; however, intake of the different food (vegetables for infants receiving a target fruit) was unchanged. These findings are in contrast to the slower changes seen in studies with preschool children, who seemed to need multiple exposures to a new food before significant increases in intake were noted (54–56). Birch et al. (53) concluded that infants may have difficulty discriminating among many foods; thus, during the first months when solid foods are introduced, acceptance of a variety of foods can be facilitated by exposing infants to a variety of foods from within "families" of similar foods.

Gerrish and Mennella (57) tested the conclusion of Birch et al. (53) with 48 formula-fed infants 4–5 months of age who had all been introduced to cereal but not vegetables or meats. There were 3 groups of infants, with 16 per group: carrot, potato, and variety (peas, potatoes, squash). The study lasted 12 days; all 48 infants were fed carrots on days 1 and 11, their "group" vegetable(s) on days 2 through 10, and pureed chicken on day 12. Results indicated that infants with repeated exposures to carrots or a variety of vegetables ate significantly more carrots on day 11 than on day 1 than infants with repeated exposures to potatoes. Furthermore, exposure to a variety of vegetables facilitated the acceptance of a novel food (i.e., pureed chicken). Gerrish and Mennella (57) concluded that their results were the first to indicate that exposure to a variety of flavors enhances acceptance of novel foods in infants. In addition, they commented that "the minimum number of exposures required to enhance acceptance appears to be more than one" because infants with repeated exposures to potatoes showed no increase in carrot acceptance on day 11 as compared to day 1. This is in contrast to Birch et al. (53), who found that a single exposure enhanced infants' intake on the second exposure, but similar to the multiple exposures needed to enhance intake among preschool children (54–56).

Skinner et al. (58) found that food-related experiences at 2–24 months of age predicted fruit and vegetable consumption at 6, 7, and 8 years of age among 70 child/mother pairs. Variety of vegetable intake in school-aged children was weakly predicted by mothers' vegetable preferences; variety of fruit intake in school-aged children was predicted by breast-feeding duration, variety of fruits consumed at 2–24 months of age, and exposure to fruits at 2–24 months of age. These results emphasize that the decisions parents and caregivers make regarding how and what to feed infants and young children have a critical and long-term impact.

Beauchamp and Mennella (59) reviewed information and studies that suggest that (1) flavors consumed by pregnant women alter the odor and presumably the flavor of their amniotic fluid, (2) the fetus is sensitive to sweet- and bitter-tasting substances, (3) newborn infants prefer sweet tastes, reject strong sour tastes, and may be indifferent to the taste of salt, (4) the chemosensory response to flavors may be influenced by an infant's nutritional needs, and (5) at least 3 volatile flavors (garlic, alcohol, and vanilla) enter human milk through the mother's diet. Beauchamp and Mennella (59) concluded that further research is needed to clarify how and to what extent specific prenatal and postnatal experiences alter the infant's perceptions and preferences and that results from research in this area "may provide a solid basis for dietary recommendations concerning intake of 'problem' flavors (e.g., sweet, salt), the difficulties, if any, of depriving the formula-fed infant of the varied flavor experience normal to all breast-fed infants, and the general value of variety in early feeding experience."

V. SUGGESTED ORDER OF INTRODUCTION

A. Iron-Fortified Infant Cereal

All but one of the sources reviewed were consistent in identifying iron-fortified infant cereal as an appropriate first solid food (2,4–7,10–12,14,17, 20,23,24,26–32); the exception (35) indicated that iron-fortified infant cereals and single-ingredient, pureed fruits and vegetables are good choices for first foods. Iron-fortified infant cereal contributes iron (2,4,6,12–14,20,26,31) and can be altered in consistency to meet the infant's developmental needs (2,4, 17,23). Most sources recommend introducing iron-fortified infant cereal between the ages of 4 and 6 months (2,4–7,9,11,12,14,20,24,27–32), although one source says 4–8 months (17).

Iron-fortified infant rice cereal is a good choice as the infant's first solid food (2,4–6,9,12,13,20,23,24,30–32) because it is least likely to cause an allergic reaction (2,4,6,12–14,17,23,24,31), although one source says that either rice or barley infant cereal can be introduced first because they are the least allergenic (20). Feed it for 2–3 days while examining the infant for symptoms of intolerance; in the absence of symptoms, increase the quantity, frequency, and consistency of the rice cereal feedings (9). After rice cereal has been accepted for several days to a week, a second infant cereal, such as oatmeal or barley, can be added (4,5,9,14,17,30), although two sources say to wait until 6 months to add these two cereals (17,20). As mentioned previously, some sources indicate waiting up to a week before introducing each new iron-fortified infant cereal. Although several sources suggest that wheat cereal should be delayed because it may cause an allergic reaction in younger infants (4,5), there are inconsistencies regarding when it can be introduced, with recommendations ranging from 6 months of age (20), to 8 months of age (4,14), to 1 year of age (17).

Infant cereal that comes premixed in a jar is convenient, but the dry varieties can be prepared in a consistency that is appropriate for the infant's developmental level (4,5,17) by mixing them with breast milk or iron-fortified infant formula (2,4,5,9,13,17,20,23–27,31,32), water (2,5,17), or, later, with juice (2,4,26,31). Satter recommends infant cereal fortified with iron as well as vitamin C because it improves iron absorption; she does not recommend mixing infant cereal with juice or water because these liquids are low in protein (23). Salt, butter, or seasonings should not be added to infant cereals (25). Adult cereals are not recommended for infants because they often contain mixed grains, they tend to contain more sodium and sugar than infant cereals, and the iron in them is not as easily absorbed by infants as is the iron in infant cereals (4).

Infant cereal should be fed with a spoon (2,4–7,9,20,27,30–32,60); it should not be added to bottles (2,4,6,7,14,17,23,26,30,31), except for medically indicated reasons, such as gastroesophageal reflux (4,5,14). Baby food nurser kits, infant feeders, and feeding bottles are also inappropriate for feeding solid foods (2,5–7,14,60). Baby food nurser kits allow solid food to filter through the bottle nipple along with the liquid (6). An infant feeder is a hard plastic container with a plunger at one end and a spout at the other end; the plunger is used to push liquid mixed with solid foods into an infant's mouth (2). Infants who are fed solid foods in a bottle or infant feeder can choke (2,4,26), are forced to eat the food (2), may consume extra calories that can lead to excessive weight gain (5,17,26), and may not learn to eat solid foods properly (2,14). Frequently, bottles are used to start infants on solid foods before they are developmentally ready to eat solid foods from a spoon (4). When developmentally ready for solid foods, infants need to learn how foods feel and taste in their mouths (31). The experience of eating from a spoon benefits infants developmentally because different tongue and lip motions are involved in sucking from a nipple than in eating from a spoon (4). Finally, infants need to become accustomed to the process of eating—sitting up, taking bites from a spoon, resting between bites, and stopping when they are full (5)—as well as the social aspects of eating solid foods (17); these early experiences will help lay the foundation for a lifetime of healthful eating habits (5).

B. Fruits and Vegetables

After infants readily accept infant cereals, fruits and vegetables may be introduced (2,5,6,9,10,14,17,20,21,24,29,31,61). Most sources recommend introducing fruits and vegetables at 6–8 months of age (4,17,20,21,30,61), although some recommend introducing them at 4–6 months (6,7,31), 4–7 months (5), around 6 months (26), or about 6–7 months of age (24). Other sources recommend introducing them at 6 months of age, after the infant readily accepts 2–3 tablespoons of infant cereal at each meal (2) or 1/3 to 1/2 cup (9). Satter recommends introducing fruits and vegetables after an infant enjoys eating thick and even lumpy infant cereal and uses the tongue to push food between his/her jaws to mash it in an up-and-down munching motion (23).

As mentioned previously, introduce one new plain fruit or vegetable at a time, wait several days to a week before introducing the next new fruit or vegetable, and watch the infant closely for reactions. Although some sources indicate that it is not critical which is introduced first (14,23,28,29), other sources recommend adding vegetables before fruits (5,7,30,31) or alternating between the two (26), because it may be harder to get infants to eat vegetables after naturally sweet fruits are given (7). However, results from a small study by Gerrish and Mennella (57) with infants 4–5 months of age indicated that the 16 infants who previously had eaten fruit daily consumed more carrots during their first feeding experience with this vegetable than the 24 infants who had never eaten fruit.

Some sources indicate that fruits and vegetables should be pureed or strained (14,20,29–31) and cooked (4,5,23,29), except for bananas, which may be mashed and fed raw (5), until the infant is ready to progress in texture to mashed and then chopped fruits and vegetables (4). Another source indicates that fresh apricots, avocado, banana, cantaloupe, mango, melon, nectarines, papaya, peaches, and plums can simply be peeled and mashed without cooking if they are ripe and soft, but apples, pears, and dried fruits usually need to be cooked in order to be pureed or mashed easily (4). On the other hand, caution has been recommended in feeding raw fruits and vegetables, except for ripe bananas, because these foods may cause choking and may be difficult for infants to digest (29).

Satter indicates that 1–2 tablespoons of fruit is a serving, although infants are generally willing to eat more because they like fruit; however, she cautions parents and caregivers to limit the amount of fruit served at first because too much fruit can cause diarrhea (23). Avoid giving infants a lot of any one type of fruit or vegetable; for example, give infants dark green and deep yellow orange vegetables no more than every other day to avoid having a yellow-tinted infant (24). This condition, called *carotenemia*, is caused by the accumulation of the yellow coloring carotene; however, it does not hurt the infant and it goes away when fewer high-carotene vegetables, including broccoli, sweet potatoes, carrots, squash, apricots, watermelon, and peaches, are fed (23).

There is concern that the level of nitrates in some vegetables may be high enough to interfere with the transport of hemoglobin through the blood of infants (17) and cause methemoglobinemia (14), also called *blue baby syndrome* (6). Unfortunately, there are substantial inconsistencies regarding numerous aspects, including which vegetables to avoid, whether both home- and commercially prepared versions should be avoided, the age at which these vegetables should be avoided, and if the risk is large enough that restrictions are needed. Several sources recommend that the following five vegetables be avoided: beets, carrots, collard greens, spinach, and turnips (2,4–6,12,14,28,29); one source specifies four of these five with carrots excluded (17), two sources specify three of these five with collard greens and turnips excluded (23,24), and one source specifies three (beets, carrots, spinach) of these five and adds broccoli (9). Two sources indicate avoiding both home- and commercially prepared versions (6,14), while other sources indicate that only home-prepared versions should be avoided (2,4,9,12,13, 17,28). Shevlov recommends using commercially instead of home-prepared versions; if home-prepared versions are used, they should be served fresh to infants and not stored, because the amount of nitrates in these foods may actually increase with storage (5). Two sources indicate limiting these vegetables to 1–2 (24) or 1–3 (23) tablespoons per serving, while another source indicates limiting them to 1–2 tablespoons but only for home-prepared versions (29). For the sources that specify the age, most indicate that infants under 6 months of age avoid these vegetables (2,4,6,12), although the AAP recommends that they not be given to "infants fed solid foods before 4 months of age." Infants are more susceptible than older children and adults to the development of methemoglobinemia (13); around 6 months of age, stomach acidity increases and nitrate overload is less of a problem (23). Some health professionals believe that the risk of methemoglobinemia is so small that restricting infants' consumption of these vegetables is not really necessary (12).

There are inconsistencies among the sources regarding when citrus fruits may be introduced. One source indicates to delay introducing citrus fruits until after 6 months of age and then to observe infants closely for reactions when they are introduced (2). However, other sources indicate that citrus fruits (17,26,29) should not be given to infants before 1 year of age because they may cause allergic reactions. One source indicates that tomatoes should not be given to infants before 1 year of age due to allergic reactions (26).

Satter recommends waiting until the infant is having two or three cereal and fruit or vegetable "meals" a day before adding another food group (23). Another source indicates that by 6 months of age, infants should be eating two meals of cereal, fruit, and vegetables each day, in addition to being breast-fed or taking formula (31).

C. Juice

Although most sources agree about delaying the introduction of juice to infants until they can drink from a cup (2,4,6,11,14,20,21,23,24,26,29–32,34,62,63), the recommended age for introducing juice varies from 4–6 months (4,31), 4–7 months (5), 6 months of age or older (2,6,26,32,63), 6–8 months (17,20,24), to 8–10 months (9). According to Satter (23), "Juice is the most abused infant food. Juice in a cup is a food and a learning device. Juice in a bottle is an abomination." The majority of sources indicate that juice should not be fed from a bottle because infants permitted to suck on a bottle of any fluid containing carbohydrates, including juice, formula, or breast milk, for prolonged periods of time are at risk for developing a pattern of early tooth decay, or nursing-bottle caries (4–6,11,12,14,20,23,26,29,31,32,63,64). Infants are ready to drink from a cup when they can sit without support and can seal their lower lip on the cup (2). A cup with two handles, a lid, and a spout is easier for an infant to use (21,22,26).

As mentioned previously, introduce one new plain juice at a time, wait several days to a week before introducing each new juice, and watch the infant closely for reactions. Juices provide vitamin C and carbohydrates, but they should not replace breast milk or infant formula (4,6,11,14,26). Juices should be 100% fruit juice (2,6,63), naturally high in vitamin C or fortified with vitamin C (2,4,23,26), and pasteurized (2,12,17,63). Either infant juice or regular adult juice with vitamin C can be offered to infants (2,17,23,26). Low-sodium vegetable juices may be offered as well (17). Fruit juice should be used as part of a meal or snack; it should not be sipped throughout the day or used to pacify an unhappy infant (63).

There are inconsistencies regarding which juices to delay and the age at which they can be introduced. Some sources indicate that orange, tangerine, grapefruit, pineapple, and tomato juice not be introduced until after 6 months of age (2,4), or around 7–8 months of age (20). One source indicates that citrus juices should be delayed until 1 year of age (17), but another source indicates that orange juice not be introduced until about the 6th month because it can make the stool acidic, which can cause a rash and pain when the infant is wiped during a diaper change (5). Juice should not be warmed, because heat destroys vitamin C (31). Avoid feeding imported canned juices to infants because the cans may have lead seams; seams of cans manufactured in the United States can no longer be made using lead solder (4). Fruit juice should not be stored in pottery containers or lead crystal containers because they may leach lead into the juices (4).

Although several sources recommend that infants not be allowed to consume excessive amounts of juice, the definition of excessive amounts varies. For example, the AAP (14) and another source (6) define excessive juice consumption for an infant as 8–10 ounces per day, while another source defines it as 8 ounces per day (11). Numerous sources place limits on the amount of juice consumed per day for infants, but the limits vary from 3 ounces (24), to 4 ounces (26), to 4–6 ounces (5,6,31,63), to 4 ounces full-strength (12,23,47), to 8 ounces half-strength (12). Excessive juice consumption can lead to diarrhea (4–6,12,14,17,47,63), displacement of breast milk or formula intake (4,9,26), which can lead to failure to thrive (12), decreased appetite for other foods (4,6,17,24,47), gas (5,47,63), abdominal pain (4,47), cramping (17), bloating (4,47), and extra calories (29). Tips to help regulate the amount of juice consumed by infants include diluting juice to 1/2 juice and 1/2 water (5,17,26) and offering infants juice with food to slow down the rate at which it is absorbed (5).

According to the AAP, there is no nutritional indication to feed juice to infants younger than 6 months of age (63). Fomon contends that the common practice of feeding juice to infants during the early months of life has no nutritional basis (13,33,34) and may be unwise, considering the adverse reactions (33,34). For example, pear juice and apple juice may cause diarrhea in infants, probably because of the combined presence of sorbitol and fructose (65); however, the adverse reactions, including diarrhea and rash, commonly observed among infants fed citrus juices and tomato juice is probably not explained by malabsorption of carbohydrate (65). Some fruit juices, such as white grape juice, may be more easily digested than other juices because they contain a balance of carbohydrates and no sorbitol (5). Juices containing sorbitol include apple, cherry, peach, pear, and prune (4).

Some of the concern regarding excessive fruit juice consumption among infants comes from results of studies regarding fruit juice consumption by young children. For example, Smith and Lifshitz (66) described failure to thrive in eight toddlers due to inadequate diets in which a disproportionate amount of calories were derived from fruit juices, especially apple juice. Dennison et al. (67) found that consumption greater than or equal to 12 fluid ounces of fruit juice per day was associated with short stature and obesity in a study with 94 children 2 years of age and 74 children 5 years of age, 97% white, and of low to middle socioeconomic status; the authors concluded that young children's consumption of fruit juice be limited to less than 12 fluid ounces per day. In contrast, Skinner et al. (68) failed to find a significant relationship between juice intake and height, body mass index, or ponderal index in a study with 105 white children 24–36 months of age and of middle to upper socioeconomic status; in addition, although intake of soda pop was negatively related to intakes of milk and juice, intakes of milk and juice were not related. Skinner et al. (68) concluded that until additional studies with a broad spectrum of children are conducted to resolve the controversies regarding fruit juice intake, no recommendations should be made to change or limit children's intake of fruit juice. In study by Skinner and Carruth (69) with 72 white children, longitudinal juice intake between 24 and 72 months of age was not associated with either short stature or overweight; the authors concluded that consumption of 100% juices by children should be encouraged by health professionals.

D. Meat and Meat Alternates

Meat and meat alternates include meat, poultry, fin fish, eggs, cheese, yogurt, and cooked dry beans and peas (2,4). Recommendations vary considerably regarding which meat or meat alternate to introduce to infants at what specific age. A few sources recommend introducing meat to infants between the ages of 6 and 8 months (4,14,20) or at 7 months (9); yogurt, cheese, cottage cheese, and egg yolk can be introduced at 9–10 months of age (20). One source indicates introducing egg yolk, meat, and poultry to infants at 7–10 months of age, and introducing yogurt, cheese, and beans to infants at 9–12 months of age (17). Another source indicates that meats may be introduced to infants between the ages of 6 and 8 months if they need more iron (21). One source indicates that meat and meat alternates are generally introduced by 8 months of age although some doctors recommend introducing them between 6 and 8 months of age (2). Another source indicates that strained meat or poultry may be introduced to infants at 7–9 months of age and cottage cheese at 10–12 months of age (31). One source indicates that strained meat, cooked dry beans, cooked finely chopped chicken, and cooked and boned fish may be introduced after vegetables and fruits are introduced at 6–8 months of age, and that mashed egg yolk, cottage cheese, yogurt, and finger foods including small pieces of cooked ground meat, chicken, or fish with all bones and tough parts removed may be introduced at 8–10 months of age (30). Another source indicates that meats, including strained beef, poultry, pork, or veal; or meat substitutes, including mild cheeses, cottage cheese, plain yogurt, and pureed beans, can be introduced to infants around 8–9 months of age (26); from 9–12 months, the infant should progress from pureed meats to ground meats, then finely chopped meats (26). Two sources indicate that after cereal has been introduced to infants at 4–6 months of age, fruits, vegetables, and meats can be offered (6,29). One source indicates that after cereal has been introduced to infants at 4–6 months of age, followed by vegetables and fruits, then meats and eggs can be introduced (10). Another source indicates that after cereal has been introduced to infants at 4 through 7 months of age, vegetables, fruits, and meats may be introduced (5). One source indicates that vegetables, fruits, meats, and bread may be introduced after the infant is used to cereal (32). Two sources indicate introducing vegetables, fruits, and meats to infants after cereal has been introduced (11,14); they state that the order of introduction is not critical, but fail to indicate a specific age range for introducing these new food groups (11,14). One source indicates that cooked and strained meat, poultry, fish, dried beans and lentils, egg yolk, and tofu may be introduced at ages 5 through 9 months (29).

According to Fomon (33), once an infant has begun to accept solid foods regularly, which generally occurs by age 5–6 months, soft-cooked red meat should be fed regularly. Feeding of meat, fish, or poultry provides iron in the heme form and enhances absorption of nonheme iron (33). Meat, fish, and poultry all enhance absorption of nonheme iron from a meal; however, red meat, which includes beef and lamb, and dark meat poultry are preferable because of their greater concentrations of heme iron (33).

Both commercial infant meats and homemade pureed meats are fine (26). Lean meat and poultry, such as strained or pureed well-cooked lean beef, pork, lamb, veal, chicken, turkey, liver, and boneless fin fish, are preferable (2). Infants may accept meat better when mixed with plain vegetables (2,17) or fruits (2), when pureed (17), or when warmed slightly (17). Additional tips for making meat and poultry more palatable for infants include cooking it with moist heat until tender, chopping or cutting it very finely against the grain, and moistening it with broth or cooking liquid from vegetables (23). Because casseroles are moist and easy to chew, they make excellent food for infants once the infants have been introduced to all the ingredients separately (23). Jarred infant dinners, combination meat and vegetable dinners, and combination or high-protein dinners should be avoided (20,26). Plain commercial infant meats offer more nutrient value, ounce for ounce, than commercial infant mixed dinners; instead of using infant mixed dinners, the desired amounts of plain infant meats and plain infant vegetables can be mixed together to make meat more acceptable to infants (4).

Cheese may be introduced to infants at 6–8 months of age (4) or 8 months of age or older (2). Yogurt, hard cheeses, and cottage cheese can be gradually introduced as occasional protein foods at 8–10 months (4) or 10–12 months of age (62); because these foods contain similar proteins as cow's milk, infants should be observed closely for reactions after eating them (2,4,62). To help decrease the risk of choking, offer small, thin slices or strips of cheese instead of chunks (2,4). Regular cheeses, such as mozzarella, Colby, natural cheddar, and cottage cheese, are better choices than cheese food, cheese spread, and pasteurized process cheese, which are generally higher in salt (2). Plain yogurt, commercially prepared from low-fat or whole milk, may be introduced in small amounts to infants 8 months of age or older (2).

Infants 8 months of age and older may be offered cooked dry beans and peas, including kidney beans, lima beans, pinto beans, and chick peas (2). Offer small amounts of 1–2 teaspoons of mashed or pureed cooked beans or peas at first (2,4); if an infant appears to have trouble digesting them, try introducing them again at a later date (4). Avoid feeding infants cooked whole beans or peas, which could cause choking (2,4). Tofu can be mashed and fed to infants. Select fresh tofu or water-packed tofu, and then boil it in clean water for about 5 minutes and allow it to cool before feeding it to infants (4).

As mentioned previously, meat and meat alternates should be introduced one at a time, waiting several days to a week between each new food, and the infant watched closely for reactions to the foods. Meat and meat alternates have a higher renal solute load than some other foods, so when these foods are fed to infants, it is appropriate to feed infants about 4–8 ounces of water each day (4).

Introducing meat and meat alternates to infants younger than 6 months of age may cause allergic reactions (4). Early introduction of nuts (2,20,29) should be avoided because of choking and/or allergic reactions. Likewise, peanut butter and other nut butters (e.g., soy nut, almond, cashew, sunflower seed) should not be fed to infants because of choking and/or allergic reactions (2,20,31).

Although most sources indicate that egg whites are a common allergen, inconsistencies exist regarding when they can be introduced. One source says to avoid giving egg whites to infants (47) and another says to avoid "early introduction" (20). Other sources say that although egg yolk may be introduced to infants at 5 through 9 months of age (29), at or after 8 months of age (2,4,5), or at 10–12 months of age (62), do not introduce egg whites and whole eggs to infants younger than 10 months of age (5) or 1 year (2,4,17,26,29,62). Infants should never be fed raw or uncooked eggs or foods that contain them, including homemade ice cream, mayonnaise, and eggnog (2,4). Although most commercial eggnog, mayonnaise, and ice cream are made with pasteurized eggs, if made with whole eggs, these products are not appropriate for infants (4). According to Satter (23), "Eggs are the mainstay of feeding children—it's difficult to feed a family without them." She indicates that unless there is a strong family tendency for allergies, infants are past the high-risk period for egg allergy by age 9 or 10 months and are ready to eat a scrambled or boiled egg (23).

One source indicates avoiding "early introduction" of seafood (20) while another indicates avoiding it until infants are 1 year of age (26). Infants should be observed closely when introducing fin fish because some infants can have allergic reactions (2,4). Remove any bones before serving fish to infants (2). Prior to feeding any freshwater sport fish to infants, consult with your state Department of Health or Natural Resources for information regarding the safety of these fish (2,4). Do not feed infants less than 1 year of age any shellfish, including shrimp, crab, lobster, crawfish, scallops, oysters, and clams; shellfish can cause severe allergic reactions in some infants (2,4,29). There is controversy regarding the safety of feeding certain types of fish to infants and young children, because some types of fish may be contaminated with appreciable concentrations of potentially hazardous organic and inorganic chemicals, such as polychlorinated biphenyls, methylmercury, dioxins, and chlorinated hydrocarbon pesticides (4). Do not feed infants or young children any of the following fish, which may contain high levels of harmful mercury: shark, swordfish, king mackerel, and tilefish (2).

Never feed raw or undercooked meat, poultry, or fish to infants (2,4). Infants should not be served home-canned meats, because they may contain harmful bacteria if improperly canned (2). Avoid feeding infants the following foods due to their high fat and/or salt content: sausage, hot dogs, bacon, bologna, luncheon meats, salami, other cured meats, fried meats, and the fat and skin trimmed from meats (2,4).

E. Grains (Other Than Iron-Fortified Infant Cereals)

As discussed previously, iron-fortified infant cereals should be the first solid foods introduced to infants at 4–6 months of age. Among the various sources, inconsistencies regarding when to introduce wheat to infants range from ages 7–10 months (23), 8 months (4), 8–9 months (2), about 10 months (24), and 1 year (30); one source says that wheat is among the foods best avoided until about 1 year of age but that it is probably okay for infants 6–8 months of age (17). Because wheat is found in many grain products, the various ages at which wheat is recommended by the different sources impacts when they recommend introducing specific grain products to infants. Most infants start teething at 6–7 months (20,26); the earliest age at which different sources indicate that teething crackers and zwieback may be introduced varies from 6 months (20,26), 7 months (6,31), 8 months (4), to 9 months (2,22). The earliest age at which toast, crackers, and dry cereals may be introduced varies from 6 months (20,26), 7 months (6,17,31), 8 months (4,5,29,30), to 9 months (2,8,22). Different sources indicate that the earliest age at which soft bread, biscuits, English muffins, and rolls may be introduced varies from 7 months (17), 8 months (2,29,47), to 9 months (20,22). Grain products such as toast, crackers, dry cereals, and bite-size pieces of soft breads may be served to infants as finger foods (8,17,20,30). The earliest age at which cooked pasta and rice may be introduced varies among the sources from 8 months (2,4,5,29), 9 months (6,22,26), to 10 months (62); two sources indicate that pasta should be mashed or finely chopped, and rice should be mashed for infants 8 and 9 months of age (2,4).

Infants should not be fed the following grain products, which pose a choking hazard: highly seasoned snack crackers and those with seeds, potato chips, corn chips, pretzels, cheese twists; breads with nuts or whole grain kernels, such as wheat berries; and whole kernels of cooked rice, barley, wheat, or other grain (4). To avoid the chances of choking on crumbs, infants should eat biscuits, small pieces of toast, or crackers only while in an upright position (4).

VI. PRACTICAL ADVICE

A. Honey

Numerous sources recommend that honey should not be added to food, water, or formula for infants younger than 12 months of age due to concern regarding infant botulism (2,12,14,23, 29,62); others make this recommendation but fail to specify an age (4,6,24). Several sources recommend that honey not be fed to infants but fail to explain why (28) or mention bacterial spores that cause food-borne illnesses, which are often fatal in infants, but fail to specify infant botulism (30). One source provides the recommendation from the AAP that honey not be given to infants younger than 12 months of age due to concern regarding infant botulism (17). Honey is sometimes contaminated with spores of a bacterium called *Clostridium botulinum* (4,12). If allowed to grow in an airtight space, these spores cause clostridium toxin, which can cause severe illness and death (23). In general, this is a problem only in nonacid foods that have been canned improperly (23). However, the young infant's intestine is also an airtight place (23) where these spores can give rise to active bacteria that can produce a toxin that can cause infant botulism (4,12). An infant's gastrointestinal tract cannot destroy these spores (4). By the time an infant reaches 1 year of age, s/he will have enough bacteria in his/ her colon to keep the *Clostridium* spores from growing (4,23); an adult's intestinal tract has the ability to prevent the growth of clostridium spores (4,17). Generally, *Clostridium* poisoning from spores is found only in infants under 6 months of age; however, to be safe, stay away from honey until infants are 1 year of age (23).

Numerous sources recommend that processed foods containing honey not be fed to infants younger than 12 months of age (6,14,24,29); one source makes this recommendation but fails to specify an age (4). Even the honey in prepared foods could cause infant botulism (2) because the spores are still viable, unless a certain temperature is reached in the preparation process (4). In contrast, one source indicates that honey is acceptable as an ingredient in such processed foods as honey graham crackers (26). Another source says not to feed infants honey alone, in cooking or baking, or in prepared foods such as cookies, bread, honey graham crackers, peanut butter with honey, or yogurt with honey (2,23). One source says that if homemade infant foods need to be sweetened, then ordinary table sugar is a better choice than honey or corn syrup (12). Pacifiers should not be dipped in honey (14,23).

There is controversy regarding whether corn syrup should be avoided as well. Some sources indicate that corn syrup should not be fed to infants (29,30,47); however, one source (4) indicates that corn syrup and other syrups currently on the market are not sources of *Clostridium botulinum* spores and are not associated with infant botulism (4). Although the consumption of corn syrup has been associated with an increased risk of infant botulism as well, this link has not been established as clearly as the association with honey, and the risk is probably very small (12); nevertheless, it is prudent to avoid giving corn syrup to infants under 1 year of age (12). The corn syrup used in some infant formulas and jarred infant foods is not of concern because these products are heated sufficiently during processing to destroy bacterial spores (12).

B. Cow's Milk

The introduction of cow's milk should be delayed until after infants are 12 months of age (2,4,6,10,12,14,17,20,22,24,28–31,33,34,47,70,71). Feeding fresh cow's milk during the first year of life may be associated with the development of iron deficiency; furthermore, the renal solute load provided by cow's milk is undesirably high (33,34). Whole cow's milk is a poor source of iron, vitamin C, and other nutrients; in addition, it contains too much protein, sodium, and other nutrients for infants (2). Raw cow's and goat's milk could be contaminated with harmful substances that can make infants sick; thus, once milk is introduced to infants at 12 months of age, only pasteurized milk products should be used (2).

C. Mealtimes

Mealtimes should be enjoyable and relaxing for infants as well as parents or caregivers (4). When solid foods are first introduced to infants, it is important for the parent or caregiver to position him- or herself so that eye contact can be maintained with the infant as each spoonful of food is offered (30,31); this allows the parent or caregiver to see signals indicating interest (e.g., opening the mouth, leaning forward) or disinterest (e.g., leaning back, turning away, sealed lips) that the infant is displaying, so that they can discontinue the feeding at the earliest sign of satiety. The parent or caregiver should sit directly in front of the infant, offer the spoon straight ahead, and wait for the infant's mouth to open before putting the spoon to the infant's lips (4). Infants should be sitting up (31) in a sturdy high chair and safely secured to prevent falls (4,17). Table 5 provides tips from the U.S. Consumer Product Safety Commission on choosing a high chair and using it safely (64).

D. Choking

Choking is a major cause of fatality in infants and young children (4). Although objects such as safety pins and coins cause choking, food is responsible for most incidents (5). Never leave an infant alone and unattended while eating (4,17,23); infants must be carefully observed when eating (14). Infants do not know their own limitations and can easily choke from eating too quickly or stuffing too much food in their mouths at one time (17). If there are older children in the house, make sure they do not try to feed an infant what they are eating (17). Avoid feeding infants or young children foods or pieces of food that are the size of a marble; foods this size can be swallowed whole and could become lodged in an infant or child's throat and cause choking (2). Soft breads such as white bread can be a hazard because they can

Table 5 Tips from the U.S. Consumer Product Safety Commission on Choosing a High Chair and Using it Safely

Choosing a high chair
- Make sure the high chair has a waist strap and a second strap that goes between the infant's legs.
- The straps should not be attached to the tray.
- The tray must lock securely.
- The legs of the high chair should be spread far enough apart at the bottom so that the high chair does not tip over easily.
- A locking device on folding high chairs will keep the chair from collapsing.

Using a high chair
- Always buckle in the infant to keep him/her from falling or sliding under the tray, where he or she could be hurt.
- Never leave an infant alone when he or she is in the high chair.
- Lock the tray securely in place after making sure the infant's hands are out of the way.

Source: Adapted from Ref. 64.

turn into a pasty glob in an infant's mouth; breads should be toasted and cut up before being given to an infant (12). A food's potential to cause choking is usually related to one or more of the following characteristics: size, shape, and consistency (4). Regarding size, both large and small pieces of food may cause choking. Small, hard pieces of food, such as nuts and seeds and small pieces of raw hard vegetables, may be swallowed before being chewed properly and may get into the airway. Larger pieces of food may be more difficult to chew and are more likely to completely block the airway if they are inhaled (4). Regarding shape, food items shaped like a cylinder or sphere, such as whole grapes, hot dog-shaped products, and round candies, are more likely to cause choking because they block the airway more completely than other shapes (4). Regarding consistency, infants can choke on foods that are (1) smooth, slippery, or firm and can slide down the throat before chewing, such as hard candy, hot dog-like products, peanuts, large pieces of fruit with skin, whole pieces of canned fruit, raw peas, and whole grapes; (2) dry or hard foods that are difficult to chew and easy to swallow whole, such as popcorn, chips, nuts, seeds, small hard pieces of raw vegetable, cookies, and pretzels; and (3) tough or sticky foods that do not break apart readily and are hard to remove from the airway, such as peanut butter, tough meat, dried fruit, and sticky candy like caramels (4,6,29).

Infants will gag when food goes to the back of their tongues before they are ready to swallow, and their gag reflex shoves the food back out again (23). Gagging is a normal part of learning to eat, and a safety mechanism to help prevent choking. An infant will probably go on eating and not get upset about gagging if the parent/caregiver does not get upset; however, if the parent/caregiver becomes alarmed and reacts, the infant can become frightened and the gagging may become worse. Although gagging is to be expected, choking is dangerous. Choking occurs when an infant takes a breath at the same time food moves past the end of the windpipe; the food plugs up the windpipe and the infant cannot breathe. If an infant is getting enough air through his/her throat to cough, s/he is probably okay; however, if an infant makes no sound or only a squeaky, whistling, inhaling sound, s/he may be choking. To help prevent choking, stay with infants while they eat, keep things calm, and have the infant sit up straight and face forward (23). Table 6 provides tips to decrease an infant's risk of choking.

E. Home-Prepared Versus Commercially Prepared Infant Foods

Infants can be fed either home-prepared or commercially prepared infant foods (2,4,6,12,14,17,23,26,28). Commercially prepared infant foods are

Table 6 Tips to Decrease an Infant's Risk of Choking

- Offer foods that are the appropriate texture for an infant's development.
- Prepare food so that it is soft and does not require much chewing; cook foods until soft enough to pierce easily with a fork.
- Puree, blend, grind, or mash and moisten food for young infants. For older infants close to 1 year old who can chew, cut foods into small pieces (cubes of food no larger than 1/4 inch) or thin slices that can be chewed easily.
- Cut round foods, such as cooked carrots, into short strips rather than round, coin-shaped pieces. Cut foods such as whole grapes, cherries, and berries into quarters, and remove the pits before feeding. Large pieces of food can become lodged in an infant's throat and cause choking.
- Remove all bones from poultry and meat and especially fish before cooking. Remove hard pits and seeds from vegetables and fruits.
- Replace foods that may cause choking with a safe substitute. For example, offer meat chopped up or mashed hamburger instead of hot dogs or pieces of tough meat.
- Cook and finely grind or mash whole grain kernels of wheat, barley, rice, etc. before feeding them to infants.
- Do not feed whole nuts or seeds or nut/seed butters to infants. Whole nuts and seeds can lodge in the throat or get caught in the windpipe. Nut/seed butters can stick to the roof of an infant's mouth.
- Closely supervise an infant's meals and snacks. Never leave an infant alone when he or she is eating.
- Make sure an infant is still and in an upright position during meals and snacks.
- Feed small portions, and encourage infants to eat slowly.
- Maintain a calm atmosphere during meals and snacks; avoid too much excitement or disruption during eating. The risk of choking increases when an infant is walking, talking, crying, laughing, or playing.
- Hold an infant when feeding him/her a bottle. Never "prop" a bottle for an infant at any age. Never leave a bottle in an infant's crib or playpen. Although older infants can hold the bottle while feeding, they should be sitting in a parent's or caregiver's arms or in a high chair or similar chair, and the bottle should be taken away when the feeding is finished.
- Make sure the hole in the nipple of the infant's bottle is not too large to prevent the liquid from flowing through too rapidly.
- Make sure that crackers, toast, or biscuits are eaten when the infant is in an upright position. An infant who eats these foods while lying down could choke on crumbs.
- Avoid giving an infant pain relief medicine for teething before mealtimes or snacks because it may interfere with chewing.
- Examples of acceptable finger foods that present a lower risk of choking include:
  - Small pieces of ripe, soft, peeled banana, peach, or pear
  - Small strips of toast or bread
  - Cooked macaroni
  - Thin slices of mild cheese

Table 6 Continued

○ Soft, cooked, chopped vegetables, such as string beans or potatoes
○ Teething biscuits
○ Soft, moist, finely chopped meat.
• In summary, do not feed infants any of the following foods:
   ○ Tough meat
   ○ Fish with bones
   ○ Hot dogs, sausages, or toddler hot dogs (unless cut into short strips, not round slices)
   ○ Large chunks of cheese
   ○ Whole beans (mash them first)
   ○ Peanuts or other nuts and seeds
   ○ Peanut butter and other nut/seed butters
   ○ Cooked or raw whole-kernel corn
   ○ Plain wheat germ
   ○ Cookies
   ○ Granola bars
   ○ Crackers or breads with seeds, nuts, or whole grain kernels such as wheat berries
   ○ Whole grain kernels
   ○ Raw vegetable pieces or hard pieces of partially cooked vegetables
   ○ Whole pieces of canned fruit (cut them up instead)
   ○ Hard pieces of raw fruit such as apple
   ○ Whole grapes, berries, cherries, melon balls, or cherry and grape tomatoes (cut into quarters and remove pits first)
   ○ Uncooked raisins and other dried fruit
   ○ Potato chips, corn chips, pretzels, cheese twists, and similar snack foods
   ○ Round, hard, or sticky candy or chewing gum
   ○ Marshmallows
   ○ Popcorn

Source: Adapted from Refs. 2 and 4.

convenient but more costly than home-prepared infant foods (23,26). Parents who prepare homemade infant foods must be especially careful to use safe food-handling and storage procedures (12). Infants should never be fed home-canned foods, because these foods may contain harmful bacteria if improperly canned (2). As discussed previously, there is concern about high levels of nitrates in certain home-prepared vegetables. One advantage to preparing infant food at home is that it exposes an infant to what the family normally eats (17). If commercially prepared infant foods are used, be sure to begin with foods for beginners, and do not offer infants food for toddlers, which often contains chunks, until they are experienced eaters (17). Tips for purchasing, serving, and storing commercially prepared infant foods are found in Table 7.

Table 7 Tips for Purchasing, Serving, and Storing Commercially Prepared Infant Foods

Remember to wash your hands before handling any food. (Refer to Table 11 for hand-washing tips.)

When you *buy* commercially prepared infant foods:
- Check the "use-by" date on infant food jars; do not buy or use the food if the date has passed.
- Buy infant food jars that are clean on the outside and do not have a broken vacuum seal. If the button on the center of the top is popped out, the seal is broken.
- More nutrition, ounce for ounce, is provided by single-ingredient infant foods, such as single vegetables, fruits, and meats, than by infant food combination dinners and infant food desserts. Plain meats and plain vegetables or fruit can be mixed together if an infant likes the taste. Serve fruit instead of an infant food dessert.
- Read the ingredient list on the infant food label to make sure that the first ingredient listed, which is present in the largest amount, is vegetable, fruit, or meat. Also, read the ingredient list to determine if salt, butter, oil, cream, sugar, or corn syrup has been added.

When you *serve* commercially prepared infant food:
- Check the "use-by" date on infant food jars; do not use the food if the date has passed.
- Wash the lid and jar of infant food before opening.
- Make sure the jar lid is sealed and has not been broken before opening it. You should hear a "pop" or "whoosh" sound when you open the lid of the jar if the seal has not been broken.
- Do not tap the jar lid or bang it to open it because this could break glass chips into the food.
- Remove enough food from the jar for one feeding and place it in a dish for feeding. If you feed directly from the jar, enzymes and bacteria from the infant's saliva contaminate the food and may cause spoilage.
- If needed, warm the infant's food on a stove or in a food warmer; stir the food and test its temperature before feeding. Do not heat infant food in jars in a microwave oven; the food can get very hot and could burn the infant's mouth.
- Once infant cereal has been mixed with liquid, serve it immediately. Do not save leftovers for another meal.
- Throw away any leftover food remaining in the dish; never save leftovers from the infant's dish for another meal.

When you *store* commercially prepared infant food:
- After opening a jar, replace the lid. Label the jar with the date and time it was opened, and place the jar in the refrigerator. Use the food within 2 days, except for infant meats and egg yolks, which should be used within 24 hours. Throw out foods not used within those times.

Table 7 Continued

- Regularly check to make sure the refrigerator temperature is cold enough, 40°F or lower, to keep the food safe.
- Check the "use-by" date on the jar when storing unopened jars. Throw out the food if the date has passed.
- Store unopened jars of infant food and boxes of infant cereal at room temperature in a cool, dry place, such as a kitchen cabinet or pantry—not in the refrigerator, car, garage, or outdoors.
- Rotate the stored jars and boxes so that you use the food previously purchased prior to using the food purchased more recently.
- Most manufacturers warn against freezing regular infant food; although it is safe to do so, it changes the texture.

Source: Adapted from Refs. 2, 12, and 17.

Tips for preparing, storing, serving, and reheating home-prepared infant foods are found in Table 8.

F. Nutrition Labels for Commercially Prepared Infant Food

Nutrition labeling is required for infant and toddler food (29). Manufacturers may include information regarding the content of additional nutrients, such as zinc, potassium, and B-complex vitamins, on the nutrition label of foods for infants and children under 2 years of age; information about other essential vitamins and minerals is mandatory only when they are added to enrich or fortify a food or when a claim is made about them on a label (2). The column for "Percent Daily Values" is not on these labels, and reference to the 2,000-calorie diet is omitted as well (29). By law, nutrition labels of foods for children less than 2 years of age cannot include information on calories from fat or on saturated fat and cholesterol (29,72). The section for "% Daily Value" at the bottom of the label shows how a food fits into the overall daily diet of the infant; it shows what percent of the nutrient is provided from one serving of the food to meet the daily dietary needs of the infant (2). The serving size is the basis on which manufacturers declare the nutrient amounts and % Daily Values on the label; it is the amount of food customarily eaten at one time (2).

G. Microwave Ovens

Adults may prefer that certain foods be served warm, but infants have no such preferences (12). Infant food should never be served hot; if it is heated at all, it should be warmed only to body temperature (12,14,17). If infant food

Table 8   Tips for Preparing, Storing, Serving, and Reheating
Home-Prepared Infant Foods

Remember to wash your hands before handling any food. (Refer to Table 11 for
hand-washing tips.)

Before you *prepare* infant food:
- Wash all bowls, utensils, pots and pans, equipment (e.g., blender, food mill, food
  processor, infant food grinder, cutting board), sink, and counters in hot, soapy
  water; rinse and sanitize them. Allow to air-dry.

When you *prepare* infant food:
- Start with good-quality food; use fresh food if possible. Check ingredients on
  the ingredient label of commercially canned or frozen foods. Prepare foods for
  an infant immediately before use, and avoid using leftover food.
- Wash fruits and vegetables well and remove peels, seeds, and pits before
  cooking. Steaming is a good cooking technique because it minimizes vitamin
  losses.
- Do not feed home-prepared beets, carrots, collard greens, spinach, or turnips
  to infants under 6 months of age.
- Remove bones, fat, skin, and gristle from meats, poultry, and fish. Meats,
  poultry, fish, dried beans or peas, and egg yolks should be well cooked. Good
  cooking methods include baking, boiling, broiling, poaching, and steaming.
  Call USDA's Meat and Poultry Hotline at 1-800-535-4555 for information
  regarding safe food handling, including what temperature to bring meat,
  poultry, and fish to during cooking. Avoid microwaving meats before pureeing
  them because the meat will become the consistency of sawdust.
- Cook foods until they are soft and tender. For younger infants, use a blender,
  food processor, fine mesh strainer, infant food grinder, or food mill to puree
  food to the appropriate texture; add breast milk, formula, cooking water, or
  water for a thinner consistency. For older infants, foods can be mashed with a
  fork or chopped finely.
- Do not add seasonings such as salt, butter, margarine, lard, oil, cream, sugar,
  syrups, gravy, sauces, or fat drippings to an infant's food.
- Never add honey to an infant's food.
- Do not use home-canned food, food from dented, rusted, bulging or leaking
  cans or jars, or food from cans or jars without labels.

When you *store* home-prepared infant food:
- Immediately after cooking, refrigerate or freeze freshly cooked food to be
  stored. Label the container with the date and time it was prepared. Do not let
  the food sit at room temperature; harmful germs can grow in the food at room
  temperature. Throw out any food left at room temperature for 2 hours or
  more, including serving time.
- Be sure to place foods to be stored in the refrigerator in a clean container with a
  tight-fitting lid. Regularly check to make sure the refrigerator temperature is
  cold enough (40°F or below) to keep food safe.

Table 8 Continued

- Use refrigerated foods within 2 days, except for meats, poultry, fish, and egg yolk, which should be used within 24 hours. Throw out foods not used within those times.
- To freeze infant food, place 1–2 tablespoons of pureed food either in spots on a clean cookie sheet or into sections of a clean ice cube tray. Cover the food with plastic wrap or foil. When frozen, place the food pieces into a covered freezer container or tightly closed plastic bag in the freezer. Label and date the containers or bags. Use frozen foods within 1 month.
- Regularly check to make sure the freezer temperature is cold enough (0°F or below) to keep food safe.

When you *serve* home-prepared infant food:
- Serve freshly cooked food to an infant right after preparing it and allowing the food to cool to lukewarm; before feeding, stir the food and test its temperature.
- Throw away any leftover food remaining in the infant's dish; do not put it back in the refrigerator or freezer.

When you *reheat* home-prepared infant food:
- Completely reheat refrigerated or frozen home-prepared infant food to at least 165°F before feeding. Allow food to cool to lukewarm. Stir the food and test its temperature to make sure it is not too hot or too cold before serving it to an infant.
- Thaw frozen foods in the refrigerator, under cold running water, or when reheating the food. Never defrost infant foods by setting them out at room temperature or in a bowl of standing water. Germs can grow in food sitting at room temperature.
- Throw out uneaten leftover food remaining in the dish.
- Do not refreeze infant food that has thawed. Label the container with the date and time it was removed from the freezer. Store thawed food in the refrigerator, and use it within 2 days, except for meats, poultry, or fish, which should be used within 24 hours. Throw out foods not used within those times.

Source: Adapted from Refs. 2 and 26.

has been heated, the parent or caregiver should use extreme caution, especially if a microwave oven is used (12). Microwave heating is very uneven and hot spots can develop within a container of food (12,17,29); even if the container remains cool, the food may become hot enough to burn an infant (12,29). Some sources indicate that infant foods, whether solid or liquid, should never be heated in a microwave oven, because uneven heating can burn an infant (6,30); one source indicates that microwave ovens should never be used to warm breast milk or infant formula (4) while another source indicates that microwave ovens can overheat breast milk which can destroy some of its protective substances (29). Some sources indicate that infant foods may be heated in a microwave oven if caution is taken. According to the AAP, infant foods may be microwaved for a few seconds at reduced power (14). During heating in a microwave oven, stir the food and turn the dish often (29); after heating, allow the food to sit for a few minutes (29). Next, the food should be stirred thoroughly to eliminate hot spots (2,4,12,14,29), and the temperature should be checked before serving (2,4,29) by touching or tasting a bit of the food (12). Very thick infant foods, such as pureed or strained meats and egg yolks, can become superheated and splatter or explode (12,17); either avoid microwaving these infant foods (12) or remove them from the jar and heat them in a microwave-safe dish (17). Some sources indicate that commercially prepared infant foods should not be left in jars to heat in a microwave oven (2,4), although one source indicates this is fine as long as the jar is opened (29).

H. Vitamin–Mineral Supplements

Some may argue that no routine supplementation should be necessary because the human race has existed over the centuries on an infant diet of breast milk (9). According to one source, healthy infants who consume breast milk or formula along with a variety of solid foods, including good sources of iron and vitamins A and C, should not need supplemental vitamins and minerals (17). However, for several nutrients this may not be entirely true of the breast-fed infant, and there are some vitamin and mineral supplemental issues for formula-fed infants (9). After a one-time intramuscular dose of vitamin K at birth for both breast-fed and formula-fed infants to protect against hemorrhagic disease of the newborn, the nutrients of concern include iron, vitamin D, and fluoride (9). As indicated in the following paragraphs, controversy exists regarding supplementation of iron, vitamin D, and fluoride for infants, especially breast-fed infants.

1. Iron

Iron deficiency is the most common nutritional deficiency in the United States; young children are the most susceptible to iron deficiency due to an increased iron requirement related to rapid growth during the first 2 years of life, along with a relatively low iron content in most infant diets when iron is not added by supplementation or fortification (73). Of greatest concern among the major consequences of iron deficiency that have been studied is the evidence that significant iron deficiency adversely affects child development and behavior; the threat of irreversible developmental delay due to a temporary nutritional deficiency emphasizes the importance of prevention (73). Another consequence of iron deficiency is enhanced lead absorption; childhood lead poisoning is a well-documented cause of neurologic and developmental deficits, and iron deficiency appears to contribute to this problem directly and indirectly through increased absorption of lead (73).

The AAP has the following recommendations for the primary prevention of iron deficiency in breast-fed infants (73):

1. By 4–6 months of age, full-term breast-fed infants need an adequate source of iron that provides approximately 1 mg/kg per day, preferably from supplemental food. Iron-fortified infant cereal is a good source of iron for the initial introduction of solid foods containing iron. An average of two servings, with a serving equal to 1/2 ounce, or 15 g, of dry cereal, is needed to meet the daily iron requirement.
2. For full-term breast-fed infants who are unable to consume sufficient iron from dietary sources after 6 months of age, elemental iron, at 1 mg/kg per day, can be used.
3. For preterm or low-birth weight infants, an oral iron supplement of elemental iron in the form of drops once a day at 2–4 mg/kg per day at 1 month should be given until 12 months of age.
4. Only iron-fortified formula should be used for weaning or supplementing breast milk for infants younger than 12 months.

In contrast, Fomon (74) contends that breast-fed infants should receive a daily iron supplement to provide 7 mg of iron per day during the first 6 months of life and 7–10 mg of iron daily from 6 to 12 months of age. His rationale is that from a public health standpoint, it seems desirable to prevent the depletion of the infant's iron stores by beginning iron supplementation during the first few weeks of life (33,34). Furthermore, the advantage of deferring iron supplementation of breast-fed infants until 4–6 months of age has not been demonstrated (74).

The AAP has the following recommendations for the primary prevention of iron deficiency in formula-fed infants (73):

1. Only iron-fortified formula should be used during the first year of life for full-term and preterm infants, regardless of the age when infant formula is started.
2. Some believe that iron-fortified formula increases gastrointestinal symptoms; however, no scientific evidence supports this belief, so the use of non-iron-fortified formula for healthy infants is not justified. No common medical indication exists for the use of a low-iron formula.

According to Fomon (34) and Shevlov (5), when infants are fed iron-forti-fied formulas, no supplementation of the diet with vitamins or minerals is required.

The AAP has the following recommendations regarding solid foods and milk for the primary prevention of iron deficiency; the first two recommen-dations are more crucial for breast-fed infants to ensure adequate iron nutri-tion (73):

1. Iron-fortified infant cereal should be introduced by 4–6 months of age or when the infant is developmentally ready (i.e., able to sit up and swallow such food).
2. A good dietary source of iron for infants beyond iron-fortified infant cereal is strained meat; it can be introduced after 6 months of age or when the infant is developmentally ready to consume such food.
3. Avoid using regular cow's milk, goat's milk, or soy milk for the milk-based part of an infant's diet before 12 months of age.

Iron-fortified infant cereals should be encouraged during the first year of life, until infants' diets include foods with good sources of heme iron (9).

2. Vitamin D

The vitamin D content of breast milk is low, and rickets can occur in deeply pigmented breast-fed infants or in those with inadequate exposure to sunlight; thus, the AAP (75) and Fomon (34) recommend that breast-fed infants receive supplemental vitamin D at 400 IU per day. However, the need for supple-mental vitamin D in exclusively breast-fed infants is controversial, and some believe it is needed only for breast-fed infants who are particularly at risk. One source defines at-risk breast-fed infants as those with limited exposure to sunlight (20). Another source defines at-risk breast-fed infants as those who live in northern urban areas especially during the winter, are dark skinned, are kept covered due to cultural practices or beliefs, have little exposure to sunlight, or have mothers with inadequate intakes of vitamin D or little exposure to sunlight (9). Most infant formulas contain more than adequate amounts of vitamin D (75). As mentioned previously, Fomon contends that no vitamin or mineral supplementation is required for infants who are fed iron-fortified infant formula (34).

3. Fluoride

The presence of fluoride in the diet is one of the two major dietary factors that influence oral health; the other is the frequency of carbohydrate consumption

(76). The cornerstone of oral health is caries prevention, beginning at 6 months of age with an evaluation of dietary fluoride intake; fluoride supplementation is indicated for breast-fed and bottle-fed infants if the primary water source is suboptimally fluoridated (76). The American Dental Association, the AAP, and the American Academy of Pediatric Dentistry have approved a fluoride supplementation schedule aimed at populations drinking suboptimally fluoridated water; the schedule begins supplementation at 6 months of age (76). Health care professionals should know the fluoride content of the primary drinking water source before prescribing supplemental dietary fluoride. For infants and children 6 months of age to 3 years of age, supplemental fluoride at 0.25 mg per day is recommended if the fluoride concentration in the local water supply is under 0.3 ppm (76). In contrast, Fomon contends that no fluoride supplements are recommended for infants (34,77).

VII. HEALTH PROMOTION AND DISEASE PREVENTION

A. Dietary Guidelines for Infants

The fifth edition of Nutrition and Your Health: Dietary Guidelines for Americans was released in 2000; it provides three basic messages and 10 guidelines to promote health for adults and children over the age of 2 years (78); these guidelines are not appropriate for infants or young children under 2 years of age. Unfortunately, it is very easy for parents and caregivers to confuse reasonable dietary guidance for adults and older children with good feeding practices for infants (35,72). Infants require separate dietary guidelines, for several reasons. The first year of an infant's life is characterized by rapid growth and changes in body composition; birth weight is doubled by 6 months of age and tripled by 1 year of age in most healthy infants (79). Although young infants have a very large energy requirement, their renal and gastrointestinal systems are not equipped to handle the addition of solid foods until 4–6 months of age (79). Breast milk and infant formulas are ideal foods for the first months of life. As an infant develops normally and moves through the transitional and modified adult periods of infant feeding (discussed in "Periods of Infant Feeding" under "Guidelines for Introducing Solid Foods" Section), there is an important need to provide developmentally appropriate and nutritious foods in positive mealtime experiences; this will enable the infant to continue to achieve normal growth and development, learn to accept and enjoy a wider variety of nutritious foods, and begin the transition from dependent to independent feeding (72,79). The Dietary Guidelines for Infants are scientifically sound as well as practical, and they offer a sensible approach to the special concerns of infant nutrition (72,79). Table 9 lists the Dietary Guidelines for Infants, along with a brief rationale for each.

Table 9 Dietary Guidelines for Infants

Build to a variety of foods.
Adults can meet their daily requirements by choosing a variety of foods from each of
the basic food groups. In contrast, infants must slowly build dietary variety as they
move from the exclusive nursing period (when they consume only breast milk or
formula) to the transitional period (when they begin to consume solid foods in
addition to breast milk or formula). Parents and caregivers who offer increasing
dietary variety as their infants are developmentally ready will help them learn to
accept and enjoy a variety of nutritious foods as they move into the modified adult
period (when most of their intake comes from table foods) and beyond.

Pay attention to your baby's appetite to avoid overfeeding or underfeeding.
An infant's appetite is the single best indicator of adequate energy intake. Parents and
caregivers who pay attention to their infant's hunger and satiety signals or cues will
avoid underfeeding or overfeeding their infant. Because eating patterns established
during infancy may carry over into later life, these guidelines emphasize helping
infants learn to follow their own internal signals of hunger and satiety.

Babies need fat.
Restricted-fat and low-fat diets are not appropriate for infants and children under the
age of 2 years. Infants have small stomachs, yet they require energy-dense foods to
support their rapid metabolic and growth rates. Fat is an excellent source of calories
and helps the brain and nervous system develop. Nutrition priorities during infancy
should reflect the promotion of growth and development instead of the prevention
of degenerative disease in later life.

Introduce fruits, vegetables, and grains, but don't overdo high-fiber foods.
The smaller stomach size of infants, along with their large requirements for energy and
minerals, demands a high-calorie, nutrient-dense diet. The bulking effect of fiber
that brings about a feeling of satiety supplies few calories and is antithetic to the
needs of rapidly growing infants. Although it is important to introduce infants to
fruits, vegetables, and grains, high-fiber foods (i.e., those with 3 + grams of fiber per
serving) should not be overdone. Infants who eat a variety of fruits, vegetables, and
grains will get all the fiber they need.

Babies need sugars in moderation.
Sugars are a readily metabolizable, efficient energy source for active, rapidly growing
infants. Parents and caregivers who consistently offer a variety of appropriate food
choices for a healthful diet will find that their children can learn to moderate their
sugar intake in the context of a varied diet and to develop healthful eating habits.

Babies need sodium in moderation.
It is neither safe nor reasonable to try to eliminate sodium from the infant diet.
However, controlling excessive sodium intake is important. Parents and caregivers
can offer a variety of seasoned and unseasoned foods so that their older infants and
children can learn to moderate their sodium intake in the context of a varied diet.

Choose foods with iron, zinc, and calcium.
Intakes of iron, zinc, and calcium are surprisingly low in the diets of many children
under 2 years of age; thus, a separate guideline that emphasizes these minerals is
warranted. Parents and caregivers should provide foods that contain bioavailable

Table 9 Continued

sources of these minerals during the first 2 years of life. Iron is found in breast milk, iron-fortified infant formula, iron-fortified infant cereals, meats and poultry, and peas, lentils, and soybeans. Nonheme iron absorption is enhanced by ascorbic acid and citric acid in juices and fruits; amino acids in meat, fish, and poultry; and heme iron in meat, fish, and poultry. Nonheme iron absorption is inhibited by polyphenols in tannins in tea; phosphates in cow's milk and egg yolk; and phytates in bran and whole grain cereals. Zinc is found in breast milk, infant formula, zinc-fortified cereals, oat cereals, meats and poultry, wheat germ, egg yolk, and cheddar cheese. Calcium is found in breast milk, infant formula, calcium-fortified infant cereals, calcium-fortified soy milk, and any dairy products.

Source: Adapted from Refs. 35 and 72.

B. Healthy People 2010 Nutrition Objectives for Infants

Table 10 includes Healthy People 2010 (80) objectives regarding nutrition for infants up to 12 months of age. The objectives address the proportion of mothers who breast-feed, growth retardation, iron deficiency, and dental caries.

C. Dental Health

Diet in early life may be seen as the foundation for a child's dental health (81). The first tooth usually erupts at about 6 months of age, which is the same time that weaning should have begun; it is well recognized that weaning may affect dental health through its influence on caries (81). *Early childhood caries* (ECC; previously called *baby bottle tooth decay* or *maxillary anterior caries*) is defined as rampant dental caries in infants and toddlers (82). ECC in infants and preschool children appear to be related to the feeding behaviors of prolonged bottle- or breast-feeding (82); it has been consistently linked to the habit of giving sweetened liquid such as formula, milk, juice, or soda pop in bottles, or giving pacifiers dipped in a sweet agent such as honey or jam (81). When an infant or toddler is routinely given a bottle filled with a sweetened liquid at bedtime or naptime, the liquid pools around the teeth during sleep, saliva flow decreases, and the child may continue to suck liquid over an extended period of time. Older infants and toddlers are also at high risk if they hold their own bottle and have access to it anytime throughout the

Table 10 Healthy People 2010 Nutrition Objectives Related to Infants Aged 0–12 Months

16-19. Increase the proportion of mothers who breast-feed their babies.

Objective	Increase in mothers who breast-feed	2010 target (%)	1998 baseline (%)
16-19a.	In early postpartum period	75	64
16-19b.	At 6 months	50	29
16-19c.	At 1 year	25	16

19-4. Reduce growth retardation (defined as height for age below the fifth percentile in the age–gender appropriate population using the 1977 NCHS/CDC growth charts) among low-income children under age 5 years.
Target: 5%   Baseline: 8%

19-12. Reduce iron deficiency among young children* and females of childbearing age.

Objective	Reduction in iron deficiency	2010 target (%)	1998 baseline (%)
19-12a.	Children ages 1–2 years	5	9
19-12b.	Children ages 3–4 years	1	4
19-12c.	Nonpregnant females ages 12–49 years	7	11

* Iron deficiency can be prevented among young children by teaching families about child nutrition, including promoting breast-feeding of infants, with exclusive breast-feeding for 4–6 months; the use of iron-fortified formulas when formulas are used; delayed introduction of cow's milk until age 12 months; and age-appropriate introduction of iron-rich solid foods, such as iron-fortified infant cereals and pureed meats, and foods that enhance iron absorption, such as vitamin C-rich fruits, vegetables, or juices.

21-1a. Reduce the proportion of young children with dental caries experience in their primary teeth.**
Target: 11%   Baseline: 18%
** The earliest opportunity to prevent dental decay occurs during prenatal counseling about diet, oral hygiene practices, appropriate use of fluorides, and the transmission of bacteria from parents to children. Early childhood caries, sometimes referred to as *baby bottle tooth decay* or *nursing caries*, can be a devastating condition, often requiring thousands of dollars and a hospital visit with general anesthesia for treatment.

Source: Adapted from Ref. 80.

day. The primary strategy to prevent ECC is education. Parents and caregivers should be encouraged not to allow infants and toddlers to drink from a bottle with any liquid that contains carbohydrates (i.e., juice, breast milk, formula) when going to sleep or for prolonged periods of time during the day (76). Breast-feeding mothers should be advised about the increased risk for dental caries if they allow the infant to sleep with them and nurse on demand

(76). Pacifers dipped in a sweet agent should not be given to infants or toddlers. The consumption and especially the frequency of sugar-containing food and drink should be reduced, regarded as "occasional" foods, and consumed at mealtimes (81).

The parent or caregiver should use an infant-sized toothbrush or a moist cloth and a simple scrubbing action on a daily basis to clean the infant's teeth that have erupted at 6 months of age; fluoridated toothpaste should not be introduced until around 2 years of age (76). Infants and young children cannot spit the toothpaste out effectively; thus, there is a potential risk of their ingesting too much fluoride, especially if large amounts of fluoridated toothpaste are used (81). As mentioned previously, a fluoride supplement is recommended for infants and children 6 months of age to 3 years of age if the fluoride in the local water supply is low (76).

D. Food Safety

Food-borne disease—what most people call *food poisoning*—is the number-one food hazard in the United States; most cases of food poisoning are attributable to mishandling or improper storage of food by the people who prepare it, either at home or in a food-service establishment (12). Microbial contamination of foods is even more of a concern for infants than it is for older children and adults (2,12). Infants tend to become more severely ill from food-borne diseases than adults, and they are at risk for dangerous, even fatal, complications (12). Unsanitary food conditions can cause serious problems; thus, general cleanliness, proper food selection, sanitary food preparation, and proper food storage are key to preventing illnesses related to food contamination in infants (2). Hand-washing is the easiest, least expensive, and most effective way to stop the spread of germs that cause illness (2). In addition to washing their own hands, it is advisable for parents and caregivers to wash an infant's hands and face before s/he eats (4). Table 11 provides tips for washing hands.

The Fight BAC!® campaign of the Partnership for Food Safety Education is a public education campaign focused on safe food handling (83). The partnership, which was formed in 1997, is a public–private coalition dedicated to educating the public about safe food handling to help reduce food-borne illness; members represent industry, government groups, consumer groups, and alliances with corporate America. The goal of the Fight BAC!® campaign is to educate consumers on four simple steps they can take to fight food-borne bacteria and reduce their risk of food-borne illness (83); Table 12 provides more details regarding these four steps.

Table 11 Hand-Washing Tips

Wash your hands thoroughly *before* you:
- Bottle-feed an infant
- Handle, prepare, serve, or touch food or bottles
- Handle food utensils and set the table
- Touch raw meat, poultry, or fish
- Eat, drink, or feed food to infants
- Put away clean dishes
- Give medication

Wash your hands thoroughly *after* you:
- Handle raw meat, poultry, fish, or eggs
- Change an infant's diaper and/or clothing
- Use the bathroom
- Handle an infant, child, or person who is ill
- Come in contact with any bodily fluids, such as soiled diapers, urine, feces, blood, vomit, mucus, spit, or breast milk
- Wipe noses, mouths, bottoms, sores, or cuts
- Get your hands dirty or have been cleaning an infant, a room, a potty chair, toys, or other objects
- Give medication
- Sneeze or cough into tissues or your hands
- Handle pets, or other animals, or garbage
- Have been playing or working outside

Follow these steps *when* washing your hands:
1. Wet your hands with warm running water. Add soap.
2. Wash all surfaces of your hands. Rub vigorously for at least 20 seconds. Wash carefully between your fingers, around the tops and palms of your hands, over your wrists, and under your nails using a clean nail brush.
3. Rinse your hands well under warm running water. Leave the water running while you dry your hands.
4. Use a clean, disposable paper towel to dry your hands.
5. Use the disposable paper towel held in your hands to turn off the faucet instead of your clean bare hands.

Source: Adapted from Ref. 2.

E. Dietary Reference Intakes

The new Dietary Reference Intakes (DRIs) replace and expand the former series of RDAs that have been published since 1941 by the Food and Nutrition Board of the National Academy Sciences and the Recommended Nutrient Intakes (RNIs) of Canada (84). To date, five reports (85–89) have

Table 12 Four Steps to Fight Food-Borne Bacteria and Reduce the Risk of Food-Borne Illness from the Fight BAC!® Campaign

Clean: Wash hands and surfaces often.
- Wash hands with hot soapy water before preparing food.
- Wash hands with hot soapy water after using the bathroom, changing diapers, or handling animals.
- To wash hands: Use warm water to moisten hands, apply soap, and rub hands together for 20 seconds before rinsing thoroughly.
- Wash countertops, cutting boards, utensils, and knives with hot soapy water after preparing each food item and before preparing the next food item.
- Use plastic or other nonporous cutting boards. Wash cutting boards in the dishwasher or in hot soapy water after use.
- Consider using paper towels to dry hands and clean kitchen surfaces. If cloth towels are used, wash them often in hot water in the washing machine.

Separate: Don't cross-contaminate.
- Keep raw meat, poultry, and seafood separate from other foods in grocery carts.
- Store raw meat, poultry, and seafood on the bottom shelf of the refrigerator so juices do not drip onto other foods.
- If possible, use one cutting board for raw meats and another for other items such as fruits, vegetables, and breads.
- Wash hands, cutting boards, dishes, and utensils with hot soapy water after they come in contact with raw meat, poultry, or seafood.
- Do not place cooked food on a plate or serving dish that previously held raw meat, poultry, or seafood.

Cook: Cook to proper temperatures.
- To make sure that meat, poultry, casseroles, etc. are cooked all the way through, use a clean meat thermometer.
- Cook roasts and steaks to at least 145°F; cook whole poultry to 180°F.
- Cook ground beef to at least 160°F. Do not eat ground beef that is still pink inside.
- Cook eggs until the white and yolk are firm, not runny.
- Do not eat foods that contain raw eggs or only partially cooked eggs.
- Cook fish until it is opaque and flakes easily with a fork.
- When microwaving foods, make sure there are no cold spots by stirring and rotating food for even heating.
- Reheat sauces, soups, and gravies to a boil. Heat other leftovers thoroughly to at least 165°F.

Chill: Refrigerate promptly.
- Set your refrigerator at 40°F and the freezer at 0°F; check them regularly to make sure they are working properly.
- Refrigerate or freeze prepared foods and leftovers within 2 hours or sooner.
- Defrost food in the refrigerator, under cold running water, or in the microwave, but never at room temperature.

Table 12 Continued

• Marinate foods in the refrigerator.
• Divide large amounts of leftovers into small, shallow containers for quick cooling in the refrigerator.
• With turkeys and other stuffed meats, remove the stuffing and refrigerate it in a separate container.
• Avoid packing the refrigerator because cool air must circulate to keep food safe.

Source: Adapted from Ref. 83.

provided DRIs for macronutrients, vitamins, and minerals, and one report has provided guidance on using the DRIs for dietary assessment (90). Table 13 provides functions, selected food sources, and DRIs for macronutrients for infants 0–6 months and 7–12 months of age. Table 14 provides functions, selected food sources, and DRIs for vitamins and minerals for infants 0–6 months and 7–12 months of age.

VIII. COMPLEMENTARY FEEDINGS OF INFANTS IN DEVELOPING COUNTRIES

The lack of access to adequate nutrition, basic sanitation, and health care in developing countries has an adverse impact on the physical and mental development of infants and young children; these inadequacies are exacerbated by poor breast-feeding and complementary feeding practices, food insecurity, and a high prevalence of diarrhea and respiratory infections (91). These issues impact recommendations for feeding infants in developing countries. The process of introducing foods other than breast milk into an infant's diet is referred to as complementary feeding (60,92–95) in developing countries. Current recommendations for infants in developing countries are to feed breast milk alone for at least 4 months and until 6 months of age if possible (60) and that the potential benefits of waiting until 6 months of age to introduce complementary foods outweigh any potential risks (92); breast-feeding is to continue until 2 years of age or later (92). The consequences of introducing complementary foods too early to infants in developing countries include increased diarrheal and allergic diseases due to intestinal immaturity, decreased breast milk production due to complementary foods displacing breast-feeding, and malnutrition due to diarrheal disease (79). The consequences of introducing complementary foods too late to infants in developing countries include growth failure because breast milk alone becomes calorically inadequate, depressed immunity due to inadequate energy and protein intake, increased diarrheal disease due to depressed immunity, mal-

Table 13 Dietary Reference Intakes for Macronutrients for Infants

Nutrient	Function	Selected food sources	0–6 months RDA/*AI*[a] (g/day)	0–6 months AMDR[b]	7–12 months RDA/*AI*[a] (g/day)	7–12 months AMDR[b]
Carbohydrate (total digestible)	RDA is based on role as primary source of energy for the brain, while AMDR[b] is based on role in maintaining body weight (in kilocalories)	The major types of carbohydrate are starch and sugar. Grains (e.g., rice, pasta, breads) and starchy vegetables (e.g., corn, potatoes) are sources of starch. Sugars are found naturally in fruits and fruit juices and are added to soft drinks, candy, and desserts	*60*	ND[c]	*95*	ND
Total fiber	Improves laxation, reduces risk of coronary heart disease, and assists in maintaining normal blood glucose levels	Includes dietary fiber naturally present in grains (e.g, oats, wheat, unmilled rice) and functional fiber synthesized or isolated from plants or animals	ND		ND	
Total fat	Energy source whose presence in the diet increases the absorption	Butter, margarine, vegetable oils, whole milk, visible fats on	*31*		*30*	

	Function	Food sources				
	of fat-soluble vitamins and their precursors, such as vitamin A and pro-vitamin A carotinoids	meat and poultry products, invisible fat in fish, shellfish, some plant products (such as seeds and nuts), and bakery products				
n-6 polyunsaturated fatty acids (linoleic acid)	Essential component of structural membrane lipids, involved with cell signaling, and precursor of eicosanoids; required for normal skin function	Nuts, seeds, and vegetable oils (e.g., soybean, safflower, corn)	4.4	ND	4.6	ND
n-3 polyunsaturated fatty acids (α-linolenic acid)	Involved in neurological development and growth; precursor of eicosanoids	Vegetable oils (e.g., soybean, canola, flaxseed), fish oils, fatty fish, and small amounts in meat and eggs	0.5	ND	0.5	ND
Saturated and *trans* fatty acids, and cholesterol	No required role in the body other than as an energy source; amounts needed by the body can be synthesized from other sources	Saturated fatty acids are present in animal fats (e.g., meat fats, butter fat) and coconut and palm kernel oils. Sources of cholesterol include animal products, especially liver and egg yolks. Sources of *trans* fatty acids include foods	ND		ND	

Table 13 Continued

Nutrient	Function	Selected food sources	0–6 months		7–12 months	
			RDA/*AI*[a] (g/day)	AMDR[b]	RDA/*AI*[a] (g/day)	AMDR[b]
		containing hydrogenated or partially hydrogenated vegetable shortenings (e.g., stick margarine)				
Protein and amino acids[d]	The major structural component of all cells in the body; functions as enzymes, in membranes, as transport carriers, and as some hormones; proteins are broken down into amino acids, which are the building blocks of	Proteins from animal sources (e.g., meat, poultry, fish, eggs, milk, cheese, yogurt) are complete proteins (i.e., they provide all nine indispensable amino acids). Proteins from plants, legumes,	*9.1*	ND	**13.5**	ND

these structural and
functional compounds;
nine of the amino acids
are indispensable (i.e.,
must be provided in the
diet); the body can make
the other amino acids
needed to synthesize
specific structures from
other amino acids

grains, nuts, seeds,
and vegetables are
incomplete proteins
(i.e., they lack one or
more of the
indispensable amino
acids)

[a] Recommended Dietary Allowances (RDAs) are in **bold** type and Adequate Intakes (AIs) are in *ital* type; both may be used as goals for individual intake.

[b] Acceptable Macronutrient Distribution Range (AMDR) is a range of intake for a particular energy source that is associated with reduced risk of chronic diseases while providing intakes of essential nutrients. If an individual consumes in excess of the AMDR, there is a potential of increasing the risk of chronic diseases and/or insufficient intakes of essential nutrients.

[c] ND = Not Determinable due to lack of data of adverse effects in this age group and concern with regard to lack of ability to handle excess amounts. Source of intake should be from food only, to prevent high levels of intake.

[d] RDA/AI is based on 1.5 g/kg/day for infants.

Source: Adapted from the Dietary Reference Intakes: Macronutrients table at www.nal.usda.gov/fnic.

Table 14 Dietary Reference Intakes for Vitamins and Minerals for Infants

Nutrient	Function	Selected food sources	0–6 months		7–12 months	
			RDA/*AI*[a]	UL[b]	**RDA**/*AI*[a]	UL[b]
Biotin	Coenzyme in synthesis of fat, glycogen, and amino acids	Liver and small amounts in fruits and meats	*5 µg/d*	ND[c]	*6 µg/d*	ND
Choline	Precursor for acetylcholine, phospholipids, and betaine	Milk, liver, eggs, and peanuts	*125 mg/d*	ND	*150 mg/d*	ND
Folate[d]	Coenzyme in the metabolism of nucleic and amino acids; prevents megaloblastic anemia	Enriched cereal grains, dark leafy vegetables, enriched and whole-grain breads and bread products, and fortified ready-to-eat cereals	*65 µg/d*	ND	*80 µg/d*	ND
Niacin[e]	Coenzyme or cosubstrate in many biological reduction and oxidation (redox) reactions—thus required for energy metabolism	Meat, fish, poultry, enriched and whole-grain breads and bread products, and fortified ready-to-eat cereals	*2 mg/d*	ND	*4 mg/d*	ND

Nutrient	Function	Food sources				
Pantothenic acid	Coenzyme in fatty acid metabolism	Chicken, beef, potatoes, oats, cereals, tomato products, liver, kidney, yeast, egg yolk, broccoli, and whole grains	1.7 mg/d	ND	1.8 mg/d	ND
Riboflavin (vitamin B_{12})	Coenzyme in numerous redox reactions	Organ meats, milk, bread products, and fortified cereals	0.3 mg/d	ND	0.4 mg/d	ND
Thiamin (vitamin B_1 or aneurin)	Coenzyme in the metabolism of carbohydrates and branched-chain amino acids	Enriched, fortified, or whole-grain products; bread and bread products; mixed foods whose main ingredient is grain; and ready-to-eat cereals	0.2 mg/d	ND	0.3 mg/d	ND
Vitamin A[f]	Required for normal vision, gene expression, reproduction, embryonic development, and immune function	Liver, dairy products, and fish	400 µg/d	600 µg/d	500 µg/d	600 µg/d

Table 14 Continued

Nutrient	Function	Selected food sources	0–6 months		7–12 months	
			RDA/*AI*[a]	UL[b]	RDA/*AI*[a]	UL[b]
Vitamin B$_6$[g]	Coenzyme in the metabolism of amino acids, glycogen, and sphingoid bases	Fortified cereals, organ meats, and fortified soy-based meat substitutes	*0.1 mg/d*	ND	*0.3 mg/d*	ND
Vitamin B$_{12}$ (cobalamin)	Coenzyme in nucleic acid metabolism; prevents megaloblastic anemia	Fortified cereals, meat, fish, and poultry	*0.4 µg/d*	ND	*0.5 µg/d*	ND
Vitamin C [ascorbic acid, dehydroascorbic acid (DHA)]	Cofactor for reactions requiring reduced copper or iron metalloenzyme and as a protective antioxidant	Citrus fruits and juices, tomatoes, tomato juice, potatoes, brussel sprouts, cauliflower, broccoli, strawberries, cabbage, and spinach	*40 mg/d*	ND	*50 mg/d*	ND
Vitamin D (calciferol)[h]	Maintains serum calcium and phosphorus concentrations	Fish liver oils, flesh of fatty fish, eggs from hens that have been fed vitamin D, fortified milk products, and fortified cereals	*5 µg/d*	25 µg/d	*5 µg/d*	25 µg/d

Nutrient	Function	Sources				
Vitamin E (α-tocopherol)[i]	A metabolic function has not yet been identified; vitamin E's major function appears to be as a nonspecific chain-breaking antioxidant	Vegetable oils, unprocessed cereal grains, nuts, fruits, vegetables, and meats	4 mg/d	ND	5 mg/d	ND
Vitamin K	Coenzyme during the synthesis of many proteins involved in blood clotting and bone metabolism	Green vegetables (collards, spinach, salad greens, broccoli), brussel sprouts, cabbage, plant oils, and margarine	2 µg/d	ND	2.5 µg/d	ND
Arsenic	No biological function in humans although animal data indicate a requirement	Dairy products, meat, poultry, fish, grains, and cereal	ND	ND	ND	ND
Boron	No clear biological function in humans, although animal data indicate a functional role	Fruit-based beverages and products, potatoes, legumes, milk, avocado, peanut butter, and peanuts	ND	ND	ND	ND
Calcium	Essential role in blood clotting, muscle contraction, nerve transmission, and bone and tooth formation	Milk, cheese, yogurt, corn tortillas, calcium-set tofu, chinese cabbage, kale, and broccoli	210 mg/d	ND	270 mg/d	ND

Table 14 Continued

Nutrient	Function	Selected food sources	0–6 months		7–12 months	
			RDA/*AI*[a]	UL[b]	RDA/*AI*[a]	UL[b]
Chromium	Helps to maintain normal blood glucose levels	Some cereals, meats, poultry, fish, and beer	*0.2 µg/d*	ND	*5.5 µg/d*	ND
Copper	Component of enzymes in iron metabolism	Organ meats, seafood, nuts, seeds, wheat bran cereals, whole-grain products, and cocoa products	*200 µg/d*	ND	*220 µg/d*	ND
Fluoride	Inhibits the initiation and progression of dental caries and stimulates new bone formation	Fluoridated water, teas, marine fish, and fluoridated dental products	*0.01 mg/d*	0.7 mg/d	*0.5 mg/d*	0.9 mg/d
Iodine	Component of the thyroid hormones; prevents goiter and cretinism	Marine origin, processed foods, iodized salt	*110 µg/d*	ND	*130 µg/d*	ND
Iron	Component of hemoglobin and numerous enzymes; prevents microcytic hypochromic anemia	*Nonheme iron sources:* Fruits, vegetables, and fortified bread and grain products such as cereal *Heme iron sources:* Meat and poultry	*0.27 mg/d*	40 mg/d	*11 mg/d*	40 mg/d

	Function	Food sources				
Magnesium	Cofactor for enzyme systems	Green leafy vegetables, unpolished grains, nuts, meat, starches, and milk	30 mg/d	ND	75 mg/d	ND
Manganese	Involved in the formation of bone as well as in enzymes involved in amino acid, cholesterol, and carbohydrate metabolism	Nuts, legumes, tea, and whole grains	0.003 mg/d	ND	0.6 mg/d	ND
Molybdenum	Cofactor for enzymes involved in catabolism of sulfur amino acids, purines, and pyridines	Legumes, grain products, and nuts	2 µg/d	ND	3 µg/d	ND
Nickel	No clear biological function in humans has been identified; may serve as a cofactor of metalloenzymes and facilitate iron absorption or metabolism in microorganisms	Nuts, legumes, cereals, sweeteners, chocolate milk powder, and chocolate candy	ND	ND	ND	ND
Phosphorus	Maintenance and pH, storage and transfer of energy and nucleotide synthesis	Milk, yogurt, ice cream, cheese, peas, meat, eggs, some cereals and breads	100 mg/d	ND	275 mg/d	ND

Table 14 Continued

Nutrient	Function	Selected food sources	0–6 months		7–12 months	
			RDA/*AI*[a]	UL[b]	RDA/*AI*[a]	UL[b]
Selenium	Defense against oxidative stress and regulation of thyroid hormone action, and the reduction and oxidation status of vitamin C and other molecules	Organ meats, seafood, and plants (depending on soil selenium content)	*15 μg/d*	45 μg/d	*20 μg/d*	60 μg/d
Silicon	No biological function in humans has been identified; involved in bone function in animal studies	Plant-based foods	ND	ND	ND	ND
Vanadium	No biological function in humans has been identified	Mushrooms, shellfish, black pepper, parsley, and dill seed	ND	ND	ND	ND

| Zinc | Component of multiple enzymes and proteins; involved in the regulation of gene expression | Fortified cereals, red meats, and certain seafood | 2 mg/d | 4 mg/d | **3 mg/d** | 5 mg/d |

[a] Recommended Dietary Allowances (RDAs) are in **bold** type and Adequate Intakes (AIs) are in *ital* type; both may be used as goals for individual intake.

[b] UL = The maximum level of daily nutrient intake that is likely to pose no risk of adverse effects. Unless otherwise specified, the UL represents total intake from food, water, and supplements. Due to lack of suitable data, ULs could not be established for thiamin, riboflavin, vitamin B_{12}, pantothenic acid, biotin, or any carotenoids. In the absence of ULs, extra caution may be warranted in consuming levels above recommended intakes.

[c] ND = Not Determinable due to lack of data of adverse effects in this age group and concern with regard to lack of ability to handle excess amounts. Source of intake should be from food only, to prevent high levels of intake.

[d] Also known as folic acid, folacin, and pteroylpolyglutamates. Given as dietary folate equivalents (DFE). 1 DFE = 1 μg food folate = 0.6 μg of folate from fortified food or as a supplement consumed with food = 0.5 μg of a supplement taken on an empty stomach.

[e] Includes nicotinic acid amide, nicotinic acid (pyridine-3-carboxylic acid), and derivatives that exhibit the biological activity of nicotinamide. Given as niacin equivalents (NE). 1 mg of niacin = 60 mg of tryptophan; 0–6 months = preformed niacin (not NE).

[f] Includes provitamin A carotenoids that are dietary precursors of retinol. Given as retinol activity equivalents (RAEs). 1 RAE = 1 μg retinol, 12 μg β-carotene, 24 μg α-carotene, or 24 μg β-cryptoxanthin. To calculate RAEs from REs of provitamin A carotenoids in foods, divide the REs by 2. For preformed vitamin A in foods or supplements and for provitamin A carotenoids in supplements, 1 RE = 1 RAE.

[g] Comprises a group of six related compounds: pyridoxal, pyridoxine, pyridoxamine, and 5'-phosphates (PLP, PNP, PMP).

[h] 1 μg calciferol = 40 IU vitamin D. The DRI values are based on the absence of adequate exposure to sunlight.

[i] As α-tocopherol includes *RRR*-α-tocopherol, the only form of α-tocopherol that occurs naturally in foods, and the 2*R*-stereoisomeric forms of α-tocopherol (*RRR*, *RSR*, *RRS*, and *RSS*-α-tocopherol) that occur in fortified foods and supplements. It does not include the 2S-stereoisomeric forms of α-tocopherol (*SRR*, *SSR*, *SRS*, and *SSS*-α-tocopherol), also found in fortified foods and supplements.

Source: Adapted from the Dietary Reference Intakes: Vitamins and Dietary Reference Intakes: Elements tables at www.nal.usda.gov/fnic.

nutrition due to inadequate calories and diarrheal disease, and micronutrient deficiencies due to inadequate dietary intake and increased needs from infection (79).

In 1992, Hendricks and Badruddin (79) provided a set of basic universal weaning recommendations for infants in developed as well as developing countries. The guidelines follow the three overlapping periods discussed previously in "Periods of Infant Feeding" under "Guidelines for Introducing Solid Foods" Section as the nursing period, the transitional period, and the modified adult period, although Hendricks and Badruddin referred to them as the exclusive breast-feeding period, the weaning period, and the modified adult period. Hendricks and Badruddin (79) commented that despite broad cultural diversity, published recommendations for weaning are remarkably consistent worldwide; however, they concluded that more research is needed in a number of areas before the recommendations can include more precise guidelines. Their basic universal weaning recommendations are provided in Table 15.

A set of guiding principles for complementary feeding of breast-fed children in developing countries during the first 2 years of life was published in 2001 (92); the guidelines can be adapted to local feeding practices and conditions in the developing countries. Table 16 lists the 10 guidelines. Food allergies appear to be less common in developing countries (92); this helps explain why there is not a guideline regarding the order of introduction for complementary foods for infants in developing countries like there is for infants in developed countries.

IX. CONCLUDING REMARKS

The introduction of solid foods plays a critical role for infants as they learn to eat when they transition from a liquid diet of only breast milk or formula to a diet that includes solid foods. Several basic guidelines apply to infants in both developed and developing countries, but some specific guidelines are more appropriate for infants in either developed or developing countries. The numerous inconsistencies in guidelines for infants in developed countries create considerable confusion. For example, information regarding the following often varies from one source to another: the length of the waiting period before introducing another new food, how long to delay wheat, when to introduce citrus fruits and citrus juices, how much juice is excessive, which high-nitrate vegetables to avoid and for how long, how long to delay various meat products, when to introduce specific grain products, whether honey should be avoided in processed foods, if corn syrup should be avoided, and heating infant foods in microwave ovens. Efforts to resolve the inconsisten-

Introducing Solid Foods to Infants

Table 15 Basic Universal Weaning Recommendations for Infants in Developed and Developing Countries

		Months																							
		0	1	2	3	4	5	6	7	8	9	10	11	12	13	14	15	16	17	18	19	20	21	22	23	24
Breast milk																										
Staple weaning food and other grains																										
Soft fruits and vegetables																										
Meats and other protein-rich foods																										

Not given	
Given regularly	
Transitional period	

1. Breast milk should be given exclusively for the first 4–6 months. In developing countries, breast-feeding should be encouraged throughout the first 2 years, even if it provides only a small part of total intake.
2. Beginning at 4 months and no later than 6 months, the infant is gradually introduced to complementary foods. The order of introduction is not precise, and schedules will vary since each infant will progress at his/her own rate. A staple food that is calorically dense and adequate in protein is important, and variety is essential in meeting nutritional needs. Iron, zinc, vitamin D, and vitamin A-rich foods should be emphasized. Initially, complementary foods are given once a day, then gradually the frequency is increased so that the infant is eating two to four meals per day by about 6 months of age. Infants over 6 months of age need to eat meals and snacks about four to six times a day in addition to breast-feeding.
3. To avoid bacterial contamination, only freshly cooked or freshly peeled or washed foods should be used. The hands of both the food provider and child should be washed before handling food.
4. Throughout the latter half of the first year of life, variety in taste and texture of diet is expanded. As the child approaches one year of age, the child should be encouraged to feed her/himself, and by 2 years of age, the child should be consuming a varied diet from the family diet with choices from each of the food groups.

Source: Adapted from Ref. 79.

Table 16 "Guiding Principles for Complementary Feeding of the
Breast-fed Child" for Infants in Developing Countries[a]

No.	Topic	Guideline
1	Duration of exclusive breast-feeding and age of introduction of complementary foods	Practice exclusive breast-feeding from birth to 6 months of age, and introduce complementary foods at 6 months of age (180 days) while continuing to breast-feed.
2	Maintenance of breast-feeding	Continue frequent, on-demand breast-feeding until 2 years of age or beyond.
3	Responsive feeding	Practice responsive feeding, applying the principles of psychosocial care. Specifically: (1) feed infants directly, and assist older children when they feed themselves, being sensitive to their hunger and satiety cues; (2) feed slowly and patiently, and encourage children to eat, but do not force them; (3) if children refuse many foods, experiment with different food combinations, tastes, textures, and methods of encouragement; (4) minimize distractions during meals if the child loses interest easily; (5) remember that feeding times are periods of learning and love—talk to children during feeding, with eye-to-eye contact.
4	Safe preparation and storage of complementary foods	Practice good hygiene and proper food handling by (1) washing caregivers' and children's hands before food preparation and eating, (2) storing foods safely and serving foods immediately after preparation, (3) using clean utensils to prepare and serve food, (4) using clean cups and bowls when feeding children, and (5) avoiding the use of feeding bottles, which are difficult to keep clean.
5	Amount of complementary food needed	Start at 6 months of age with small amounts of food, and increase the quantity as the child gets older while maintaining frequent breast-feeding. The energy needs from complementary foods for infants with "average" breast milk intake in developing countries are approximately 200 kcal per day at 6–8 months of age, 300 kcal per day at 9–11 months of age, and 550 kcal per day at 12–23 months of age. In industrialized countries these estimates differ somewhat (130, 310, and 580 kcal/d at 6–8, 9–11 and 12–23 months, respectively) because of differences in average breast milk intake.

able 16 Continued

o.	Topic	Guideline
6	Food consistency	Gradually increase food consistency and variety as the infant gets older, adapting to the infant's requirements and abilities. Infants can eat pureed, mashed and semisolid foods beginning at 6 months. By 8 months most infants can also eat "finger foods" (foods that can be eaten by children alone). By 12 months, most children can eat the same types of foods as consumed by the rest of the family (keeping in mind the need for nutrient-dense foods, as explained in Principle 8). Avoid foods that may cause choking (i.e., items that have a shape and/ or consistency that may cause them to become lodged in the trachea, such as nuts, grapes, raw carrots).
7	Meal frequency and energy density	Increase the number of times that the child is fed complementary foods as he/she gets older. The appropriate number of feedings depends on the energy density of the local foods and the usual amounts consumed at each feeding. For the average healthy breast-fed infant, meals of complementary foods should be provided two to three times per day at 6–8 months of age and three to four times per day at 9–11 and 12–24 months of age, with additional nutritious snacks (such as a piece of fruit or bread or chapatti with nut paste) offered one to two times per day, as desired. Snacks are defined as foods eaten between meals—usually self-fed, convenient, and easy to prepare. If energy density or amount of food per meal is low or if the child is no longer breast-fed, more frequent meals may be required.
8	Nutrient content of complementary foods	Feed a variety of foods to ensure that nutrient needs are met. Meat, poultry, fish, or eggs should be eaten daily or as often as possible. Vegetarian diets cannot meet nutrient needs at this age unless nutrient supplements or fortified products are used (see Principle 9). Vitamin A-rich fruits and vegetables should be eaten daily. Provide diets with adequate fat content. Avoid giving drinks with low nutrient value, such as tea and coffee, and sugary drinks such as soda. Limit the amount of juice offered so as to avoid displacing more nutrient-rich foods.

Table 16 Continued

No.	Topic	Guideline
9	Use of vitamin–mineral supplements or fortified products for infants and mother	Use fortified complementary foods or vitamin–mineral supplements for the infant, as needed. In some populations, breast-feeding mothers may also need vitamin–mineral supplements or fortified products, both for their own health and to ensure normal concentrations of certain nutrients (particularly vitamins) in their breast milk.
10	Feeding during and after illness	Increase fluid intake during illness, including more frequent breast-feeding, and encourage the child to eat soft, varied, appetizing, favorite foods. After illness, give food more often than usual and encourage the child to eat more.

[a] These guidelines were developed from discussions at several technical consultations and from documents on complementary feeding. The target group for these guidelines is breast-fed children during the first 2 years of life. The guidelines do not cover specific feeding recommendations for non-breast-fed children, although many of the guidelines are also appropriate for such children (except for the recommendations regarding meal frequency and nutrient content of complementary foods). In addition, these guidelines apply to normal, term infants (including low-birth weight infants born at >37 weeks gestation). Infants or children recovering from acute malnutrition or serious illnesses may need specialized feeding. Preterm infants may also need special feeding. However, these guidelines can be used as the basis for developing recommendations on complementary feeding for these subgroups. *Source*: Adapted from Ref. 92.

cies, including additional research when appropriate, are needed to decrease the confusion. In contrast, the emphasis in most sources regarding the following is very encouraging: the importance of developmental readiness to determine when to introduce solid foods, the critical role of the feeding relationship, and the need to avoid forced feeding. In many ways, how solid foods are introduced is as important as which solid foods are introduced, because the eating patterns learned in infancy and continued throughout childhood can last a lifetime.

ACKNOWLEDGMENTS

Appreciation is expressed to Michelle L. Baglio, RD, LD, for her extensive help in obtaining references and preparing tables for this chapter. The following people are appreciated for providing feedback on earlier versions of this chapter: Michelle L. Baglio, RD, LD, Caroline H. Guinn, RD, LD, and Nicole M. Shaffer, RD, LD.

REFERENCES

1. Webster's II New College Dictionary. Boston: Houghton Mifflin, 2001.
2. Feeding Infants: A Guide for Use in the Child Nutrition Programs. FNS-258. Washington, DC: U.S. Department of Agriculture, Food and Nutrition Service, 2001. Available at http://www.fns.usda.gov/tn/Resources/feeding_infants.pdf.
3. University of Kentucky Cooperative Extension Service. Parent Express, A Guide for You and Your Baby: 6 Months Old. 2001. Available at http://www.ca.uky.edu/agc/pubs/fcs3/fcs3136/FCS3136.pdf (accessed on November 19, 2002).
4. Infant Nutrition and Feeding: A Reference Handbook for Nutrition and Health Counselors in the WIC and CSF Programs. FNS-288. Washington, DC: U.S. Department of Agriculture, Food and Nutrition Service, 1993.
5. Shelov SP, ed. Your Baby's First Year. New York: Bantam Books, 1998.
6. Story M, Holt K, Sofka D, eds. Bright Futures in Practice: Nutrition. 2d ed. Arlington, VA: National Center for Education in Maternal and Child Health, 2002. (Available at www.brightfutures.org.)
7. University of Kentucky Cooperative Extension Service. Nourishing the Older Infant: Four to Twelve Months. 1997. Available at http://www.ca.uky.edu/agc/pubs/fcs3/fcs3149/fcs3149.pdf (accessed on November 19, 2002).
8. University of Kentucky Cooperative Extension Service. Parent Express, A Guide for You and Your Baby: 9 Months Old. 2001. Available at http://www.ca.uky.edu/agc/pubs/fcs3/fcs3139/FCS3139.pdf (accessed on November 19, 2002).
9. Akers SM, Groh-Wargo SL. Normal nutrition during infancy. In: Samour PQ, Helm KK, Lang CE, eds. Handbook of Pediatric Nutrition. Gaithersburg, MD: Aspen, 1999:65–97.
10. Heird WC. Nutritional requirements during infancy. In: Ziegler EE, Filer LJ, eds. Present Knowledge in Nutrition. Washington, DC: International Life Sciences Institute Press, 1996:396–403.
11. Hall RT, Carroll RE. Infant feeding. Pediatr Rev 2000; 21:191–199.
12. Meister K. Feeding Baby Safely: Facts, Fads and Fallacies. The American Council on Science and Health. 1998. Available at http://www.acsh.org/publications/booklets/feedingbaby.pdf (accessed on April 18, 2003).
13. Fomon SJ. Cow milk and beikost. In: Fomon SJ, ed. Nutrition of Normal Infants. St. Louis, MO: Mosby—Year Book, 1993:443–454.
14. Committee on Nutrition, American Academy of Pediatrics. Supplemental foods for infants. In: Kleinman RE, ed. Pediatric Nutrition Handbook. 4th ed. Elk Grove Village, IL: American Academy of Pediatrics, 1998:43–53.
15. Parkinson KN, Drewett RF. Feeding behavior in the weaning period. J Child Psychol Psych 2001; 42:971–978.

16. Fomon SJ. History. In: Fomon SJ, ed. Nutrition of Normal Infants. St. Louis, MO: Mosby, 1993:6–14.
17. Dietz WH, Stern L, eds. Guide to Your Child's Nutrition. New York: Villard Books, 1999.
18. Fomon SJ. Trends in infant feeding since 1950. In: Fomon SJ, ed. Nutrition of Normal Infants. St. Louis, MO: Mosby, 1993:15–35.
19. Fomon SJ. Nutrition of Normal Infants. St. Louis, MO: Mosby, 1993.
20. Smaha MB. Nutrition management of the full-term infant. In: Williams CP, ed. Pediatric Manual of Clinical Dietetics. Chicago: American Dietetic Association, 1998:49–66.
21. U.S. Department of Agriculture, U.S. Department of Education, U.S. Department of Health and Human Services. Healthy Start, Grow Smart, Your Six-Month-Old. Washington, DC, 2002. Available at http://www.ed.gov/offices/OESE/earlychildhood/healthystart/sixmonth.pdf.
22. U.S. Department of Agriculture, U.S. Department of Education, U.S. Department of Health and Human Services. Healthy Start, Grow Smart, Your Nine-Month-Old. Washington, DC, 2002. Available at http://www.ed.gov/offices/OESE/earlychildhood/healthystart/.
23. Satter E. Child of Mine: Feeding with Love and Good Sense. Palo Alto, CA: Bull, 2000.
24. Bobroff LB. Introducing Solid Foods. University of Florida Cooperative Extension Service. 2000. Available at http://edis.ifas.ufl.edu/BODY-HE965 (Accessed on April 18, 2003).
25. University of Kentucky Cooperative Extension Service. Parent Express, A Guide for You and Your Baby: 4 Months Old, 2001. Available at http://www.ca.uky.edu/agc/pubs/fcs3/fcs3134/FCS3134.pdf (Accessed on November 19, 2002).
26. Tamborlane WV, Weiswasser JZ, Fung T, Held NA, Liskov TP, eds. The Yale Guide to Children's Nutrition. New Haven, CT: Yale University Press, 1997.
27. U.S. Department of Agriculture, U.S. Department of Education, U.S. Department of Health and Human Services. Healthy Start, Grow Smart, Your Four-Month-Old. Washington, DC, 2002. Available at http://www.ed.gov/offices/OESE/earlychildhood/healthystart/fourmonth.pdf.
28. Johnson DB. Nutrition in infancy: evolving views on recommendations. Nutrition Today 1997; 32:63–69.
29. Hedstrom N. Feeding Your Baby. University of Maine Cooperative Extension. 1998. Available at http://www.umext.maine.edu/onlinepubs/PDFpubs/4061.pdf (accessed on November 19, 2002).
30. Archuleta M. Feeding Your Baby: The First Year. New Mexico State University Cooperative Extension Service. 2003. Available at http://cahe.nmsu.edu/pubs/_e/e-135.pdf (accessed on April 18, 2003).
31. International Food Information Council Foundation. Starting Solids: A Guide for Parents and Child Care Providers. 2000. Available at http://ific.org/proactive/newsroom/release.vtml?id = 17565 (accessed on November 18, 2002).
32. Pescara L. Solid Food: Ready or Not? Ohio State University Cooperative Extension. 1999. Available at http://ohioline.osu.edu/mob-fact/0005.html (accessed on April 18, 2003).

33. Fomon SJ. Feeding normal infants: rationale for recommendations. J Am Diet Assoc 2001; 101:1002–1005.

34. Fomon SJ. Recommendations for feeding normal infants. In: Fomon SJ, ed. Nutrition of Normal Infants. St. Louis, MO: Mosby—Year Book, 1993:455–458.

35. Kleinman RE, Fomon SJ, Greenspan S, Lauer RM, Baker SS, Glinsmann WH, Beauchamp GK, Finberg L, Lonnerdal B. Dietary guidelines for infants. Pediatric Basics 1994; 69:1–29.

36. Harris G, Thomas A, Booth DA. Development of salt taste in infancy. Dev Psychol 1990; 26:534–538.

37. Harris G. Determinants of the introduction of solid food. J Reprod Infant Psychol 1988; 6:241–249.

38. Skinner JD, Carruth BR, Houck K, Moran J, Coletta F, Cotter R, Ott D, McLeod M. Transitions in infant feeding during the first year of life. J Am Coll Nutr 1997; 16:209–215.

39. Nevling W, Carruth BR, Skinner J. How do socioeconomic status and age influence infant food patterns? J Am Diet Assoc 1997; 97:418–420.

40. Bronner YL, Gross SM, Caulfield L, Bentley ME, Kessler L, Jensen J, Weathers B, Paige DM. Early introduction of solid foods among urban African-American participants in WIC. J Am Diet Assoc 1999; 99:457–461.

41. Heath A-LM, Tuttle CR, Simons MSL, Cleghorn CL, Parnell WR. A longitudinal study of breast-feeding and weaning practices during the first year of life in Dunedin, New Zealand. J Am Diet Assoc 2002; 102:937–943.

42. Underwood BA. Weaning practices in deprived environments: the weaning dilemma. Pediatrics 1985; 75:194–198.

43. University of Kentucky Cooperative Extension Service. Parent Express, A Guide for You and Your Baby: 10 Months Old. 2001. Available at http://www.ca. uky.edu/agc/pubs/fcs3/fcs3140/FCS3140.pdf (accessed on November 19, 2002).

44. Lundy B, Field T, Carraway K, Hart S, Malphurs J, Rosenstein M, Pelaez-Nogueras M, Coletta F, Ott D, Hernandez-Reif M. Food texture preferences in infants versus toddlers. Early Child Devel Care 1998; 146:69–85.

45. Northstone K, Emmett P, Nethersole F, ALSPAC Study Team. The effect of age of introduction to lumpy solids on foods eaten and reported feeding difficulties at 6 and 15 months. J Hum Nutr Dietetics 2001; 14:43–54.

46. Satter EM. The feeding relationship. J Am Diet Assoc 1986; 86:352–356.

47. U.S. Department of Agriculture, U.S. Department of Education, U.S. Department of Health and Human Services. Healthy Start, Grow Smart, Your Eight-Month-Old. Washington, DC, 2002. Available at http://www.ed.gov/offices/OESE/earlychildhood/healthystart/eightmonth.pdf.

48. Fomon SJ, Bell EF. Energy. In: Fomon SJ, ed. Nutrition of Normal Infants. St. Louis, MO: Mosby—Year Book, 1993:103–120.

49. Adair LS. The infant's ability to self-regulate caloric intake: A case study. J Am Diet Assoc 1984; 84:543–546.

50. Birch LL, Fisher JO. Development of eating behaviors among children and adolescents. Pediatrics 1998; 101:539–549.

51. Sullivan SA, Birch LL. Infant dietary experience and acceptance of solid foods. Pediatrics 1994; 93:271–277.

52. Mennella JA, Beauchamp GK. Mothers' milk enhances the acceptance of cereal during weaning. Pediatr Res 1997; 41:188–192.
53. Birch LL, Gunder L, Grimm-Thomas K, Laing DG. Infants' consumption of a new food enhances acceptance of similar foods. Appetite 1998; 30:283–295.
54. Birch LL, Marlin DW. I don't like it; I never tried it: effects of exposure to food on two-year-old children's food preferences. Appetite 1982; 3:353–360.
55. Birch LL, McPhee L, Shoba BC, Pirok E, Steinberg L. What kind of exposure reduces children's food neophobia? Appetite 1987; 9:171–178.
56. Sullivan SA, Birch LL. Pass the sugar, pass the salt: experience dictates preference. Dev Psychol 1990; 26:546–551.
57. Gerrish CJ, Mennella JA. Flavor variety enhances food acceptance in formula-fed infants. Am J Clin Nutr 2001; 73:1080–1085.
58. Skinner JD, Carruth BR, Bounds W, Ziegler P, Reidy K. Do food-related experiences in the first 2 years of life predict dietary variety in school-aged children? J Nutr Educ Behav 2002; 34:310–315.
59. Beauchamp GK, Mennella JA. Early feeding and the acquisition of flavor preferences. In: Boulton J, et al., eds. Long-Term Consequences of Early Feeding. Nestlé Nutrition Workshop Series. Vol 36. Philadelphia: Vevey/Lippincott-Raven, 1996:163–177.
60. World Health Organization, Department of Nutrition for Health and Development. Complementary Feeding: Family Foods for Breast-Fed Children. WHO/NHD/00.1 WHO/FCH/CAH/00.6, 2000, p 52.
61. U.S. Department of Agriculture, U.S. Department of Education, U.S. Department of Health and Human Services. Healthy Start, Grow Smart, Your Seven-Month-Old. Washington, DC, 2002. Available at http://www.ed.gov/offices/OESE/earlychildhood/healthystart/sevenmonth.pdf.
62. U.S. Department of Agriculture, U.S. Department of Education, U.S. Department of Health and Human Services. Healthy Start, Grow Smart, Your 10-Month-Old. Washington, DC, 2002. Available at http://www.ed.gov/offices/OESE/earlychildhood/healthystart/.
63. Committee on Nutrition, American Academy of Pediatrics. The use and misuse of fruit juice in pediatrics. Pediatrics 2001; 107:1210–1213. Available at http://pediatrics.aappublications.org/cgi/reprint/107/5/1210.
64. U.S. Department of Agriculture, U.S. Department of Education, U.S. Department of Health and Human Services. Healthy Start, Grow Smart, Your Five-Month-Old. Washington, DC, 2002. Available at http://www.ed.gov/offices/OESE/earlychildhood/healthystart/fivemonth.pdf.
65. Fomon SJ. Carbohydrate. In: Fomon SJ, ed. Nutrition of Normal Infants. St. Louis, MO: Mosby—Year Book, 1993:176–191.
66. Smith MM, Lifshitz F. Excess fruit juice consumption as a contributing factor in nonorganic failure to thrive. Pediatrics 1994; 93:438–443.
67. Dennison BA, Rockwell HL, Baker SL. Excess fruit juice consumption by preschool-aged children is associated with short stature and obesity. Pediatrics 1997; 99:15–22.

68. Skinner JD, Carruth BR, Moran J, Houck K, Coletta F. Fruit juice intake is not related to children's growth. Pediatrics 1999; 103:58–64.

69. Skinner JD, Carruth BR. A longitudinal study of children's juice intake and growth: the juice controversy revisited. J Am Diet Assoc 2001; 101:432–437.

70. U.S. Department of Agriculture, U.S. Department of Education, U.S. Department of Health and Human Services. Healthy Start, Grow Smart, Your 12-Month-Old. Washington, DC, 2002. Available at http://www.ed.gov/offices/OESE/earlychildhood/healthystart/.

71. University of Kentucky Cooperative Extension Service. Parent Express, A Guide for You and Your Baby: 12 Months Old. 2001. Available at http://www.ca.uky.edu/agc/pubs/fcs3/fcs3142/FCS3142.pdf (accessed on November 19, 2002).

72. Glinsmann WH, Bartholmey SJ, Coletta F. Dietary guidelines for infants: a timely reminder. Nutr Rev 1996; 54:50–57.

73. Committee on Nutrition, American Academy of Pediatrics. Iron deficiency. In: Kleinman RE, ed. Pediatric Nutrition Handbook. 4th ed. Elk Grove Village, IL: American Academy of Pediatrics, 1998:233–246.

74. Fomon SJ. Iron. In: Fomon SJ, ed. Nutrition of Normal Infants. St. Louis, MO: Mosby—Year Book, 1993:239–260.

75. Committee on Nutrition, American Academy of Pediatrics. Vitamins. In: Kleinman RE, ed. Pediatric Nutrition Handbook. 4th ed. Elk Grove Village, IL: American Academy of Pediatrics, 1998:267–281.

76. Committee on Nutrition, American Academy of Pediatrics. Nutrition and oral health. In: Kleinman RE, ed. Pediatric Nutrition Handbook. 4th ed. Elk Grove Village, IL: American Academy of Pediatrics, 1998:523–529.

77. Fomon SJ. Fluoride. In: Fomon SJ, ed. Nutrition of Normal Infants. St. Louis, MO: Mosby—Year Book, 1993:299–310.

78. Nutrition and Your Health: Dietary Guidelines for Americans. 5th ed. Home and Garden Bulletin No. 232. Washington, DC: U.S. Department of Agriculture and U.S. Department of Health and Human Services, 2000.

79. Hendricks KM, Badruddin SH. Weaning recommendations: the scientific basis. Nutr Rev 1992; 50:125–133.

80. U.S. Department of Health and Human Services. Healthy People 2010: With Understanding and Improving Health and Objectives for Improving Health. 2nd ed. Washington, DC: U.S. Government Printing Office, 2000.

81. Holt RD. Weaning and dental health. Proc Nutr Soc 1997; 56:131–138.

82. American Dietetic Association. Position of the American Dietetic Association: oral health and nutrition. J Am Diet Assoc 2003; 103:615–625.

83. Partnership for Food Safety Education. Fight BAC! Available at http://www.fightbac.org/main.cfm (accessed on May 27, 2003).

84. Trumbo P, Schlicker S, Yates AA, Poos M. Dietary reference intakes for energy, carbohydrate, fiber, fat, fatty acids, cholesterol, protein, and amino acids. J Am Diet Assoc 2002; 102:1621–1630.

85. Institute of Medicine. Dietary Reference Intakes for Calcium, Phosphorus, Magnesium, Vitamin D, and Fluoride. Washington, DC: Food and Nutrition Board, National Academy Press, 1997.

86. Institute of Medicine. Dietary Reference Intakes for Thiamin, Riboflavin, Niacin, Vitamin B6, Folate, Vitamin B12, Pantothenic Acid, Biotin, and Choline. Washington, DC: Food and Nutrition Board, National Academy Press, National Academy Press, 1998.

87. Institute of Medicine. Dietary Reference Intakes for Vitamin C, Vitamin E, Selenium, and Carotenoids. Washington, DC: Food and Nutrition Board, National Academy Press, 2000.

88. Institute of Medicine. Dietary Reference Intakes for Vitamin A, Vitamin K, Arsenic, Boron, Chromium, Copper, Iodine, Iron, Manganese, Molybdenum, Nickel, Silicon, Vanadium, and Zinc. Washington, DC: Food and Nutrition Board, National Academy Press, 2001.

89. Institute of Medicine. Dietary Reference Intakes for Energy, Carbohydrate, Fiber, Fat, Fatty Acids, Cholesterol, Protein and Amino Acids. Washington, DC: Food and Nutrition Board, National Academy Press, 2002.

90. Institute of Medicine. Dietary Reference Intakes: Applications in Dietary Assessment. Washington, DC: Food and Nutrition Board, National Academy Press, 2000.

91. Lutter CK. Macrolevel approaches to improve the availability of complementary foods. Food Nutr Bull 2003; 24:83–103.

92. Dewey K. Guiding Principles for Complementary Feeding of the Breast-Fed Child. Washington, DC: Pan American Health Organization, World Health Organization, 2001. Available at http://www.who.int/child-adolescent-health/New_Publications/NUTRITION/guiding_principles.pdf.

93. World Health Organization, UNICEF. Complementary Feeding of Young Children in Developing Countries: A Review of Current Scientific Knowledge. 1998. Available at www.who.int/en/ (accessed on May 5, 2003).

94. World Health Organization. Report of Informal Meeting to Review and Develop Indicators for Complementary Feeding. Washington, DC, 2002. Available at http://www.who.int/child-adolescent-health/New_Publications/NUTRITION/Informal-meeting-for-CF.pdf.

95. World Health Organization. Nutrition: Infant and Young Child—Complementary Feeding. Available at http://www.who.int/child-adolescent-health/NUTRITION/complementary.htm (accessed on April 18, 2003).

11
Growth During the First Year of Life

Jon A. Vanderhoof
University of Nebraska Medical Center, Omaha, Nebraska, U.S.A.

Carol Lynn Berseth
Mead Johnson Nutritionals, Evansville, Indiana, U.S.A.

I. INTRODUCTION

The first year of life is characterized by very rapid growth (1). The fetus grows at a rapid rate in utero, but the growth rate declines shortly before birth. After a few days of no growth or even weight loss, rapid weight gain and linear growth resume. During the first 6 months of life, the average infant increases in weight by about 115%, in body length by approximately 34%, and in head circumference by approximately 22%. For infants whose body weight is low at birth, weight gain will be greater on a percentage basis. An overweight infant will increase weight less rapidly. For example, an infant at the 5th percentile will increase its weight by 135% by 6 months of age, whereas an infant with a birth weight at the 95th percentile will only achieve, on average, a 105% weight gain by 6 months of age. The rate of growth is greatest during the initial 4–6 months and tapers off after that time. The average infant achieves a weight gain of approximately 1.1–1.2 kg/mo during the first 6 months tapering down to approximately 0.4–0.5 kg/mo during the second 6 months. Linear growth similarly is greatest during the first 6 months, tapering off somewhat thereafter. Length increases about 3.5–3.9 cm/mo during the first 4 months, down to about 1.8 cm/mo at 6 months of age.

II. MEASURING GROWTH

Accurate and reproducible measurements are important in comparing the growth rates of infant groups and assessing the growth progress in individual patients. Numerous established techniques have been published regarding appropriate means of collecting these data. These techniques have been utilized to collect much of the growth data contained in many reference groups, including the Third National Health and Nutrition Examination Survey, or NHANES III, as well as the World Health Organization's Multicenter Growth Reference Study.

Ideally, growth measurements should be collected by two technicians. One technician is usually needed to position the infant and obtain the correct measurement, while a second technician is available to assist in positioning the infant and recording the data. Repeat measurements by the same technicians, but switching roles, will increase the accuracy of the measurements. However, in a clinical setting it is not always possible to obtain measurements in this ideal fashion. Even when optimally obtained, some variation in measurement is to be anticipated, and this variation must be considered in interpretation of growth data. As any experienced clinician knows, this is especially true in evaluating the growth progress of an individual infant. When the two technicians are available and growth measurements have been obtained twice, differences that appear too great should be reconfirmed by repeat measurements. In individual patients, for monitoring of progressive growth, measurements suggesting significant changes in the growth patterns should definitely be verified by repeat examination. Measurements should be obtained without clothing to exclude the possibility of variation in the weight of clothing on subsequent measurements.

Commercially available electronic scales are ideal for weighing an infant. The infant can also be weighed while being held by the mother and the mother's weight subsequently subtracted to obtain the infant weight, provided the electronic scale is accurate. Some scales can automatically subtract the mother's weight. Obviously, the procedure will be more accurate if the mother can remove shoes and heavy garments before weighing the infant. Spring balances and even beam balances are not very appropriate for measuring the weight of infants, for these measurements are more subjective and not as reproducible. When it is difficult to remove the infant's diaper, 100 grams should be deducted from the measured weight.

Several commercially available pieces of equipment are available to measure an infant's length. Two people are usually required to successfully complete this task. The lower orbits of the eyes and the ear canals should be placed in the same vertical plane, with the child's head positioned against the end of the measuring apparatus. The shoulders and buttocks should rest on the board and the shoulders and hips should be aligned at right angles to the long axis of the body. The head board should be carefully positioned with the infant looking straight up. A second technician can best position the infant appropriately on the device. Legs must be straightened and the footboard positioned against the soles of the infant's feet. One person must hold the infant to maintain his or her position and ensure that the head remains against the vertical head board. Care must be taken to make certain that the infant is not arching the spine or flexing the knees. The measurement is then obtained with the child's heels against the footboard, using slight pressure on the ankles to ensure that the legs are straight and the spine is fully extended.

Head circumference is measured with a flexible tape, preferably one that is not elastic. The tape is positioned just above the eyebrows at a level across the front of the head. The greatest circumference may be determined by moving the tape across the back of the head and pulling it tight to obtain an appropriate reading. The tape should be tightened to compress the hair and the measurement obtained to the nearest millimeter. Head circumference can often best be obtained with the infant seated in the mother's lap.

Weight, length, and head circumference are the most important measurements in monitoring infant growth. Other pieces of data are occasionally useful (Table 1). Crown–rump length, chest circumference, and limb length have all been utilized to monitor growth. Skinfold thickness is occasionally determined to assess adequacy of weight gain and nutritional status. Skinfold thickness is a crude measurement of subcutaneous fat, which often reflects a child's caloric intake and energy reserves. The high degree of variability in assessing skinfold thickness limits the usefulness of this technique, especially in small infants. All of these measurements are subjected to a higher degree of interobserver variation, making them less reliable for clinical studies and certainly less reliable in monitoring an individual infant's progress. Experience utilizing these techniques is also somewhat limited, which adds to the variability problem. In some instances limb length can be utilized in place of

Table 1 Useful Measurements
in Monitoring Growth

Weight
Length
Head circumference
Skin fold thickness
Limb length
Crown–rump length
Chest circumference

Table 2 Methods to Evaluate Growth
and Body Composition

Isotopic dilution
DEXA (dual energy x-ray absorptiometry)
TOBEC (total body electrical conductivity)
CT (computerized tomography)
MRI (magnetic resonance imaging)

---

linear growth when linear growth data is difficult to obtain. Crown–rump length and chest circumference are occasionally used to monitor prenatal nutrition but are of limited value in evaluating the infant's growth. More recently, imaging techniques such as the DEXA and MRI have been utilized to measure subcutaneous fat and total body fat content (Table 2).

Comparison of weight relative to length is an easy way to estimate the relative degree of fat vs. lean body mass. A high weight percentile versus length percentile determination suggests a greater degree of adiposity. A mathematical variant of this is the body mass index, in which the weight in kilograms is divided by the square of the length in centimeters. While its use has been popularized in adults, it has seen relatively little application in children under 2 years of age. Perhaps the greatest value of this parameter in older children is to assess the risk of obesity-related diseases. In infants, the usefulness of body mass index has not been well established.

Frequency of assessment of growth parameters in individual children in a clinical setting is often determined by local or regional practice standards. Normally, at least three measurements should be obtained during the first 6 months. This is especially true for clinical studies. At least one measurement should be obtained shortly after birth, especially before 2 months of age, and a subsequent measurement should be obtained after weight gain slows down, around 4 months of age. One-, 2-, 4-, and 6-month measurements are ideal. Because growth is most rapid during the first 4 months, more frequent measurements during this period of time are required. During this interval, weight is perhaps the most important measurement that can be obtained, because it changes most rapidly and is most reproducible. It is also the most acute indicator of nutritional adequacy.

III. PLOTTING GROWTH

Normally, growth is assessed using standardized growth charts (Figs. 1 and 2). These provide a quick and easy means of identifying problems or deviations

Birth to 36 months: Boys
Length-for-age and Weight-for-age percentiles

NAME _____

RECORD # _____

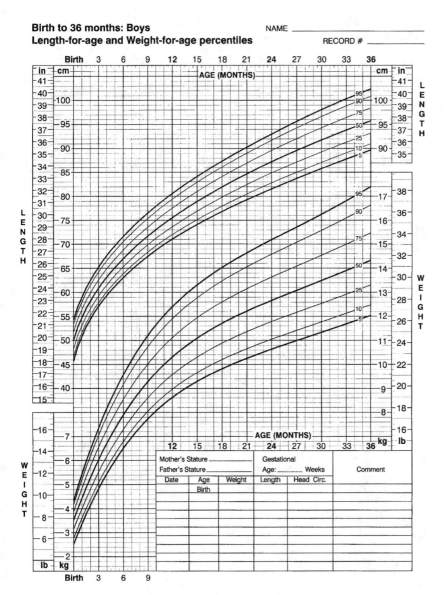

Figure 1 Standard male infant growth curve. (From the National Center for Health Statistics in collaboration with the National Center for Chronic Disease Prevention and Health Promotion. Modified April 20, 2001. www.cdc.gov/growthcharts.)

Birth to 36 months: Girls   NAME _____
Length-for-age and Weight-for-age percentiles   RECORD # _____

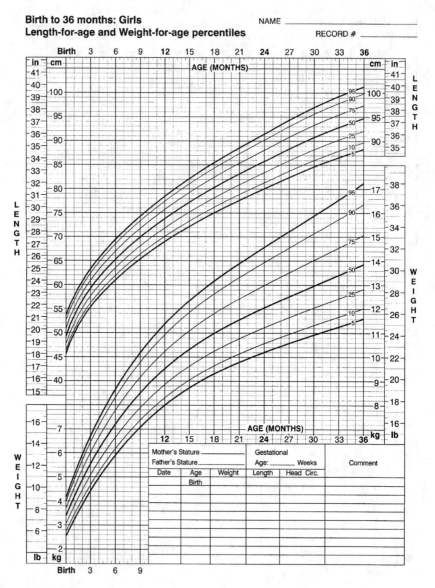

Figure 2 Standard female infant growth curve. (From the National Center for Health Statistics in collaboration with the National Center for Chronic Disease Prevention and Health Promotion. Modified April 20, 2001. www.cdc.gov/growthcharts.)

from normal growth. Revised growth charts from the Centers for Disease Control National Center for Health Statistics are most frequently consulted at the present time. Use of gender-specific growth charts is important, because the growth rate in girls is somewhat slower than that in boys. Growth velocity measurements may also be useful in monitoring an infant's growth progress. Naturally, multiple measurements over time are required to adequately assess growth velocity. Standard deviation scores or Z scores can be computed, eliminating the need to analyze boys and girls separately. Measurements taken at different ages can be converted to Z scores and combined for data analysis. Such techniques are often useful in population studies but usually not helpful in evaluating the growth progress of an individual infant. Z scores have the advantage of allowing combined analysis of children of different genders for evaluation of populations, and they permit measurements taken at different ages to be combined for data analysis.

It is also important to make certain that the database utilized to construct the growth curve is relevant to the population for which the growth curve is utilized. For example, many commonly used growth curves are developed from data collected predominantly from middle-class white children and subsequently applied to different racial and socioeconomic groups. Recent attempts have been made to improve the quality of growth curves by broadening the sample and making them more relevant to today's population. The infant growth charts originally developed by the National Center for Health Statistics in 1977 used data from the Fels Research Institute collected in Yellow Springs, Ohio, between 1929 and 1975 (2). While this data provided much comprehensive information about children's growth, the sample is very limited in geographical, cultural, socioeconomic, and genetic variability. As a result, the Centers for Disease Control and Prevention released a revision of the 1977 growth charts in May 2000. These revised growth charts were developed from databases more accurately reflecting the current geographic, ethnic, and socioeconomic distribution in the United States. These revised charts also reflect a higher percentage of breast-feeding, which is common in today's population. Neither base was limited to healthy children; consequently, both databases likely include some infants who are inappropriately fed or have a chronic illness. Nonetheless, the newer growth curves are considered to reflect the current standard of care in pediatric practice. Further data will soon be available from the World Health Organization based on the growth of infants throughout the world and may give us even more insight into the growth rates of normal children.

While body composition can be estimated from a comparison of height and weight data, more accurate techniques are available to make these assessments (see Table 2). Measurement of total body water, total body potassium, and body density can be obtained by isotopic dilution. More recently, the total body electrical conductivity (TOBEC) and bioelectrical impedance analysis have been employed for this purpose. Unfortunately, these techniques are not widely available (3–6). Bone mineral content and fat-free mass can now be easily assessed the through the use of dual-energy X-ray absorptiometry (DEXA) (7). DEXA provides precise quantification for a three-compartment model of body composition. This includes bone mineral content, a critical measure of peak bone mass in children, lean tissue mass, and fat-free mass (8). Minimal radiation exposure is required. While these techniques are widely available, appropriate software for infants is not. Consequently, many commercially available studies on bone mineral density in infants are unreliable. Because this technique has the advantage of also being able to measure bone mineral density, fat-free body mass, and body fat content, it will probably become the technique of choice for body composition studies in the near future. This is exemplified by the recent publication by Butte et al. (9) describing the composition of gestational weight gain using DEXA as well as other techniques.

IV. GROWTH PATTERNS

Monitoring growth is important to assess the overall health and well-being of the infant and to determine whether the infant is receiving adequate nutritional intake. It is during the first 4 months of life that growth is most rapid and infants are most susceptible to nutritional deprivation. Numerous diseases and disorders may produce abnormal growth patterns that will require further evaluation. Most infants with failure to thrive exhibit a growth pattern characterized by normal head circumference, a slight length reduction, and weight reduction out of proportion to length reduction. This is the classical pattern seen with nutritional deprivation of any cause. It may suggest gastrointestinal disease with malabsorption or poor oral intake, or it may indicate impaired nutritional intake because of some other disease process. Most commonly, inadequate feeding of the infant is the cause of this type of growth pattern.

Infants who demonstrate this type of growth curve should first be evaluated to determine if caloric intake is adequate. Breast-fed infants should be weighed before and after nursing to determine the appropriate volume received. Mothers frequently perceive that infants have achieved much greater caloric intake, because they themselves feel chronically engorged. Offering supplemental formula feeding at the conclusion of breast-feeding or giving the child a short trial of formula feeding to assess weight gain are other means of evaluating this problem. Formula-fed infants are much easier to evaluate for nutrient intake. Care must be exercised to make certain parents are correctly mixing and diluting formula. Unless the cause of the child's poor intake can be immediately identified, verification of intake by an independent observer, occasionally requiring hospitalization, may be very enlightening.

Excess caloric losses may result from malabsorption of nutrients, but this is a relatively infrequent occurrence. More commonly, marginal intake or chronic emesis is at fault. Additionally, a hypermetabolic state such as congenital heart disease with heart failure or renal or liver disease may increase metabolic utilization enough to produce a failure-to-thrive pattern that is suggestive of nutrient deprivation.

Two other abnormal growth patterns may be identified. The first is subnormal head circumference with height and weight proportionally reduced. These children often have peculiar facies and demonstrate microcephaly, developmental retardation, and occasionally seizures. Perinatal insults or intrauterine infections are not uncommon causes. Chromosomal or genetic anomalies may fit into this pattern as well. A third category of poor growth includes children with normal or enlarged head circumference and weight that is either proportional to height or only slightly reduced. These children are often referred to as *constitutional dwarfs*. Endocrine disorders and structural dystrophies are found in this group. Hypopituitarism and hypothyroidism may present with this type of growth curve, although such findings may not be detected during the first year of life because growth rates many decelerate toward the latter part of the first year.

V. FEEDING AND GROWTH

The type of infant feeding may influence growth patterns significantly. Agostoni et al. highlighted different growth patterns between breast-fed and formula-fed infants that appeared most pronounced during the first 6 months of life (10). Breast-fed infants had significantly higher growth indices at 1 month, 2 months, and 3 months of age. However, their indices were also highest at birth. Formula-fed infants had significantly higher weight for age measurements at several intervals during the first 6 months. The growth indices progressively increased for the formula-fed infants and declined for the breast-fed infants over the 12-month interval. In other words, the second 6 months was characterized by progressive decline in growth rate in breast-fed infants relative to the formula-fed infants.

Butte et al. explored both differences in weight gained and body composition in breast-fed versus formula-fed infants (11). During early infancy, fat-free mass was lower and fat mass and percent body fat were higher in breast-fed versus formula-fed infants between 3 and 9 months of age. Differences in body composition diminished once complementary feedings were added. Previous studies of pooled data from the World Health Organization analysis of growth data on breast-fed infants from the United States, Canada, and Europe have demonstrated a consistent downward trend in weight-for-age, length-for-age, and weight-for-length Z score after 2–3 months of age. A more rapid decline in growth in breast-fed relative to formula-fed infants during the latter part of the first year of life has been observed. Differences in weight were most pronounced in girls during the second 6 months of age, coincidental with the reduced energy intake of breast-fed relative to formula-fed infants during that interval. In the DARLING study, skinfold thickness in breast-fed infants was less than that of formula-fed infants from 9 to 17 months of age (12). Exclusivity of breast-feeding in this study was associated with a lower weight-for-age and weight-for-length Z score at 12 months. However, in today's society, late weaning from the breast is a relatively rare occurrence.

Energy utilization between breast-fed and formula-fed infants may be different as well. Breast-fed infants have been shown to have a reduced energy expenditure relative to formula-fed infants during the first year of life (13). On the contrary, De Bruin et al. simultaneously measured energy intake, total daily intake, energy expenditure, and body composition in individual infants, with subsequent direct calculation of energy requirements (14). Healthy infants exclusively breast-fed or formula-fed for the first 4 months of age differed significantly between feeding groups, but these differences were not followed by accompanying differences in energy expenditure growth or body composition.

Ong et al. examined the relationship between maternal smoking, maternal parity, and breast or bottle feeding and size at birth and childhood growth between birth and 5 years of age in a large representative birth cohort (15). Infants of maternal smokers were small at birth but showed complete catch-up growth over the first 12 months. Primiparas had infants who were small at birth but caught up rapidly. Breast-fed infants were similar in size at birth to bottle-fed infants but grew more slowly during infancy. However, when the data for boys and girls were analyzed separately, breast-fed girls differed in growth status and body composition at 4 and 8 months of age as a result of lower weight gain between 2 and 4 months of age. At 2–4 months of age, the formula-fed girls were found to have higher weight gains. This resulted in a higher amount of total body fat and fat premass at 4 and 8 months of age. This correlates with previous data as well as animal studies that also showed that such feeding effects appeared to be more common in females (16–19). Whether or not any of these differences relate to energy concentration differences in breast milk vs. formula are difficult to assess, but most of the data suggest that they are relatively comparable. Measuring energy content of breast milk may be somewhat difficult. Significant differences in the literature exist (14,20).

Issues related to whether or not breast-feeding during infancy has any significant beneficial effect on long-term growth issues are hotly debated. Some evidence suggests that obesity may be more common in children who were breast-fed as infants. Long-term effects of breast-feeding on body habitus has also been recently evaluated. Armstrong and Reilly tested the hypothesis that breast-feeding is associated with a reduced risk of obesity in a population-based sample of 32,200 children. These children were studied between 39 and 42 months of age (21). The prevalence of obesity was significantly lower in children previously breast-fed as compared to formula-fed, and the association persisted after adjustment for socioeconomic status, birth weight, and gender. Liese et al. observed a markedly lower prevalence of obesity among breast-fed than non-breast-fed children in two different German cities (22). Gillman and colleagues also have reported some beneficial effects of breast-feeding in the reduction of obesity (23).

In contrast, Hediger et al. found an inconsistent relationship between breast-feeding and obesity (24). These investigators found a significant 37% reduction in being at risk of overweight (85th to 95th percentile) among children who had been breast-fed for any time at all as compared with those who were never breast-fed. However, there was only a 16% reduction in actually being overweight, as defined by being greater than the 95th percentile. They also found no strong dose-dependent effect of the duration of breast-feeding on overweight status in early childhood, nor could they demonstrate an apparent threshold effect or reduction in risk with full breast-feeding for 3 months or more or 6 months or more. Children who were fully breast-fed for 3 months or longer had about a 30% decreased risk for overweight. Duration of full breast-feeding as an independent variable showed only a weak linear association with the child's body mass index. Poulton and Williams in a small study found a small reduction in risk of overweight during late childhood and adolescence in previously breast-fed infants (25). While the data are still inconclusive, there is a suggestion that breast-fed infants are not as likely to become obese. Confounding variables are difficult to eliminate. Likewise, it is difficult to sort out those factors related to the process of breast-feeding from the actual nutrient content or constituents of the breast milk.

VI. LOW-BIRTH-WEIGHT INFANTS

The growth and development of extremely- and/or very-low-birth-weight infants with severe intrauterine growth retardation during the first year of life is also a major area of investigation. Perhaps the most important parameter evaluated in this age group is head circumference. There is quite a close relationship between head circumference growth and estimated brain weight and development during the first 2 years of life (26–27). The majority of children in this category appear to have complete or almost complete head circumference catch-up growth, although a significant amount of data suggests that head circumference growth is suboptimal. Recent evidence holds that head circumference catch-up growth in small-for-gestational-age very-low-birth-weight infants is heavily related to the energy intake available during the first 10 days of postnatal life (28). Infants who had normal head circumference catch-up growth appear to have had a very high caloric intake, which is quite different from those who do not manifest adequate catch-up growth. Likewise, early feeding practices appear to be closely associated with IQ in very-low-birth-weight infants (29–30). It appears that postnatal energy requirements for rapidly growing infants between 30 weeks' gestation and 6 months after term, which correlates with the growth spurt and head circumference growth, have been generally underestimated, especially for small-for-gestational-age very-low-birth-weight infants.

Intrauterine growth retardation in term children, especially if associated with microcephaly, may be accompanied by delayed growth as well as neurodevelopmental disturbances (31–32). However, studies on long-term outcome on small-for-gestational-age very-low-birth-weight infants have found no difference in cognitive functioning or in the rate of cerebral palsy if one controls for a variety of perinatal and demographic factors (33). Postnatal growth appears to have a favorable predictive value in intellectual functioning for small-for-gestational-age term-born male adolescents (34). However, small-for-gestational-age status does appear to be associated with impaired psychomotor development if adequate catch-up growth is not achieved (34). All of these data point to the importance of aggressive provision of adequate nutrition very early in life to ensure optimal outcome.

VII. LONG-CHAIN POLYUNSATURATED FATTY ACIDS

The recent inclusion of long-chain polyunsaturated N-3 fatty acids to infant formulas has stimulated a great deal of research in the growth effects of these fatty acids on both term and preterm infants (35). A minority of studies, all in preterm infants, have shown that infants fed formulas enriched with N-3 long-chain polyunsaturated fatty acids had some parameter of decreased growth relative to infants fed a control formula (36–40). However, a clear majority of studies, in fact, suggest that N-3 LC PUFAs have no adverse effect on infant growth. There are a number of reasons why one might postulate an effect of N-3 LC PUFAs on growth, including effects on eicosanoid production, altered membrane characteristics, and direct influence on molecular events governing gene expression (41). Even more speculative is the possibilities that N-3 LC PUFAs may, in fact, reduce fat deposition and that N-6 PUFAs, as well as saturated fatty acids, may induce adipogenesis. There is certainly a significant amount of experimental data to suggest that N-3 LC PUFAs and N-6 LC PUFAs act differently in this regard (42). Unfortunately, all epidemiologic studies comparing formula-fed vs. breast-fed infants to rates of obesity have been done in infants consuming formulas that did not contain N-3 LC PUFAs. This certainly leaves the door open for some speculation that N-3 LC PUFAs in breast milk may be responsible, at least partially, for the differences in weight gain and obesity observed between breast-fed and formula-fed infants.

SUMMARY

Growth patterns during the first year of life have been well described and converted to standard growth curves. While initial growth curves were heavily based on very homogeneous populations, more recent data have permitted the development of curves that more clearly reflected the heterogeneity of today's society. Monitoring growth during the first year of life relative to these growth curves is an important means of not only defining the child's nutritional adequacy but identifying significant medical problems. Some differences between breast-fed and formula-fed infants may be apparent at times during the first year of life, but they typically normalize after that period of time. More data need to be collected on the effects of breast-feeding and the subsequent development of obesity, especially in light of the recent inclusion of LC PUFAs in infant formula.

REFERENCES

1. Guo SM, Roche AF, Fomon SJ, et al. Reference data on gains in weight and length during the first two years of life. J Pediatr 1991; 119(3):355–362.
2. Roche AF. Growth, maturation, and body composition: the Fels Longitudinal Study 1929–1991. Cambridge, UK: University Press, 1992.
3. deBruin NC, Luijendijk IHT, Visser HKA, Degenhart HJ. Effect of alterations in physical and chemical characteristics on TOBEC-derived body composition estimates: validation with nonhuman models. Phys Med Biol 1994; 39:1143–1156.
4. Fiorotto ML. Measurements of total body electrical conductivity for the estimation of fat and fat-free mass. In: Whitehead RG, Prentice A, eds. New Techniques in Nutritional Research. San Diego: Academic Press, 1991:281–301.

5. Fiorotto ML, de Bruin NC, Brans YW, et al. Total body electrical conductivity measurements: an evaluation of current instrumentation for infants. Pediar Res 1995; 37:94–100.

6. deBruin NC, Westerperp KR, Degenhart HJ, Visser HKA. Measurement of fat-free mass in infants. Pediatr Res 1995; 38:411–417.

7. Hogler W, Brody J, Woodhead HJ, et al. Importance of lean mass in the interpretation of total-body densitometry in children and adolescents. J Pediatr 2003; 143:81–88.

8. Ogle GD, Allen JR, Humphries IR, et al. Body-composition assessment by dual-energy x-ray absorptiometry in subjects aged 4–26 y. Am J Clin Nutr 1995; 61:746–753.

9. Butte NF, Ellis KJ, Wong WW, Hopkinson JM, Smith OE, et al. Composition of gestational weight gain impacts maternal fat retention and infant birth weight. Am J Obstet Gynecol 2003; 189:1423–1432.

10. Agostoni C, Grandi F, Gianni ML, et al. Growth patterns of breast-fed and formula-fed infants in the first 12 months of life: an Italian study. Arch Dis Child 1999; 81(5):395–399.

11. Butte NF, Wong WW, Hopkinson JM, et al. Infant feeding mode affects early growth and body composition. Pediatrics 2000; 106(6):1355–1366.

12. Dewey KG, Peerson JM, Heinig MJ, et al. Growth of breast-fed and formula-fed infants from 0 to 18 months: the DARLING Study. Pediatrics 1992; 89(6 Pt 1):1035–1041.

13. Butte N, Heinz C, Hopkinson J, et al. Fat mass in infants and toddlers: comparability of total body water, total body potassium, total body electrical conductivity, and dual-energy x-ray absorptiometry. J Pediatr Gastroenterol Nutr 1999; 29(2):184–189.

14. de Bruin NC, Degenhart HJ, Gal S, et al. Energy utilization and growth in breast-fed and formula-fed infants measured prospectively during the first year of life. Am J Clin Nutr 1998; 67(5):885–896.

15. Ong KK, Preece MA, Emmett PM, et al. Size at birth and early childhood growth in relation to maternal smoking, parity and infant breast-feeding: longitudinal birth cohort study and analysis. Pediatr Res 2002; 52(6):863–867.

16. Dewey KG, Heinig MJ, Nommsen LA, et al. Breast-fed infants are leaner than formula-fed infants at 1 y of age: the DARLING study. Am J Clin Nutr 1993; 57:140–145.

17. Dewey KG, Heinig MJ, Nommsen LA, Lonnerdal B. Adequacy of energy intake among breast-fed infants in the DARLING study: relationships to growth velocity, morbidity and activity levels. J Pediatr 1991; 119:538–547.

18. Butte NJ, Wong WW, Garza C. Energy requirements of breast-fed infants. J Am Coll Nutr 1991; 10:190–195.

19. Lewis DS, Bertrand HA, McMahan CA, et al. Effect of interaction of sex and energy intake on lean body mass and fat mass gain in infant baboons. J Nutr 1984; 114:2021–2026.

20. Lucas A, Ewing G, Roberts SB, Coward WA. How much energy does the breast-fed infant consume and expend? Br Med J 1987; 295:72–77.

21. Armstrong J, Reilly JJ. Breastfeeding and lowering the risk of childhood obesity. Lancet 2002; 359(9322):2003–2004.
22. Liese AD, Hirsch T, von Mutius E, et al. Inverse association of overweight and breast feeding in 9- to 10-y-old children in Germany. Int J Obes Relat Metab Disord 2001; 25(11):1644–1650.
23. Gillman MW, Rifa-Shiman SL, Camargo CA, et al. Risk of overweight among adolescents who were breastfed as infants. Jama 2001; 285(19):2461–2467.
24. Hediger ML, Overpeck MD, Kuczmarski RJ, Ruan WJ. Association between infant breastfeeding and overweight in young children. Jama 2001; 285(19): 2453–2460.
25. Poulton R, Williams S. Breastfeeding and risk of overweight. JAMA 2001; 286(12):1448–1449.
26. Dobbing J, Sands J. Head circumference, biparietal diameter and brain growth in fetal and postnatal life. Early Hum Dev 1978; 2:81–87.
27. Brandt I. Brain growth, fetal malnutrition, and clinical consequences. J Perinat Med 1981; 9:3–26.
28. Brandt I, Sticker EJ, Lentze MJ. Catch-up growth of head circumference of very-low-birth-weight, small-for-gestational-age preterm infants and mental development to adulthood. J Pediatr 2003; 142:463–468.
29. Morley R, Lucas A. Randomized diet in the neonatal period and growth performance until 7.5–8 y of age in preterm children. Am J Clin Nutr 2000; 71:822–828.
30. Lubchenco LO, Delivoria-Papadopoulos M, Butterfield LJ, et al. Long-term follow-up studies of prematurely born infants, I: relationship of handicaps to nursery routines. J Pediatr 1972; 80:501–508.
31. Strauss RS, Dietz WH. Growth and development of term children born with low birth weight: effects of genetic and environmental factors. J Pediatr 1998; 133:67–72.
32. Larroque B, Bertrais S, Czernichow P, Leger J. School difficulties in 20-year-olds who were born small for gestational age at term in a regional cohort study. Pediatrics 2001; 108:111–115.
33. Laa-Hajnal B, von Siebenthal K, Kovari H, et al. Postnatal growth in VLBW infants: significant association with neurodevelopmental outcome. J Pediatr 2003; 143:163–170.
34. Lundgren EM, Cnattingius S, Jonsson B, Tuvemo T. Intellectual and psychological performance in males born small for gestational age with and without catch-up growth. Pediatr Res 2001; 50:91–96.
35. Lapillonne A, Carlson SE. Polyunsaturated fatty acids and infant growth. Lipids 2001; 36:901–911.
36. Carlson SE, Cooke RJ, Werkman SH, Tolley EA. First-year growth of preterm infants fed standard compared to marine oil n-3 supplemented formula. Lipids 1992; 27:901–907.
37. Carlson SE, Werkman SH, Tolley EA. Effect of long-chain n3 fatty acid supplementation on visual acuity and growth of preterm infants with and without bronchopulmonary dysplasia. Am J Clin Nutr 1996; 63:687–697.

38. Ryan AS, Montalto MB, Groh-Wargo S, et al. Effect of DHA-containing formula on growth of preterm infants to 59 weeks postmenstrual age. Am J Hum Biol 1999; 11:457–467.

39. Vanderhoof J, Gross S, Hegyi T. A multicenter long-term safety and efficacy trial of preterm formula supplemented with long-chain polyunsaturated fatty acids. J Pediatr Gastroenterol Nutr 2000; 31:121–127.

40. O'Connor DL, Hall R, Adamkin D, et al. Growth and development in preterm infants fed long-chain polyunsaturated fatty acids: a prospective, randomized controlled trial. Pediatrics 2001; 108:359–371.

41. Fewtrell MS, Morley R, Abbot RA, et al. Double-blind, randomized trial of long-chain polyunsaturated fatty acid supplementation in formula fed to preterm infants. Pediatrics 2002; 110:73–82.

42. Gibson RA, Chen W, Makides M. Randomized trials with polyunsaturated fatty acid interventions in preterm and term infants: functional and clinical outcomes. Lipids 2001; 36:873–883.

12

Prenatal and Infant Nutrition in the Pathogenesis of Type 1 Diabetes
Implications for Diagnosis and Therapy

Andrew Muir and Jin-Xiong She
Medical College of Georgia, Augusta, Georgia, U.S.A.

I. INTRODUCTION

The concept of type 1 diabetes as a disease of childhood and adolescence is being challenged by studies that relate islet autoimmunity to prenatal and infantile determinants (1–5). Recent discoveries that increased maternal age (6,7), ABO incompatibility (8), and rapid postnatal growth (9–11) are all diabetes risk factors suggest that the pathogenic process starts very early in life. Interactions among protective and predisposing genes, environmental exposures, and immunological responses all appear necessary for the initiation and propagation of autoimmune T-lymphocyte responses that destroy the insulin-producing pancreatic beta cells. This chapter will review the current understanding of the pathogenesis of type 1 diabetes and highlight the contribution of infant nutrition to the initiation of progression of autoimmunity.

A. Immunology

Autoimmune reactions arise because of deficiencies in either central (intrathymic) tolerance or peripheral tolerance (12–16). In an intrathymic process called *negative selection*, apoptosis is usually induced in T-lymphocyte clones that avidly bind antigen presented by antigen-presenting cells in the context of self human leukocyte antigen (HLA) molecules. Normally, a small number of potentially self-reactive clones escape negative selection in the thymus and are rendered harmless by peripheral tolerance processes. These include the induction of anergy, activation-induced cell death, immunoregulation (suppression) by soluble mediators, and immunological ignorance.

Immunological insult to the pancreatic beta cells in type 1 diabetes begins months or, more typically, years before hyperglycemia and the symptoms of the disease appear (17–20). This delay occurs because islet cell mass must be substantially depleted before a state of clinically significant insulin deficiency occurs. Preclinical lesions include infiltration of islets by mononuclear immune cells. Based on limited human studies and intensive evaluation of experimental animal models of autoimmune diabetes, it appears that the earliest cells to infiltrate the islets are macrophages and dendritic cells. These cells can act as antigen-presenting cells, either within the islet or in draining lymph nodes. Infiltration of CD4 + and then CD8 + cells follows. B-lymphocytes appear to be important mediators of the autoimmune response, probably through their antigen-presenting function (21–25). The autoantibodies made by autoimmune B-lymphocytes do not, however, appear to be pathogenic.

Our understanding of autoimmune beta-cell destruction is derived from extensive studies with experimental animal models. Human studies are restricted by the difficulty of identifying patients before islet destruction is nearly complete and by limited access to target tissues and pathogenic immune cells. Nonetheless, two important hypotheses of tolerance are particularly important to the current understanding of diabetes. First, reduced avidity of the binding between the antigen-presenting cell and the T-lymphocyte may result in abnormal persistence of autoimmune lymphocyte clones (13,15,26,27). Changes in antigen structure, HLA function, or accessory signaling could cause persistence and activation of self-reactive lymphocytes. Second, opposing effector and regulatory functions exist among immune cells that comprise the immune response in the lymph nodes and at the site of inflammation. In a simplified view, for example, Th1 CD4 + helper T-lymphoctyes are identified by their inflammatory actions. They appear to be important in promoting beta-cell destruction, whereas Th2 CD4 + T-lymphocytes appear to limit the harm (28–32).

B. Genetics

1. Inherited Risk of Diabetes

Inherited determinants of type 1 diabetes were demonstrated by family studies reporting concordance for the monozygotic twin of an affected patient between 35% and 50% (33,34). This compared to a disease prevalence among the general population in the United States of 2–3 per 1000 (34). The healthy sibling of a child with diabetes has a 5% risk of developing the disease. This empirically determined risk can be further defined by examining specific risk genes. Identity of HLA genotypes between siblings carries a 15–20% risk of concordance for disease, whereas the risk of diabetes in siblings sharing a single HLA haplotype is about 4%. A healthy individual who shares no HLA genes with a sibling with diabetes has a disease risk of only 1%.

The high frequency of other autoimmune conditions among patients with type 1 diabetes and their family members hints that genetic influences are both disease-specific and nonspecific (35–38). One class of autoimmune susceptibility genes may provide a biological milieu that promotes the generation or perpetuation of self-reactive lymphocyte clones, irrespective of their particular antigen specificity. These genes could involve any part of the immune response, including antigen processing and presentation, accessory signaling, lymphocyte activation and regulation, production of soluble mediators of immunity, and cell death processes. A second class of genes may determine target organ specificity, perhaps by: (1) defining which self-antigens generate autoimmune responses, (2) controlling responses to environmental agents that either precipitate or exacerbate autoimmunity, or (3) influencing end-organ susceptibility to immune-mediated damage. A third class of autoimmunity genes exerts effects that prevent autoimmune disease. These genes may prevent the initiation or propagation of autoimmunity or encode products that protect target organs from autoreactive immune cells and soluble mediators of immunity (Table 1).

2. HLA Genes in Diabetes

Genes within the HLA complex have the strongest known genetic influence on type 1 diabetes (39). The genes comprise a series of polymorphic loci that are in linkage disequilibrium; i.e., selective pressures have maintained nonrandom associations among alleles of neighboring loci. As shown in Table 2, the

Table 1 Classes of Autoimmunity Genes

Gene class	Function	Example
1	General susceptibility to autoimmunity	HLA DR3, DR4, DQB1*0302, CTLA-4
2	Target tissue/organ specificity	INS (insulin), ?HLA DR3/4 (αβ transcomplementary heterodimers)
3	Protection from autoimmunity	DQB1*0602, DRB1*0403, DRB1*0406

Table 2 HLA-Encoded Susceptibility to Type 1 Diabetes

DR-DQB1/DR-DQB1 genotype	Prevalence in general population (%)	Prevalence in diabetes patients (%)	Absolute risk
03-0201/04-0302 (DR 3/4)	1.8	35	1/15
04-0302/04-0302 (DR 4/4)	0.7	10	1/20
03-0201/03-0201 (DR 3/3)	1.5	9.0	1/40
04-0501/04-0301 (DR 1/4)	0.6	2.0	1/60
15-0602/X (DR15/X)	50.7	20	1/15,000

X = any other HLA haplotype.

DR and DQ loci impart strong influences on diabetes susceptibility. Whereas DQB1*0302 and *0201 are susceptibility alleles, dominant protection from disease is conferred by the DQB1*0602 allele. When one dissects out the effects of linkage disequilibrium, islet autoimmunity is also controlled by the DR locus. The DR3 and DR4 alleles (except DRB1*0403 and DRB1*0406) confer high risk for type 1 diabetes. The HLA molecules bind fragments of endocytosed antigens so that they may be presented in a recognizable form at the surface of antigen-presenting cells to CD4+ T-lymphocytes. HLA mediation of diabetes susceptibility is believed to result from variations of the antigen species bound by the molecules (acting as a class 2 organ-specific effect). The exceptionally high risk conferred to individuals who are heterozygous for DR3/4 haplotypes may result from transcomplementary association of the αβ components of the molecule, i.e., the dimeric DR protein is composed of one maternally derived and one paternally derived peptide that have unique avidity for an autoantigen. HLA type may also influence the signal generated within T-lymphocytes in response to their interactions with antigen-presenting cells (acting as a class 1 autoimmune gene effect) (40).

The higher concordance of diabetes among monozygotic twins as compared to HLA-identical siblings illustrates a role of non-HLA genes in the elimination of pancreatic beta cells. Linkage studies have identified over 20 genetic intervals that may contain one or more susceptibility genes each (41). The influence of any one of these loci is much smaller than that of the HLA genes. Susceptible alleles do not therefore have to be expressed at all of the genes that influence type 1 diabetes. It is presumed that disease predisposition is influenced by both the number of susceptibility genes and the magnitude that each of the genes exerts on the autoimmune phenotype.

3. Non-HLA Genes in Diabetes

The 5' noncoding region of the insulin gene (INS) was the first gene outside of the HLA complex to be identified as a diabetes susceptibility gene. It is currently believed that alleles that promote lower levels of insulin expression in the thymus during the establishment of immunological tolerance to the hormone allow the escape of autoreactive clones (13,42). This suggests that INS functions as a class 2 susceptibility gene. The CTLA-4 T-lymphocyte accessory molecule is a mediator of immunoregulatory communication between antigen-presenting cells. As the only known gene within the narrowly mapped IDDM12 region, it is likely that CTLA-4 functions as a class 1 susceptibility gene in diabetes. The gene is also reported to influence susceptibility to Graves disease, rheumatoid arthritis, multiple sclerosis, and celiac disease (36).

C. Environment

A role for environmental agents in the etiology of diabetes is indicated by (1) the lack of complete concordance for diabetes among monozygotic twins, (2) seasonal periodicity of both the onset of symptomatic disease and the birth month of people with diabetes, and (3) varied prevalence of type 1 diabetes among countries, i.e., high in Finland and Sardinia, low in Iceland and Japan) (34,38,43). Despite a multitude of proposed agents, proof of their roles has been elusive (see Table 3).

Dietary components may directly provoke responses of the mucosal immune system against their antigenic components, may "redirect" harmless immune responses to harmful ones, or may include toxins (e.g., nitrosamines, Bafilomycin A) that inflict an initial insult to beta cells (44–47). Diet issues related to infants will be discussed in more detail in Section II.

Congenital rubella infection is a cause of diabetes, but successful immunization programs have made this an uncommon occurrence today. Inconsistent results characterize the multitude of studies that have examined

Table 3 Some Proposed Environmental Agents Influencing Type 1 Diabetes

Type of stimulus	Example
Diet	Cow milk (casein), omega-3 fatty acids, vitamin D, antioxidants (vitamin E, zinc, others)
Infection	Prenatal, postnatal enteroviruses (especially Coxsackie), rotavirus, congenital rubella
Immunizations	None widely suspected
Toxins	Dietary-*n*-nitroso compounds, Bafilomycin A, patulin

the association of type 1 diabetes with many other viral infections. Evidence of an association between diabetes and enteroviruses and, in particular, Coxsackie viruses continues to accumulate (3,48). A high frequency of Coxsackie viremia but not other viruses at the time of diabetes diagnosis in children suggests that the infection accelerates the loss of insulin production (49–51). Prospective studies of infants have temporally linked enterovirus infections to the appearance of autoantibodies against the islet components, insulin, the 65-kDa isoform of glutamic acid decarboxylase (GAD65), and the membrane tyrosine phosphatase, called IA-2. The presence of these autoantibodies predicts the appearance of frank diabetes. Given the known tropism of Coxsackie viruses for islets, the absence of autoimmunity before these infections, and the very young age of these seroconverters, these studies suggest that enterovirus infections may actually initiate the autoimmune response (52).

Significant public attention was brought to studies suggesting that routine childhood immunizations against *Haemophilus influenzae* and the measles/mumps/rubella combination caused type 1 diabetes. Multicenter studies have not confirmed any of these associations (53–55). Given the low level of confidence in the incriminating data and the profound negative impact that immunization withdrawal would have on public health, no routine immunization schedules should be modified, even in children at high risk for diabetes.

Interestingly, while stimulation of immune responses against infectious agents has been implicated as a cause of diabetes, so too has been the lack of immune stimulation brought about by advances of modern society. The hygiene hypothesis builds on data that indicate that normal memory responses and immune regulation require frequent stimulation of the immune system. An unintended consequence of water purification, sewage treatment, antibiotics, and immunizations may be the rise in many autoimmune diseases that is currently being documented (56).

II. DIET AS AN ENVIRONMENTAL TRIGGER OF AUTOIMMUNITY

A. Macronutrients

1. Cow Milk Proteins and Breast-Feeding

Diabetes was reduced in susceptible animals (BB rats) by feeding them diets free of milk proteins (57). The observation fueled epidemiologic studies of the role of cow milk in human diabetes. Associations between diabetes and cow milk introduction into the diet were indeed found, both in case-control studies and in ecological population studies (1,58,59). A series of reports suggested that early introduction of formula with a cow milk base, short duration of breast-feeding, and early introduction of solid foods increased the risk for diabetes. The associations were not universally observed, but a meta-analysis of these studies concluded that the relative risk for diabetes related to early cow milk consumption was about 1.5 (60). Subsequently, it was suggested that the risk may be attributable to recall or participation biases (61). Early reports from prospective studies of cow milk exposure in infants at high risk for developing diabetes in the United States, Australia, and Germany have been unable to associate cow milk exposure or breast-feeding history with the appearance of diabetes-related autoantibodies, but the studies have not followed enough subjects for a sufficient period to draw conclusions about overt diabetes (54,62,63). A prospective trial from Finland has yielded a conclusion that is subtly different from the others. Whereas different feeding patterns were not associated with the presence or absence of islet autoimmunity, a short duration of breast-feeding or early cow milk introduction was related to progression of islet autoantibody status to higher risk categories (64).

The cow milk hypothesis draws support from immunological observations. Immune responses to cow milk proteins have been carefully studied. Insulin autoimmunity is believed to be important in the pathogenesis of diabetes (65). Therefore, humoral and cellular responses against bovine insulin were examined in infants with varying exposures to cow milk products. Both specific IgG responses and T-lymphocyte proliferation responses were higher at 3 months of age in children that had received cow milk formula as compared to those that had been exclusively breast-fed (66). In a separate study, immune responses against bovine insulin among the children of a group of 78 mothers who avoided cow milk, egg white, and fish in their own diets during the first 3 months of breast-feeding were examined. Compared to the children of 45 mothers who did not follow the restricted diet, the level of antibodies against bovine insulin at 18 months of age were higher in the children of the mothers on the restrictive diet. The authors suggested that presentation of antigens as a component of breast milk may favor tolerance, whereas the same antigen introduced in formula may result in immune sensitization (67). Although insulin is an important autoantigen in diabetes, the link between responses to bovine insulin, human insulin, and diabetes is yet to be substantiated.

Others have noted that specific isoforms of beta casein (A1 and B) may provoke immune responses that are associated with type 1 diabetes but not with other autoimmune conditions (i.e., multiple sclerosis, thyroiditis) (68). Differences in the prevalence of type 1 diabetes in Nordic countries (especially between the high level in Finland and the low level in Iceland) have been associated with differences in the predominant isoform of the countries' beta casein content in commercial milk (69). Catabolism of the A1 and B variants of beta casein results in the production of an opioid, beta-casomorphin-7, whereas enzymatic breakdown of the A2 variant does not. The opioid metabolite can inhibit intestinal lymphocyte proliferation in vitro and could therefore influence immune responses generated by the mucosal immune system of the gut (70). Indeed, one report of experiments in NOD mice, an inbred strain that spontaneously develops autoimmune diabetes, suggests that exacerbating effects of A1 casein on diabetes are reversed by adding naloxone to the drinking water (71). The gut-associated lymphoid tissue controls tolerance responses to ingested antigens as well as the clearance of ingested pathogens. Alteration of intestinal lymphocyte activity could therefore alter diabetes risk by reducing tolerance to diabetogenic antigens or changing the response to enterovirus infections (2,72). Interestingly, celiac disease, a condition found more frequently than expected among patients with diabetes, is also associated with beta casein A1 and B consumption (68).

The definitive answer to the cow milk/breast-feeding controversy is expected from the ongoing Trial to Reduce IDDM in the Genetically at Risk (TRIGR). This international, multicenter, prospective trial is designed to provide conclusive evidence of the role of cow milk formula in the pathogenesis of type 1 diabetes. Infants have been randomly assigned to receive either cow milk formula or protein hydrolysate in the first 6 months of life, once the mother has decided to reduce or stop breast-feeding. The size of the study group is expected to provide 90% power to detect a 33% reduction of type 1 diabetes in the treatment group as compared to the control group (65,66).

2. Polyunsaturated Fatty Acids

The recent introduction of docosahexaenoic acid (DHA) to commercial infant formula to improve neurological and visual development has heightened interest in the potential antiinflammatory properties of omega-3 fatty acids. Addition of a mixture of omega-3 and omega-6 fatty acids to the chow of Wistar rats prevented their susceptibility to alloxan-induced diabetes (73). This disease is toxin-mediated rather than autoimmune. The effect is therefore likely to reflect a change in pancreatic beta cells rather than in the immune system. Similar success has not been reported in experimental animal models of autoimmune islet destruction.

Nonetheless, a population-based, retrospective case-control study from Norway reported a negative association between childhood diabetes and maternal cod liver oil treatment during pregnancy (74). In questionnaires answered by mothers 1–17 years after their pregnancy, the cod liver oil effect was independent of the use of other vitamin supplements, particularly vitamin D. Other potential confounders, including the study center, the children's ages and gender, duration of breast-feeding, and mothers' educational levels, did not alter the cod liver oil association. Interestingly, an association between diabetes and postnatal cod liver oil ingestion was not observed in this study. This intriguing observation is consistent with an important effect of omega-3 fatty acid supplementation in prenatal life but a smaller effect thereafter. It is important to recall, however, that the design of the study is liable to recall bias, similar to that implicated as a problem in studies of breast-feeding and cow milk exposure in children with diabetes. In addition, specific information about dose and timing of ingestion was not obtained. If confirmatory data are derived from ongoing epidemiologic studies, then the antiinflammatory effects of omega-3 fatty acids and the relative safety of administering them in pharmacological doses may prove compelling enough to generate a prospective controlled trial of omega-3 fatty acids for diabetes prevention.

B. Micronutrients

1. Vitamin D

Vitamin D has recently become a popular candidate therapy for diabetes prevention, because of a convergence of genetic, epidemiological, and experimental animal model data. Polymorphisms of the vitamin D receptor (VDR) have been associated with susceptibility to type 1 diabetes in European and Asian populations (75–78). Additionally, immunomodulating effects of vitamin D on antigen-presenting cells and lymphocytes are well described (79). Investigations of the 1,25-dihydroxy vitamin D as a preventive agent for type 1 diabetes have been published in an important experimental animal model. Both insulitis and diabetes were reduced in NOD mice by very high dose 1,25-dihydroxy vitamin D treatment (80,81). Hyperglycemia in mice receiving alternate-day 0.5-ug intraperitoneal doses of the potent vitamin D metabolite was reduced to about one-third the rate observed in mice receiving a placebo injection. Trials of vitamin D analogues with and without combination immunosuppressive therapy suggest autoimmune beta-cell destruction can be limited even when treatment is started after islet infiltration by lymphocytes has occurred. Further NOD mouse investigations suggest that the vitamin D treatment increases a population of CD4 +, CD25 + regulatory T-lymphocytes in pancreatic lymph nodes by altering the function of antigen-presenting dendritic cells. The problem of hypercalcemia caused by the high-dose vitamin D therapy may be effectively subverted by use of synthetic vitamin-D receptor-altered ligands that exert minimal effects on calcemia (82).

Important supporting data for a role for vitamin D in diabetes prevention has also arisen from human studies. A multicenter, retrospective, case-control European study of 820 children with diabetes by age 15 years and 2335 controls showed a relative risk of 0.67 for disease among children who received vitamin D supplements during their first year of life as compared to those who did not receive supplements (83). More recently, a prospective study from Finland recorded both dose and duration of vitamin D treatment in almost 11,000 children whose mothers completed a dietary questionnaire after the child's first birthday. The group reported a lower risk of type 1 diabetes by age 30 years among those children who received the Finnish minimum recommended daily dose of 2,000 IU/day (84).

The observational studies in humans and the promising results of vitamin D receptor ligand therapy in NOD mice suggest a trial of vitamin D or an analogue is likely to be launched someday. A trial of vitamin D at current recommended daily allowance levels of 400 IU/day is not supported by the animal studies, but it offers a high degree of safety. Trials of higher vitamin D doses or synthetic analogues may offer a better chance of diabetes prevention, but most protocols will first need to be proven safe in children.

2. Antioxidants

Oxidative stress contributes to the destruction of beta cells in the evolution of autoimmune diabetes in experimental animals, and treatment with antioxidants prevents diabetes and reduces autoimmune infiltration of the islets (85–87). In addition, oxidative modification of proteins may contribute to their ability to stimulate the immune system (88). The only human trials of antioxidant therapy for prevention of human diabetes have examined the effect of nicotinamide. Results from small trials have returned inconsistent results, but a definitive multicenter, prospective, placebo-controlled trial reported that nicotinamide at a dose of 1.2 g/m^2 of body surface area did not reduce the progression to diabetes among nondiabetic subjects who had circulating islet autoantibodies (89–91).

III. SCREENING

An ideal screening test is accurate, reliable, easy to perform, and acceptable to patients and physicians. It should also diagnose a condition that cannot be recognized clinically and for which there is an acceptable therapy that will improve the patient's quality of life or prognosis. Technical and biological advances through the 1990s dramatically improved many of the features of diabetes as a candidate disease for screening. The identification of specific islet autoantigens (insulin, GAD65, IA-2 being most frequently tested) have been the major advances in this regard. Nonetheless, screening for type 1 diabetes remains practical only for research, because a safe and effective intervention has not yet been found.

A. Genetic

Initial screening efforts for patients with asymptomatic islet autoimmunity began with a genetic screen, in that relatives of patients were studied. As a result of those prospective studies and their limited extension to the general populations, it has become possible to use HLA types to assign absolute risks for diabetes among children in the general population and those who have a relative with diabetes (17,18,92,93). When fully realized, genetic risks will be based on typing all loci according to either susceptibility to or protection from diabetes. The current understanding of the relative strengths of gene influences and the interactions among the many susceptibility and protective genes does not yet allow such complex risk assignment. Research programs that have assessed genetic risk currently combine family history and HLA typing to assess genetic risk. The addition of INS (insulin) genotyping can improve the absolute risk assessment slightly.

Practically, only children with the highest-risk HLA genotypes can be prospectively followed to characterize the preclinical phases of diabetes. The Prospective Assessment of Newborn Diabetes Autoimmunity (PANDA) and the Diabetes Autoimmune Study in the Young (DAISY) are American infant diabetes screening programs that use DNA from infant blood samples to determine HLA type. The Environmental Determinants of Diabetes in the Young (TEDDY) is a prospective, international study that launched in 2004. The protocol calls for a long-term monitoring program of newborns who are found to be at high risk for diabetes on neonatal genetic screening tests.

B. Autoantibodies

The list of autoantigens associated with diabetes includes as many as 10 or more species (94). Most of these are not routinely measured in research or clinical laboratories. This discussion focuses on the four autoantigens used most frequently.

1. Islet Cell Autoantibodies

These autoantibodies are detected by their binding to islets in frozen sections of normal human pancreas. They are present in about 80% of patients at the time of their diabetes onset. Visualized by indirect immunofluorescence, islet cell autoantibody assays are subjective and difficult to standardize. Extensive workshops have been unable to demonstrate acceptable reproducibility among different laboratories (95). They remain in limited use today, because when performed in the world's premier laboratories, islet cell autoantibodies distinguish a minority of people at high risk for diabetes who would be considered at low risk by the cumulative results of other autoantibody tests (18,96).

2. Insulin Autoantibodies

Among high-risk children followed from birth, the first autoantigen to stimulate antibody production is most frequently insulin (97,98). Insulin autoreactivity may be associated with HLA DR4 and is more frequent among those whose diabetes onset is at an early age (99). It has been considered to be of particular importance in the pathogenesis of diabetes, because T-lympho-cyte clones isolated from islets of NOD mice most frequently recognize insulin peptides (100). Insulin-reactive clones have been isolated from peripheral blood of patients with diabetes (101). Immunotherapy with insulin is able to arrest diabetes in NOD mice (102–104). Similar success has not been realized yet in human trials, albeit the most promising mouse immunotherapies are still undergoing basic safety evaluations in humans. Recent workshop data show that insulin autoantibody assays are, technically, the most challenging of the commonly used modern assays.

3. Glutamic Acid Decarboxylase 65 (GAD65) Autoantibodies

Autoantibodies against GAD65 are present in some 70% of patients with newly diagnosed diabetes. GAD65 is the rate-limiting enzyme in the synthetic pathway of the neurotransmitter, gamma-aminobutyric acid (GABA). The autoantigen is present in small quantities in pancreatic beta cells. Now measured by immunoprecipitation of synthetic antigen, the detection of autoantibodies to GAD65 has become a highly reliable assay. It is currently available in commercial labs, but it does not have approval by the Federal Drug Administration for clinical use.

4. IA-2/ICA-512 Autoantibodies

Autoantibodies to a membrane tyrosine phosphatase were discovered in the sera of diabetic patients by immunoprecipitation of human islet expression libraries (105). The function of IA-2 remains unknown. Some assays for this autoantibody use a recombinant fragment of the whole length of protein called ICA-512. Minimal differences exist in the predictive capacity of assays that use the whole protein or the ICA-512 fragment. Up to 50–60% of patients with newly diagnosed diabetes have autoantibodies against IA-2. Natural history studies have repeatedly demonstrated that the autoantibody appears later than the others, and it adds specificity to the prediction for future diabetes.

C. First-Phase Insulin Loss

In response to an intravenous glucose challenge, insulin is released in two phases. The first-phase release begins virtually immediately, reflecting initial degranulation of stored insulin from beta cells. Experimentally, the first-phase insulin response is defined as the sum of the serum insulin concentrations drawn 1 and 3 minutes after the completion of a 3-minute, 500-mg/kg intravenous glucose infusion (maximum dose of 35 g) (106).

Blunting or loss or the first-phase insulin response is an important predictor of diabetes in patients with circulating autoantibodies, because it reflects significant loss of beta-cell mass. The response is also reduced in patients with chronic hyperglycemia from type 2 diabetes. As with other predictive tests of diabetes, applications of the first-phase insulin response are currently limited to research. In many of the coming diabetes prevention trials, a participant's first-phase insulin response may determine whether beta-cell destruction has progressed to the point where an intervention with a moderate risk for adverse events could be ethically administered. Because of this application and because young children normally have lower first-phase insulin responses than older children, age-specific data from the Diabetes Prevention Trial-1 may prove invaluable in accurately assigning diabetes risk.

D. Screening in the Future

Screening for diabetes among the general population will become important when a preventive treatment becomes available. The TrialNet is a consortium sponsored by the National Institutes of Health that will be coordinating all federally funded trials of diabetes prevention agents in the United States for the foreseeable future (107). It will be important for ideal screening strategies to be defined should a successful prevention treatment be identified either in a TrialNet-coordinated effort or elsewhere.

The predictive abilities and limitations of current autoantibody assays are well understood. In the U.S. Diabetes Prevention Trial-1, 5.9% of relatives of patients with type 1 diabetes tested positive for at least one autoantibody and 2.9% had more than one circulating autoantibody (18). Specificity continues to be the limiting characteristic of these assays. The most specific autoantibody pairs (e.g., ICA and IA-2) have specificity for diabetes near 90% but sensitivity below 50%. On the other hand, sensitive autoantibody outcomes (e.g., positive for ICA or GAD65 alone) have specificities of 65–70% (95,96). When one allows for the relatively low prevalence of type 1 diabetes in the general population, the positive predictive value of autoantibody assays is acceptable for many research purposes but is often too low to justify the introduction of potentially toxic intervention therapies. Tests that can better define which autoantibody-positive individuals will develop diabetes and can better define the time until islet cell failure will result in hyperglycemia will be helpful. Additionally, tests that can identify future cases before autoantibodies become positive may allow the application of preventive treatments that block the initiation of autoimmunity. It is hypothesized that treatments that interfere with the initiation or the early propagation of autoimmune responses will be less toxic than treatments that must arrest well-established autoimmune responses.

Genomic and proteomic techniques hold promise for accomplishing these goals. Very small blood sample volumes (taken either from cord blood or capillary blood sample) provide information on the expression of thousands of proteins. Our group has demonstrated the feasibility of automated microarray screening and has defined a high-risk gene expression profile (She et al., in preparation). The utility of this profile must still be defined by prospective testing in large populations of children who have no detectable autoantibodies at the time of their first sampling. We are therefore pursuing a population-based screening strategy that defines high-risk children based on their HLA type and the presence or absence of relatives with diabetes.

One biological limitation of screening for diabetes is the heterogeneity of leukocytes in peripheral blood samples. Most circulating cells are not relevant to the autoimmune process. The tissue samples that are enriched for relevant cells (pancreas, draining lymph nodes) are currently inaccessible for routine testing, although endoscopic pancreas biopsies have been performed in selected cases (24). Cell-enrichment techniques for identifying the nature of potentially relevant cell populations in blood are currently possible, but they require impractically large volumes of blood. Finally, proteomic techniques measure concentrations of a large number of circulating proteins that may be released from inflammatory or target cells.

IV. PREVENTION

A. Risk of Disease vs Risk of Intervention

As outlined earlier, the future of diabetes prevention therapies will depend on the accuracy of predictive strategies, the pathological processes that are interrupted by the treatment, and the toxicity of that therapy. Treatments that have minimal or no significant adverse effects are likely to have clinical application to patients who have sustained little or no target cell damage. These interventions can be widely applied, even if they offer only partial protection from type 1 diabetes or its complications. With increasing complexity of the autoimmune response (more autoantigens, more extensive islet destruction), efficacious therapies are likely to carry more risk (e.g., immunosuppression). As the toxicity of proposed treatments increase, the accuracy of diagnosis must also increase. Currently, the confidence in diabetes predictions necessary to allow toxic therapies to be ethically investigated cannot be attained until beta-cell mass is markedly reduced and diabetes onset is near.

B. Infant Interventions

Two intervention trials have been launched in infants. As noted earlier, the TRIGR study is an international, multicenter trial of cow milk avoidance (66). Children at high genetic risk for diabetes were assigned to receive a formula based on either cow milk or a protein hydrolysate. Mothers were encouraged to breast-feed for as long as they desired, and formula was only initiated at the mother's request.

The preventive potential of inhaled insulin in genetically at-risk children who have developed autoantibodies is being examined in the DIPP study (108). The insulin is proposed in this trial to work by an effect on the nasal-associated lymphoid tissue and induction of immune tolerance to insulin. Autoantibodies to insulin typically appear before autoantibodies to other defined antigens. Based on animal studies, it is hoped that the induction of tolerance to insulin will prevent the progression of early phases of islet autoimmunity to more advanced and destructive phases.

Prevention trials of other dietary interventions for infants that are in the planning phases include dietary supplementation of omega-3 fatty acids and vitamin D. More potentially toxic interventions (e.g., transient depletion of CD3+ T-lymphocytes and other forms of T-lymphocyte toxicity, cytokine blockade) are unlikely to be tested in infants for many years (109,110). These treatments are likely to require initial testing in children with newly diagnosed diabetes to determine whether their "honeymoon"—the period after diagnosis during which recovery of endogenous insulin secretion contributes to good blood glucose control—can be prolonged. Success in these trials could then proceed to testing in older children who have a specifically defined 5-year diabetes risk.

V. CONCLUSIONS

Type 1 diabetes is increasingly being considered a disease of infancy and may well have prenatal determinants. Genetic predispositions are increasingly being defined and are now useful for screening large infant populations for systematic studies of disease pathogenesis and diabetes prevention. Environmental interactions with high-risk genes and immune responses are potential doorways to new prediction strategies and therapeutic interventions. Associations of diabetes with increased maternal age, ABO incompatibility, rapid growth, dietary components, and viral infections are being pursued in this regard. Agents that will be investigated for diabetes prevention will focus on antigen avoidance, modulation of autoimmune responses, and target organ sensitivity to immune attack. Ultimate success of prediction research will be reached when presymptomatic tests will be considered as diagnostic. Genomic and proteomic approaches offer the hope of attaining this goal. The ideal application of prediction strategies will be realized when preventive treatments become available.

REFERENCES

1. Kostraba JN, Cruickshanks KJ, Lawler-Heavner J, Jobim LF, Rewers MJ, Gay EC, Chase HP, Klingensmith G, Hamman RF. Early exposure to cow's milk and solid foods in infancy, genetic predisposition, and risk of IDDM. Diabetes 1993; 42:288–295.
2. Harrison LC, Honeyman MC. Cow's milk and type 1 diabetes: the real debate is about mucosal immune function. Diabetes 1999; 48:1501–1507.
3. Salminen K, Sadeharju K, Lonnrot M, Vahasalo P, Kupila A, Korhonen S, Ilonen J, Simell O, Knip M, Hyoty H. Enterovirus infections are associated with the induction of beta-cell autoimmunity in a prospective birth cohort study. J Med Virol 2003; 69:91–98.
4. Viskari HR, Roivainen M, Reunanen A, Pitkaniemi J, Sadeharju K, Koskela P, Hovi T, Leinikki P, Vilja P, Tuomilehto J, Hyoty H. Maternal first-trimester enterovirus infection and future risk of type 1 diabetes in the exposed fetus. Diabetes 2002; 51:2568–2571.
5. Hawa MI, Leslie RD. Early induction of type 1 diabetes. Clin Exp Immunol 2001; 126:181–183.
6. Stene LC, Magnus P, Lie RT, Sovik O, Joner G. Maternal and paternal age at delivery, birth order, and risk of childhood onset type 1 diabetes: population-based cohort study. BMJ 2001; 323:369.
7. Wagener DK, LaPorte RE, Orchard TJ, Cavender D, Kuller LH, Drash AI. The Pittsburgh diabetes mellitus study. 3: An increased prevalence with older maternal age. Diabetologia 1983; 25:82–85.
8. Berzina L, Ludvigsson J, Sadauskaite-Kuehne V, Nelson N, Shtauvere-Brameus A, Sanjeevi CB. DR3 is associated with type 1 diabetes and blood group ABO incompatibility. Ann NY Acad Sci 2002; 958:345–348.
9. DiLiberti JH, Carver K, Parton E, Totka J, Mick G, McCormick K. Stature at time of diagnosis of type 1 diabetes mellitus. Pediatrics 2002; 109:479–483.
10. Scheffer-Marinus PD, Links TP, Reitsma WD, Drayer NM. Increased height in diabetes mellitus corresponds to the predicted and the adult height. Acta Paediatr 1999; 88:384–388.
11. Songer TJ, LaPorte RE, Tajima N, Orchard TJ, Rabin BS, Eberhardt MS, Dorman JS, Cruickshanks KJ, Cavender DE, Becker DJ, et al. Height at diagnosis of insulin dependent diabetes in patients and their nondiabetic family members. Br Med J (Clin Res Ed) 1986; 292:1419–1422.
12. Bach JF, Chatenoud L. Tolerance to islet autoantigens in type 1 diabetes. Annu Rev Immunol 2001; 19:131–161.

13. Chentoufi AA, Polychronakos C. Insulin expression levels in the thymus modulate insulin-specific autoreactive T-cell tolerance: the mechanism by which the IDDM2 locus may predispose to diabetes. Diabetes 2002; 51:1383–1390.

14. Flodstrom M, Shi FD, Sarvetnick N, Ljunggren HG. The natural killer cell—friend or foe in autoimmune disease? Scand J Immunol 2002; 55:432–441.

15. Ohashi PS, DeFranco AL. Making and breaking tolerance. Curr Opin Immunol 2002; 14:744–759.

16. Rosmalen JG, van Ewijk W, Leenen PJ. T-cell education in autoimmune diabetes: teachers and students. Trends Immunol 2002; 23:40–46.

17. Schatz D, Krischer J, Horne G, Riley W, Spillar R, Silverstein J, Winter W, Muir A, Derovanesian D, Shah S, Malone J, Maclaren N. Islet cell antibodies predict insulin-dependent diabetes in United States school-age children as powerfully as in unaffected relatives. J Clin Invest 1994; 93:2403–2407.

18. Krischer JP, Cuthbertson DD, Yu L, Orban T, Maclaren N, Jackson R, Winter WE, Schatz DA, Palmer JP, Eisenbarth GS. Screening strategies for the identification of multiple antibody-positive relatives of individuals with type 1 diabetes. J Clin Endocrinol Metab 2003; 88:103–108.

19. Rosmalen JG, Leenen PJ, Pelegri C, Drexhage HA, Homo-Delarche F. Islet abnormalities in the pathogenesis of autoimmune diabetes. Trends Endocrinol Metab 2002; 13:209–214.

20. Liu E, Eisenbarth GS. Type 1A diabetes mellitus-associated autoimmunity. Endocrinol Metab Clin North Am 2002; 31:391–viii.

21. Jansen A, Homo-Delarche F, Hooijkaas H, Leenen PJ, Dardenne M, Drexhage HA. Immunohistochemical characterization of monocytes–macrophages and dendritic cells involved in the initiation of the insulitis and beta-cell destruction in NOD mice. Diabetes 1994; 43:667–675.

22. Foulis AK, Liddle CN, Farquharson MA, Richmond JA, Weir RS. The histopathology of the pancreas in type 1 (insulin-dependent) diabetes mellitus: a 25-year review of deaths in patients under 20 years of age in the United Kingdom. Diabetologia 1986; 29:267–274.

23. Foulis AK, McGill M, Farquharson MA. Insulitis in type 1 (insulin-dependent) diabetes mellitus in man—macrophages, lymphocytes, and interferon-gamma containing cells. J Pathol 1991; 165:97–103.

24. Imagawa A, Hanafusa T, Tamura S, Moriwaki M, Itoh N, Yamamoto K, Iwahashi H, Yamagata K, Waguri M, Nanmo T, Uno S, Nakajima H, Namba M, Kawata S, Miyagawa JI, Matsuzawa Y. Pancreatic biopsy as a procedure for detecting in situ autoimmune phenomena in type 1 diabetes: close correlation between serological markers and histological evidence of cellular autoimmunity. Diabetes 2001; 50:1269–1273.

25. Moriwaki M, Itoh N, Miyagawa J, Yamamoto K, Imagawa A, Yamagata K, Iwahashi H, Nakajima H, Namba M, Nagata S, Hanafusa T, Matsuzawa Y. Fas and Fas ligand expression in inflamed islets in pancreas sections of patients with recent-onset type 1 diabetes mellitus. Diabetologia 1999; 42:1332–1340.

26. Hanninen A, Martinez NR, Davey GM, Heath WR, Harrison LC. Transient blockade of CD40 ligand dissociates pathogenic from protective mucosal immunity. J Clin Invest 2002; 109:261–267.

27. Turley SJ. Dendritic cells: inciting and inhibiting autoimmunity. Curr Opin Immunol 2002; 14:765–770.

28. Wilson SB, Kent SC, Patton KT, Orban T, Jackson RA, Exley M, Porcelli S, Schatz DA, Atkinson MA, Balk SP, Strominger JL, Hafler DA. Extreme Th1 bias of invariant Valpha24JalphaQ T cells in type 1 diabetes. Nature 1998; 391:177–181.

29. Flohe SB, Wasmuth HE, Kerad JB, Beales PE, Pozzilli P, Elliott RB, Hill JP, Scott FW, Kolb H. A wheat-based, diabetes-promoting diet induces a Th1-type cytokine bias in the gut of NOD mice. Cytokine 2003; 21:149–154.

30. Halminen M, Juhela S, Vaarala O, Simell O, Ilonen J. Induction of interferon-gamma and IL-4 production by mitogen and specific antigens in peripheral blood lymphocytes of type 1 diabetes patients. Autoimmunity 2001; 34:1–8.

31. Kallmann BA, Lampeter EF, Hanifi-Moghaddam P, Hawa M, Leslie RD, Kolb H. Cytokine secretion patterns in twins discordant for type I diabetes. Diabetologia 1999; 42:1080–1085.

32. Rapoport MJ, Mor A, Vardi P, Ramot Y, Winker R, Hindi A, Bistritzer T. Decreased secretion of Th2 cytokines precedes up-regulated and delayed secretion of Th1 cytokines in activated peripheral blood mononuclear cells from patients with insulin-dependent diabetes mellitus. J Autoimmun 1998; 11:635–642.

33. Redondo MJ, Yu L, Hawa M, Mackenzie T, Pyke DA, Eisenbarth GS, Leslie RD. Heterogeneity of type I diabetes: analysis of monozygotic twins in Great Britain and the United States. Diabetologia 2001; 44:354–362.

34. Gale EA. The rise of childhood type 1 diabetes in the 20th century. Diabetes 2002; 51:3353–3361.

35. Cooper GS, Miller FW, Pandey JP. The role of genetic factors in autoimmune disease: implications for environmental research. Environ. Health Perspect 1999; 107(suppl 5):693–700.

36. Kristiansen OP, Larsen ZM, Pociot F. CTLA-4 in autoimmune diseases—a general susceptibility gene to autoimmunity? Genes Immun 2000; 1:170–184.

37. Heward J, Gough SC. Genetic susceptibility to the development of autoimmune disease. Clin Sci (Lond) 1997; 93:479–491.

38. Akerblom HK, Vaarala O, Hyoty H, Ilonen J, Knip M. Environmental factors in the etiology of type 1 diabetes. Am J Med Genet 2002; 115:18–29.

39. She JX. Susceptibility to type I diabetes: HLA-DQ and DR revisited. Immunol Today 1996; 17:323–329.

40. Ettinger RA, Nepom GT. Molecular aspects of HLA class II alpha-beta heterodimers associated with IDDM susceptibility and protection. Rev Immunogenet 2000; 2:88–94.

41. Pociot F, McDermott MF. Genetics of type 1 diabetes mellitus. Genes Immun 2002; 3:235–249.

42. Vafiadis P, Bennett ST, Todd JA, Nadeau J, Grabs R, Goodyer CG,

Wickramasinghe S, Colle E, Polychronakos C. Insulin expression in human thymus is modulated by INS VNTR alleles at the IDDM2 locus. Nat Genet 1997; 15:289–292.

43. Nystrom L, Dahlquist G, Rewers M, Wall S. The Swedish childhood diabetes study. An analysis of the temporal variation in diabetes incidence 1978–1987. Int J Epidemiol 1990; 19:141–146.

44. Verger P, Garnier-Sagne I, Leblanc JC. Identification of risk groups for intake of food chemicals. Regul Toxicol Pharmacol 1999; 30:S103–S108.

45. Myers MA, Mackay IR, Rowley MJ, Zimmet PZ. Dietary microbial toxins and type 1 diabetes—a new meaning for seed and soil. Diabetologia 2001; 44:1199–1200.

46. Helgason T, Jonasson MR. Evidence for a food additive as a cause of ketosis-prone diabetes. Lancet 1981; 2:716–720.

47. Longnecker MP, Daniels JL. Environmental contaminants as etiologic factors for diabetes. Environ Health Perspect 2001; 109(suppl 6):871–876.

48. Lonnrot M, Korpela K, Knip M, Ilonen J, Simell O, Korhonen S, Savola K, Muona P, Simell T, Koskela P, Hyoty H. Enterovirus infection as a risk factor for beta-cell autoimmunity in a prospectively observed birth cohort: the Finnish Diabetes Prediction and Prevention Study. Diabetes 2000; 49:1314–1318.

49. Andreoletti L, Hober D, Hober-Vandenberghe C, Fajardy I, Belaich S, Lambert V, Vantyghem MC, Lefebvre J, Wattre P. Coxsackie B virus infection and beta cell autoantibodies in newly diagnosed IDDM adult patients. Clin Diagn Virol 1998; 9:125–133.

50. Yin H, Berg AK, Tuvemo T, Frisk G. Enterovirus RNA is found in peripheral blood mononuclear cells in a majority of type 1 diabetic children at onset. Diabetes 2002; 51:1964–1971.

51. Craig ME, Howard NJ, Silink M, Rawlinson WD. Reduced frequency of HLA DRB1*03-DQB1*02 in children with type 1 diabetes associated with enterovirus RNA. J Infect Dis 2003; 187:1562–1570.

52. Sadeharju K, Hamalainen AM, Knip M, Lonnrot M, Koskela P, Virtanen SM, Ilonen J, Akerblom HK, Hyoty H. Enterovirus infections as a risk factor for type I diabetes: virus analyses in a dietary intervention trial. Clin Exp Immunol 2003; 132:271–277.

53. Graves PM, Barriga KJ, Norris JM, Hoffman MR, Yu L, Eisenbarth GS, Rewers M. Lack of association between early childhood immunizations and beta-cell autoimmunity. Diabetes Care 1999; 22:1694–1697.

54. Hummel M, Fuchtenbusch M, Schenker M, Ziegler AG. No major association of breast-feeding, vaccinations, and childhood viral diseases with early islet autoimmunity in the German BABYDIAB Study. Diabetes Care 2000; 23:969–974.

55. DeStefano F, Mullooly JP, Okoro CA, Chen RT, Marcy SM, Ward JI, Vadheim CM, Black SB, Shinefield HR, Davis RL, Bohlke K. Childhood vaccinations, vaccination timing, and risk of type 1 diabetes mellitus. Pediatrics 2001; 108:E112.

56. Kukreja A, Maclaren NK. NKT cells and type-1 diabetes and the "hygiene

hypothesis" to explain the rising incidence rates. Diabetes Technol Ther 2002; 4:323–333.

57. Daneman D, Fishman L, Clarson C, Martin JM. Dietary triggers of insulin-dependent diabetes in the BB rat. Diabetes Res 1987; 5:93–97.

58. Dahl-Jorgensen K, Joner G, Hanssen KF. Relationship between cow's milk consumption and incidence of IDDM in childhood. Diabetes Care 1991; 14:1081–1083.

59. Virtanen SM, Laara E, Hypponen E, Reijonen H, Rasanen L, Aro A, Knip M, Ilonen J, Akerblom HK. Cow's milk consumption, HLA-DQB1 genotype, and type 1 diabetes: a nested case-control study of siblings of children with diabetes. Childhood diabetes in Finland study group. Diabetes 2000; 49:912–917.

60. Gerstein HC. Cow's milk exposure and type I diabetes mellitus. A critical overview of the clinical literature. Diabetes Care 1994; 17:13–19.

61. Norris JM, Scott FW. A meta-analysis of infant diet and insulin-dependent diabetes mellitus: Do biases play a role? Epidemiology 1996; 7:87–92.

62. Norris JM, Beaty B, Klingensmith G, Yu L, Hoffman M, Chase HP, Erlich HA, Hamman RF, Eisenbarth GS, Rewers M. Lack of association between early exposure to cow's milk protein and beta-cell autoimmunity. Diabetes Autoimmunity Study in the Young (DAISY). JAMA 1996; 276:609–614.

63. Couper JJ, Steele C, Beresford S, Powell T, McCaul K, Pollard A, Gellert S, Tait B, Harrison LC, Colman PG. Lack of association between duration of breast-feeding or introduction of cow's milk and development of islet autoimmunity. Diabetes 1999; 48:2145–2149.

64. Kimpimaki T, Erkkola M, Korhonen S, Kupila A, Virtanen SM, Ilonen J, Simell O, Knip M. Short-term exclusive breastfeeding predisposes young children with increased genetic risk of type I diabetes to progressive beta-cell autoimmunity. Diabetologia 2001; 44:63–69.

65. Gottlieb PA, Eisenbarth GS. Insulin-specific tolerance in diabetes. Clin Immunol 2002; 102:2–11.

66. Paronen J, Knip M, Savilahti E, Virtanen SM, Ilonen J, Akerblom HK, Vaarala O. Effect of cow's milk exposure and maternal type 1 diabetes on cellular and humoral immunization to dietary insulin in infants at genetic risk for type 1 diabetes. Finnish Trial to Reduce IDDM in the Genetically at-Risk Study Group. Diabetes 2000; 49:1657–1665.

67. Paronen J, Bjorksten B, Hattevig G, Akerblom HK, Vaarala O. Effect of maternal diet during lactation on development of bovine insulin-binding antibodies in children at risk for allergy. J Allergy Clin Immunol 2000; 106: 302–306.

68. Monetini L, Cavallo MG, Manfrini S, Stefanini L, Picarelli A, Di Tola M, Petrone A, Bianchi M, La Presa M, Di Giulio C, Baroni MG, Thorpe R, Walker BK, Pozzilli P. Antibodies to bovine beta-casein in diabetes and other autoimmune diseases. Horm Metab Res 2002; 34:455–459.

69. Birgisdottir BE, Hill JP, Harris DP, Thorsdottir I. Variation in consumption of cow milk proteins and lower incidence of type 1 diabetes in Iceland vs the other 4 Nordic countries. Diabetes Nutr Metab 2002; 15:240–245.

70. Elliott RB, Harris DP, Hill JP, Bibby NJ, Wasmuth HE. Type I (insulin-dependent) diabetes mellitus and cow milk: casein variant consumption. Diabetologia 1999; 42:292–296.

71. Kolb H, Pozzilli P. Cow's milk and type I diabetes: the gut immune system deserves attention. Immunol Today 1999; 20:108–110.

72. Vaarala O. The gut immune system and type 1 diabetes. Ann NY Acad Sci 2002; 958:39–46.

73. Mohan IK, Das UN. Prevention of chemically induced diabetes mellitus in experimental animals by polyunsaturated fatty acids. Nutrition 2001; 17:126–151.

74. Stene LC, Ulriksen J, Magnus P, Joner G. Use of cod liver oil during pregnancy associated with lower risk of type I diabetes in the offspring. Diabetologia 2000; 43:1093–1098.

75. Fassbender WJ, Goertz B, Weismuller K, Steinhauer B, Stracke H, Auch D, Linn T, Bretzel RG. VDR gene polymorphisms are overrepresented in german patients with type 1 diabetes compared to healthy controls without effect on biochemical parameters of bone metabolism. Horm Metab Res 2002; 34:330–337.

76. Chang TJ, Lei HH, Yeh JI, Chiu KC, Lee KC, Chen MC, Tai TY, Chuang LM. Vitamin D receptor gene polymorphisms influence susceptibility to type 1 diabetes mellitus in the Taiwanese population. Clin Endocrinol (Oxf) 2000; 52:575–580.

77. Yokota I, Satomura S, Kitamura S, Taki Y, Naito E, Ito M, Nisisho K, Kuroda Y. Association between vitamin D receptor genotype and age of onset in juvenile Japanese patients with type 1 diabetes. Diabetes Care 2002; 25:1244.

78. Guja C, Marshall S, Welsh K, Merriman M, Smith A, Todd JA, Ionescu-Tirgoviste C. The study of CTLA-4 and vitamin D receptor polymorphisms in the Romanian type 1 diabetes population. J Cell Mol Med 2002; 6:75–81.

79. DeLuca HF, Cantorna MT. Vitamin D: its role and uses in immunology. FASEB J 2001; 15:2579–2585.

80. Mathieu C, Laureys J, Sobis H, Vandeputte M, Waer M, Bouillon R. 1,25-Dihydroxyvitamin D3 prevents insulitis in NOD mice. Diabetes 1992; 41:1491–1495.

81. Mathieu C, Waer M, Laureys J, Rutgeerts O, Bouillon R. Prevention of autoimmune diabetes in NOD mice by 1,25 dihydroxyvitamin D3. Diabetologia 1994; 37:552–558.

82. Zella JB, DeLuca HF. Vitamin D and autoimmune diabetes. J Cell Biochem 2003; 88:216–222.

83. Vitamin D supplement in early childhood and risk for type I (insulin-dependent) diabetes mellitus. The EURODIAB Substudy 2 Study Group. Diabetologia 1999; 42:51–54.

84. Hypponen E, Laara E, Reunanen A, Jarvelin MR, Virtanen SM. Intake of vitamin D and risk of type 1 diabetes: a birth-cohort study. Lancet 2001; 358:1500–1503.

85. Rabinovitch A, Suarez-Pinzon WL, Strynadka K, Lakey JR, Rajotte RV.

Human pancreatic islet beta-cell destruction by cytokines involves oxygen free radicals and aldehyde production. J Clin Endocrinol Metab 1996; 81:3197–3202.

86. Murata Y, Amao M, Hamuro J. Sequential conversion of the redox status of macrophages dictates the pathological progression of autoimmune diabetes. Eur J Immunol 2003; 33:1001–1011.

87. Ho E, Bray TM. Antioxidants, NFkappaB activation, and diabetogenesis. Proc Soc Exp Biol Med 1999; 222:205–213.

88. Trigwell SM, Radford PM, Page SR, Loweth AC, James RF, Morgan NG, Todd I. Islet glutamic acid decarboxylase modified by reactive oxygen species is recognized by antibodies from patients with type 1 diabetes mellitus. Clin Exp Immunol 2001; 126:242–249.

89. Gale EA, Bingley PJ, Emmett CL, Collier T, European Nicotinamide Diabetes Intervention Trial (ENDIT) Group. European Nicotinamide Diabetes Intervention Trial (ENDIT): a randomised controlled trial of intervention before the onset of type 1 diabetes. Lancet 2004; 363:925–931.

90. Elliott RB, Pilcher CC, Fergusson DM, Stewart AW. A population-based strategy to prevent insulin-dependent diabetes using nicotinamide. J Pediatr Endocrinol Metab 1996; 9:501–509.

91. Lampeter EF, Klinghammer A, Scherbaum WA, Heinze E, Haastert B, Giani G, Kolb H. The Deutsche Nicotinamide Intervention Study: an attempt to prevent type 1 diabetes. DENIS Group. Diabetes 1998; 47:980–984.

92. Ilonen J, Sjoroos M, Knip M, Veijola R, Simell O, Akerblom HK, Paschou P, Bozas E, Havarani B, Malamitsi-Puchner A, Thymelli J, Vazeou A, Bartsocas CS. Estimation of genetic risk for type 1 diabetes. Am J Med Genet 2002; 115:30–36.

93. Gillespie KM, Gale EA, Bingley PJ. High familial risk and genetic susceptibility in early-onset childhood diabetes. Diabetes 2002; 51:210–214.

94. Yoon JW, Jun HS. Cellular and molecular pathogenic mechanisms of insulin-dependent diabetes mellitus. Ann NY Acad Sci 2001; 928:200–211.

95. Verge CF, Stenger D, Bonifacio E, Colman PG, Pilcher C, Bingley PJ, Eisenbarth GS. Combined use of autoantibodies (IA-2 autoantibody, GAD autoantibody, insulin autoantibody, cytoplasmic islet cell antibodies) in type 1 diabetes: Combinatorial Islet Autoantibody Workshop. Diabetes 1998; 47:1857–1866.

96. Maclaren N, Lan M, Coutant R, Schatz D, Silverstein J, Muir A, Clare-Salzer M, She JX, Malone J, Crockett S, Schwartz S, Quattrin T, DeSilva M, Vander VP, Notkins A, Krischer J. Only multiple autoantibodies to islet cells (ICA), insulin, GAD65, IA-2 and IA-2beta predict immune-mediated (Type 1) diabetes in relatives. J Autoimmun 1999; 12:279–287.

97. Rewers M, Norris JM, Eisenbarth GS, Erlich HA, Beaty B, Klingensmith G, Hoffman M, Yu L, Bugawan TL, Blair A, Hammam RF, Groshek M, McDuffie RS Jr. Beta-cell autoantibodies in infants and toddlers without IDDM relatives: diabetes autoimmunity study in the young (DAISY). J Autoimmun 1996; 9:405–410.

98. Ziegler AG, Hummel M, Schenker M, Bonifacio E. Autoantibody appearance and risk for development of childhood diabetes in offspring of parents with type 1 diabetes: the 2-year analysis of the German BABYDIAB Study. Diabetes 1999; 48:460–468.

99. Yu L, Cuthbertson DD, Eisenbarth GS, Krischer JP. Diabetes Prevention Trial 1: prevalence of GAD and ICA512 (IA-2) autoantibodies by relationship to proband. Ann NY Acad Sci 2002; 958:254–258.

100. Wegmann DR, Norbury-Glaser M, Daniel D. Insulin-specific T cells are a predominant component of islet infiltrates in prediabetic NOD mice. Eur J Immunol 1994; 24:1853–1857.

101. Schloot NC, Willemen S, Duikerken G, de Vries RR, Roep BO. Cloned T cells from a recent-onset IDDM patient reactive with insulin B-chain. J Autoimmun 1998; 11:169–175.

102. Bregenholt S, Wang M, Wolfe T, Hughes A, Baerentzen L, Dyrberg T, von Herrath MG, Petersen JS. The cholera toxin B subunit is a mucosal adjuvant for oral tolerance induction in type 1 diabetes. Scand J Immunol 2003; 57:432–438.

103. Aspord C, Thivolet C. Nasal administration of CTB-insulin induces active tolerance against autoimmune diabetes in nonobese diabetic (NOD) mice. Clin Exp Immunol 2002; 130:204–211.

104. Muir A, Peck A, Clare-Salzler M, Song YH, Cornelius J, Luchetta R, Krischer J, Maclaren N. Insulin immunization of nonobese diabetic mice induces a protective insulitis characterized by diminished intraislet interferon-gamma transcription. J Clin Invest 1995; 95:628–634.

105. Lan MS, Wasserfall C, Maclaren NK, Notkins AI. IA-2, a transmembrane protein of the protein tyrosine phosphatase family, is a major autoantigen in insulin-dependent diabetes mellitus. Proc Natl Acad Sci USA 1996; 93:6367–6370.

106. Bingley PJ. Interactions of age, islet cell antibodies, insulin autoantibodies, and first-phase insulin response in predicting risk of progression to IDDM in ICA + relatives: the ICARUS data set. Islet Cell Antibody Register Users Study. Diabetes 1996; 45:1720–1728.

107. Bluestone JA, Matthews J. The Immune Tolerance Network: tolerance at the crossroads. Philos Trans R Soc Lond B Biol Sci 2001; 356:773–776.

108. Hahl J, Simell T, Kupila A, Keskinen P, Knip M, Ilonen J, Simell O. A simulation model for estimating direct costs of type 1 diabetes prevention. Pharmacoeconomics 2003; 21:295–303.

109. Herold KC, Burton JB, Francois F, Poumian-Ruiz E, Glandt M, Bluestone JA. Activation of human T cells by FcR nonbinding anti-CD3 mAb, hOKT3gamma1(Ala-Ala). J Clin Invest 2003; 111:409–418.

110. Herold KC, Hagopian W, Auger JA, Poumian-Ruiz E, Taylor L, Donaldson D, Gitelman SE, Harlan DM, Xu D, Zivin RA, Bluestone JA. Anti-CD3 monoclonal antibody in new-onset type 1 diabetes mellitus. N Engl J Med 2002; 346:1692–1698.

13

Adolescent Nutrition and Preconception During Pregnancy

Jane Blackwell and Lawrence D. Devoe
Medical College of Georgia, Augusta, Georgia, U.S.A.

I. BACKGROUND AND SCOPE OF THE PROBLEM

The Department of Health and Human Services (DHHS) estimates that 900,000 pregnancies occur each year among women aged 15–19 and that most (85%) of these pregnancies are unintended, with many ending in abortion (1,2). The personal and public financial impact of adolescent (teen) pregnancies in the United States is estimated in the billions of dollars annually (3). Teen pregnancy rates have declined steadily over the past decade, with the largest declines (by race) in African Americans (37%), non-Hispanic whites (7%), Asians (5%), and Hispanics (2%) (4). The DHHS (2) reported that from 1991 to 2001, the birth rate for the 15- to 19-year-old population declined from a 62.1 to 45.9 per 1000. Although all 50 states reported declining teenage birth rates, there was considerable variability among the states, ranging from 50% in Vermont to 6% in Georgia.

Numerous factors have contributed to the decreased numbers of births to adolescents, including welfare reform and special programs providing greater access to contraceptive information and abstinence education. (5). Schools, television, teen-oriented magazines, newspapers, and movies have increased teen awareness regarding the health hazards associated with pregnancy and sexually transmitted diseases.

The decreasing age of menarche from 15 to 12.5 years, coupled with changes in parenting and greater exposure to sexually explicit information, has influenced adolescent approaches to sexuality (6–8). Teenagers are becoming sexually active and achieving pregnancy at a much younger age.

Although the numbers of pregnancies in the 10- to 14-year-old age group are not comparable to those in the 15- to 19-year-old group, their unique nutritional, physical, and developmental needs have not been adequately differentiated. In 1990, the Centers for Disease Control (CDC) reported birth rates for children 10–14 as 11,657, reaching a decade high of 12,901 in 1994 and falling to 9462 in 1998. (9) Consequently, special concerns must be addressed to this subset of very young pregnant teens, as programs concerning sex education and birth control are rarely available to them.

Adverse pregnancy outcomes in teens are commonly related to unrecognized social barriers, knowledge deprivation, and/or biologic immaturity (10). Adolescents, especially those between 10 and 14 years of age, are at higher risk for pregnancy-induced hypertension, abnormally high or low weight gain, anemia, preterm labor, obstructed labors, severe asthma (10–12), and newborn attachment disorders. The Scottish Needs Assessment Program found that among adolescents, the risk of spontaneous abortion was highest in girls 13–15 years of age. Olausson et al. (13) found high preterm birth rates, <32 weeks, increasing significantly with decreasing maternal age. Very young pregnant women may also have greater exposure and yet lack immunity to common childhood diseases, such as rubella, parvovirus, and varicella (14), all of which may exert adverse effects on fetal–placental development and growth. Premature (delivery at less than 38 weeks' gestation) and low-birthweight (<2500 grams) newborns are twice as common in adolescent pregnancies when compared with adult pregnancies (10). In the past decade, rates of neonatal mortality and morbidity have decreased by 23% in adult pregnancies but have actually risen in adolescent pregnancies.

Adolescent behaviors account for much of the higher risks associated with teen pregnancy. Teens are more likely to smoke when pregnant, be unmarried, or fail to receive timely prenatal care and enter pregnancy without prepregnant nutritional preparation (15). Tobacco, drug, and alcohol use along with accidents, physical fighting, suicidal ideation, and sexually transmitted diseases are more prevalent in adolescent populations and can significantly increase developmental risks to the teenager and her fetus (8).

System barriers such as poverty, lack of food, negative attitudes, and inadequate refrigeration typify some of the environmental disadvantages for pregnant adolescents (16). Programs such as the Special Supplemental Nutrition Program for Women, Infant and Children (WIC) supplies economically disadvantaged teens and others with nutrient support by providing food sources high in protein and needed vitamins (17). However, these supplements are often shared with family members living in the same household and not exclusively available to the pregnant teen. Access to healthy foods is limited, and typical teen diets are high in sugar and saturated fats. Therefore, adolescents may enter pregnancy with malnutrition and poor nutrient stores at a time when energy and nutrient needs are their greatest.

Adolescents who are significantly under- or overweight need intensive nutritional care throughout gestation (18) The earlier the pregnant adolescent can initiate care, the more opportunities exist to identify and abate risk behaviors, assess nutrient intake, monitor weight gain, and treat underlying nutritional deficiencies. Unfortunately, adolescents are more likely to have late or no prenatal care (19,20). Blankson et al. (21) suggest that adolescents, especially those younger than 15, have even more sporadic antenatal clinic attendance in second pregnancies (10). In summary, the adolescent who is at risk for pregnancy presents challenges for their special developmental nutritional needs during pregnancy. The foci of nutrition during adolescence

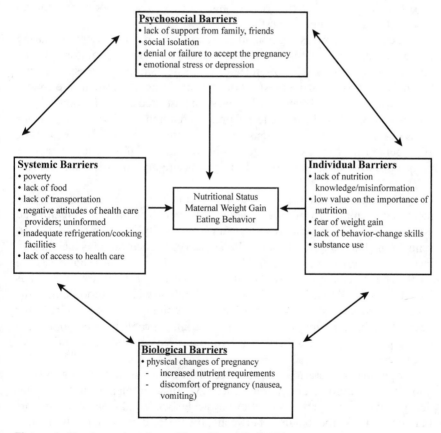

Figure 1 Barriers to good nutrition. (From Ref. 13.)

and adolescent pregnancy are as follows (10,16):(1) targeted nutrient intake, (2) appropriate weight gain, (3) elimination of harmful social factors, and (4) addressing psychological, biological, individual, and system barriers to good nutrition (Fig. 1).

II. PRECONCEPTIONAL PREPARATION FOR PREGNANCY

While health care planning prior to pregnancy is a well-accepted intervention in adult populations, it is problematic for adolescents whose pregnancies are largely unplanned. Optimal prepregnancy preparation involves the active pursuit of good health and health behaviors while avoiding substances and drugs known to be harmful to the fetus or the potential mother. This is important, since adolescents commonly abuse alcohol. Cornelius et al. (22) reported that binge drinking (five or more drinks/session) occurred among 37% of teens in the first trimester.

Teenagers express significant concerns about their weight, relating weight to image rather than to graphs that depict normal or abnormal age–sex weight percentiles. This often leads to unsafe dieting practices (anorexia, bulimia) and severe nutrient restrictions when additional nutrients are greatly needed for growth and energy (23). The strongest predictors of infant weight, after gestational length, are maternal pregravid weights and pregnancy weight gains (24–26). Underweight teens with a body mass index (BMI) below the 10th percentile for sex and age at the beginning of pregnancy will be predisposed to deliver infants that are premature and/or of low birthweight (LBW) (25).

During the past decade, obesity, defined as a BMI above 29, has increased dramatically among adolescent women. The National Health and Nutrition Examination Survey (27) examined obesity in children and adolescents in the United States between 1988 and 1994. Their findings included an increase in obesity in children 6–11 years of age from 4% in 1965 to 13% in 1999. The percentage of overweight adolescents 12–19 years of age has increased from 5% in 1970 to 14% in 1999. Obesity in childhood places the child at increased risk for obesity as an adult, with higher associated risks for heart disease, hypertension, diabetes, breathing problems, and joint pain during pregnancy and higher cholesterol and predisposition to certain types of cancers as adults.

Special considerations may be needed for certain metabolic diseases that appear in childhood and adolescence. As an example, juvenile insulin-dependent diabetes presents a set of physical, social, and dietary risk factors that complicate the balance between glucose and insulin requirements. Growth in adolescence is associated with increased insulin levels, and at the same time there is an increase in insulin resistance in both adolescence and pregnancy (28,29). Consequently, adolescents with diabetes who do become pregnant have a higher rate of spontaneous abortion, ranging from 6% to 29% (30). As in adults, these early losses are often in children with poor glycemic control in the early conceptual time period. Once pregnant, the teen will need to be monitored not only for associated early pregnancy loss, but also for commonly associated pyelonephritis, preterm labor, polyhydramnios, and fetal macrosomia.

In summary, teens who are planning to become pregnant should have a preconceptional exam by their care provider. They should be evaluated and have the following items attended to: (1) any dietary deficiencies, (2) a nonimmune rubella status, (3) necessary changes in treatment regimen for pre-existing illness, (4) lifestyle habits such as imbibing illicit drugs, smoking, and alcohol ingestion, and (5) desire for weight loss or weight gain before conception.

III. ADOLESCENT NUTRITION

Adolescence is a time of rapid physical and mental growth in which teens gain 50% of their adult weight, 50% of their skeletal mass, and 20% of their adult height (31). The U.S. Department of Agriculture's annual survey suggests that typical diets of teens do not meet the minimum requirements on the Food Guide Pyramid. Knopp (29) provides an extensive review of hormone-mediated nutrient metabolism in pregnancy and clearly identifies that large gaps continue to exist in our knowledge as to the adaptive changes seen in adolescent pregnancy.

Giddens et al. (32) studied the intake of selected nutrients and energy substrates by 59 pregnant adolescents and 97 pregnant adults and found that all were below reference values for vitamins D and E, calcium, magnesium, zinc, iron, fiber, and folate. Other studies (18,31,33–35) support these findings. Mean copper intake was decidedly below the estimated safe and adequate dietary intake. The mean intake of protein, thiamin, riboflavin, niacin, phosphorus, selenium, and vitamins B_6, B_{12}, and C met or exceeded reference values in both adolescence and adults. Among the adolescent subjects, only 79% reported high compliance in taking prescribed prenatal multivitamin and mineral supplements.

Most adolescents depend on an adult family member to purchase and prepare food. Meal patterns in this age group have also been examined. In one study of food activities among 50 adolescents, 22 (44%) participated in meal planning, 18 (36%) purchased most of their food, and 27 (54%) reported responsibility for meal preparation. Therefore, family, as well as individual education and guidance on appropriate nutrient intake during adolescent pregnancy is necessary. Guidance should focus on food sources found to be deficient in teen diets. The incorporation of more vegetables, fruits, whole grains, fortified cereals, and dairy products into meals and snacks will improve the dietary intake of these nutrients.

Iron-deficiency anemia reduces physical work capacity, learning, memory, and physical performance (36,37) and is the most common anemia of pregnancy. Infants born to iron-deficient mothers have a higher prevalence of anemia in the first 6 months of life (36). Iron-deficiency anemia in early pregnancy has been associated with low-birthweight infants and preterm delivery (38). The needs of the adolescent for iron are greatest during periods of increased muscle mass and blood volume (29,31). This demand is accentuated in pregnancy and then superimposed on the adolescents' baseline growth needs. The peak incidence of iron-deficiency anemia for girls is between the ages of 15 and 19 years (39), a time coinciding with increasing teen pregnancy rates. Most teens cannot meet this increased nutritional need without iron supplementation. Poverty and poor nutrition contribute significantly to high rates of anemia in teen pregnancies. The National Health Examination Survey (NHANES) II found that 8.7% of females aged 16–19 living below the poverty level had iron-deficiency anemia as compared to 3% of females living above the poverty level (40).

Multivitamin use in adolescent pregnancy is recommended and should provide at least 800 µg of foliate for 3 months prior to conception to reduce the risk of neural-tube defects. In 1996, the Health Education Authority launched the public component of a campaign to draw attention to the benefits of preconception vitamin supplementation in reducing the risk of neural-tube defects. Edwards et al. (41) studied teenagers' beliefs surrounding vitamin supplementation and found that 72% thought vitamin tablets were "good for the baby," 8% thought they were "bad for the baby," and 15% believed that vitamins "didn't make a difference to the health of the baby." Those adolescents who thought vitamins were "bad" for the baby were concerned there might be unknown side effects or allergies that might develop as a result of taking them for such a long period of time. They also felt that vitamins, as pills, were unnatural and determined that pills were for sick people and might unbalance their system. Another pilot survey by the same group found that adolescents believed that folic acid might cause birth defects, since they believed that acids might be corrosive. Therefore, when counseling adolescents in the use of vitamins and folic acid, care must be taken to address misconceptions that could affect subsequent dietary compliance (42).

Calcium-poor diets are common among nonpregnant and pregnant adolescents. It is the mineral for bone growth and homeostasis, with 99% of total body calcium being deposited in the bone (43). Bone growth continues until adulthood; at term, the fetus contains 25–30 mg of calcium (44).

Adaptive changes in pregnancy enhance calcium absorption, storage, and diversion to the fetus (29). Calcium absorption is greatest from 30 weeks' gestation to term, with the primary source being maternal bone calcium (29). If the mother has sufficient calcium intake, her skeleton is spared. However, when diets are poor in calcium, as they often are in teens, the needs of the fetus would supercede those of the mother (45,46). The continued bone growth during adolescence is also reflected by higher intake levels of magnesium (335 mg) and phosphorus (4,000 mg) when compared to those of adults (magnesium and phosphorus at 290 and 580 mg, respectively) (32). Variations in calcium intake during adolescence may account for as much as 5–10% of adult peak bone mass, placing this group at risk for the subsequent development of osteoporosis (31,47).

The reference value for calcium intake in children greater than 10 years of age is between 1200 and 1300 mg daily (10,32). In pregnancy, the National Institute of Health recommends this value be increased to a range of 1,500–2,000 mg per day, or about 50% higher than in nonpregnant states. Increased values persist if the mother will breast-feed after delivery. Only about 20% of adolescents are aware of the recommended dietary allowance (RDA) for calcium, and only 10% know the calcium content of various food sources (31). Excellent food sources of calcium are calcium-fortified orange juice, nonfat skim milk, yogurt, tofu, canned salmon with edible bones, cheese, cottage cheese, ice cream, and turnip greens.

IV. CALORIC INCREASES AND RECOMMENDED WEIGHT GAIN

Fast-growing, active teens have tremendous energy needs. However, adolescent caloric needs vary depending on their rate of growth, degree of physical maturation, body composition, and overall athletic activity. Little is known about the endocrinological and metabolic maladaptations of the growing adolescent mother during pregnancy (29). Prenatal weight gain is the most important predictor of newborn weight in adolescence. Studies that examined weight gains among pregnant adolescents demonstrated wide variances, with the very young mothers showing the lowest weight gains (32,48,49). A weight gain of 15.9 kg confers the lowest incidence of low-birthweight infants (50,51).

Caloric intake during pregnancy should be based on pregravid patient weights. Separate recommended dietary allowances have not been established for teen versus adult pregnancy, except for calcium, phosphorus, and magnesium (Table 1). Total weight gain in pregnancy ranges from 28 to 40 pounds for BMIs that are under 19.8; 25–35 pounds for BMIs of 19.8–26.0;

Table 1   Recommended Dietary Allowances for Adult Nonpregnant Women and Women Pregnant with Singletons, and Estimated Dietary Requirements for Women Pregnant with Twins, Triplets, and Quadruplets

Nutrient	Nonpregnant	Singleton pregnancy	Twin pregnancy	Triplet or quadruplet pregnancy	Dietary sources
Calories	2,200 kcal	2,500 kcal	3,500 kcal	4,500 kcal	Proteins, fats, carbohydrates
Protein (20%)	110 g	126 g	176 g	225 g	Meats, seafood, poultry, dairy products
Carbohydrate (40%)	220 g	248 g	350 g	450 g	Breads, cereals, pasta, dairy, fruits
Fat (40%)	98 g	112 g	155 g	200 g	Dairy products, nuts, oils
Folic acid	180 µg	400 µg	800 µg	1,200 µg	Dark green vegetables, citrus fruits
Niacin	15 mg	17 mg	25 mg	35 mg	Meats, nuts, beans
Riboflavin	1.3 mg	1.6 mg	3.0 mg	4.0 mg	Meats, liver, breads, cereals, pasta
Thiamin	1.1 mg	1.5 mg	3.0 mg	4.0 mg	Pork, meats, breads, cereals, pasta
Vitamin A	800 µg RE	800 µg RE	1,000 µg RE	1,200 µg RE	Dark green, orange, or yellow produce; liver
Vitamin B_6	1.6 mg	2.2 mg	4.4 mg	6.0 mg	Meats, liver, breads, cereals, pasta
Vitamin B_{12}	2.0 µg	2.2 µg	3.0 mg	4.0 mg	Meats, poultry
Vitamin C	60 mg	70 mg	150 mg	200 mg	Citrus fruits
Vitamin D	5 µg	10 µg	15 µg	20 µg	Fortified dairy products
Vitamin E	8 mg	10 mg	14 mg	16 mg	Nuts, oils, enriched grains
Calcium	800 mg	1,200 mg	2,000 mg	3,000 mg	Milk, cheese, ice cream
Iodine	150 µg	175 µg	300 µg	400 µg	Iodized salt, seafood
Iron	15 mg	30 mg	60 mg	90 mg	Meats, eggs, breads, cereals, pasta
Magnesium	280 mg	320 mg	500 mg	750 mg	Seafood, beans, breads, cereals, pasta
Phosphorus	800 mg	1,200 mg	2,000 mg	3,000 mg	Meats
Selenium	55 µg	65 µg	75 µg	90 µg	Breads, cereals
Zinc	12 mg	15 mg	30 mg	45 mg	Meats, seafood, eggs

Source: National Research Council, Food and Nutrition Board. Recommended Dietary Allowances. 10th ed. Washington, DC: National Academy Press, 1999.

and 15–25 pounds for BMIs over 26.0–29.0 (Table 2). Very young and African American teens are advised to aim for pregnancy weight gains toward the upper end of normal for their BMI, while teens with short stature (<157 cm) should be encouraged to have total weight gain at the lower end of the normal range (52). Excessive weight gain in adolescent pregnancy has been linked to obesity in adulthood (53) and risk of other chronic diseases such as diabetes and heart disease (54)

Birthweights associated with the highest infant survival in adolescents do not appear to be different from those found in adult pregnancies (55,56). Rees et al. (57) found that in the United States, the lowest neonatal mortality was associated with infants that weighted at least 3000 grams. Cultural and ethnic differences in birthweights have also been identified. In their study, they found that 41% of African American babies and 27% of babies born to Caucasian adolescents weighed less than 3000 grams and that young gravidas required more weight gain than did older adolescents or adults to produce the infants of the same birthweight. Inadequate early weight gains of less than 4.3 pounds by 24 weeks' gestation have been associated with increased risk of low-birthweight babies. Excessive weight gains above the 75th percentile are associated with macrodome, or infants weighing 4000 or more grams.

It should be remembered that teens continue to grow late into adolescence (49). Roche and Davila (58) found that the median age of adult stature attainment in Caucasians was 17.3 years; therefore, nearly 50% of females continued to grow after this time. Even after menarche, there is continued slow growth, with significant changes in fat deposition and weight increments.

Table 2 Recommended Total Weight Gain Ranges for Pregnant Women,[a] by Prepregnancy Body Mass Index (BMI)[b]

Weight-for-height category	Recommended total gain	
	Kilograms	Pounds
Low (BMI < 19.8)	12.5–18	28–40
Normal (BMI 19.8–26.0)	11.5–16	25–35
High[c] (BMI > 26.0–29.0)	7–11.5	15–25

[a] Young adolescents and black women should strive for gains at the upper end of the recommended range. Short women (<157 cm, or 62 in.) should strive for gains at the lower end of the range.
[b] BMI is calculated using metric units.
[c] The recommended target gain for obese women (BMI > 29.0) is at least 6.8 kg (15 lb).
Source: Nutrition During Pregnancy, p. 10 (1999), by the National Academy of Sciences.

The Camden Nutritional Study (49) and the Rowett Research Institute (59–61) performed pioneering work in nutrient partitioning in adolescence. Wallace et al. (62) suggest that similarities exist between adolescent and ovine pregnancy. Their data suggest a hierarchy of nutrient partitioning in young pregnant growing females. Further, they define nutrient partitioning and competition as altered physiological states promoting the growth of maternal tissues at the expense of the fetus and mammary gland. The Camden Nutritional Study also showed preferential distribution of nutrients in adolescent pregnancies to support continued maternal growth rather than fetal growth. The Camden Nutritional Study concluded that for adolescents, the recommended caloric intake per day is between 2200 and 2500 calories, or between 250 and 300 calories beyond the nonpregnant dietary requirement.

V. PROMOTING GOOD NUTRITION THROUGH THE USE OF DEVELOPMENTAL STRATEGIES

Nutritional counseling and needs identification in the current health care system are aimed principally at women whose cognitive and developmental processes are located between 20 and 35 years of age. Prenatal appointments are generally brief, leaving little time to discuss or encourage healthful nutritional practices. In addition, contemporary care practices assume that the pregnancy is wanted and that eventually mothers will connect with their fetus and, once instructed, will eat a healthy diet and adopt a healthy lifestyle. These assumptions cannot be made for pregnant teens, who may have little emotional, physical, or financial support and whose pregnancies may be unintended.

Effective nutritional strategies must address the social, environmental, and attitudinal barriers present in contemporary teen life. Further research is needed that incorporates developmentally appropriate activities and learning styles of both the very young pregnant teen and her older counterpart. Very young pregnant teens display operational and concrete thought processes. This means that children in this age group have difficulty understanding and integrating what they cannot touch, see, hear, or smell. Successful nutritional programs will be those that develop strategies that incorporate hands-on project learning in nutrition that includes some sort of reward that the teen would value.

Pregnant teenagers have traditionally had nutritional counseling, if at all, in the context of a traditional antenatal clinic. Junior high and high school courses such as home economics are usually elective. Nutrition in today's family is something experienced, not learned. To identify channels and barriers to nutrition education for pregnant adolescents, Janas and Hymans

(63) studied an all-woman focus group consisting of schoolteachers, school nurse, dietician, high school economics teacher, and adolescent representatives from the community at large. They were able to divide the nutritional obstructions into two main categories: implementation and impact barriers. They found that the negative attitudes regarding the development of a school-based nutrition program were fears that such a program would encourage teens to become pregnant, that school was not an appropriate place for such programs, and that classes on nutrition would interfere with academic class attendance. Impact barriers were poor reading skills, serious problems with families, finances, substance abuse, and difficulty in finding convenient times to meet.

Long et al. (64) developed a six-lesson nutrition curriculum consisting of presentations, discussion, and hands-on activity for teens called the Great Beginnings Program. The study demonstrated that a limited number of weekly lessons using comprehensive information about nutrition does make a difference in birth outcome and complemented the WIC program in which participants were also enrolled. The experimental group had significantly better outcomes in nutrition knowledge, maintenance of diet quality, mean maternal weight gain, and mean infant birthweight. Hunt et al. (51) found similar results when an 8-week course on nutrition was implemented for a group whose ages ranged from 14 to 19 years.

When resources are limited, teens with special nutritional problems should be identified and a comprehensive assessment made. In this way a nutrient-targeted nutritional rehabilitation program can be designed. Criteria for referral for nutritional counseling (Table 3) are those teens that are underweight, under the 10th percentile in weight-for-height, or overweight, over the 20th percentile for weight-for-height. Other problems that require referral are excessive vomiting accompanied by weight loss, significant medical problems that impact nutrition, such as diabetes, alcoholism, drug use, lactose intolerance, and anemia and prior history of low-birthweight infants. Pica or other aberrant cravings are surprisingly prevalent and not uncommon, especially in the southern United States. For some families, ice, dirt, clay, and laundry starch are looked upon as being healthy for the gastrointestinal system. Dirt, clay, and starch coat the intestinal tract and block the absorption of nutrients, especially iron. Teens that engage in these dietary practices usually have severe iron-deficiency anemia and malnutrition.

More research is needed in nutritional program development for teens that includes activities that incorporate the teaching of nutrition through play, role-playing, self-awareness, body control, rewards, acceptance, art therapy, puppetry, trust, and the like. Emotionally pregnant teens, in order to care about their fetus, need to engage in activities with health care providers that help them to care about themselves and to develop positive self-esteem,

Table 3 Criteria for Referral for Nutrition Counseling

I. Weight or growth problems
  A. Infant
    1. Previous low-birthweight infant
    2. Present intrauterine growth retardation or small for gestational age
  B. Mother
    1. Overweight
      a. Pregravid obesity (20% weight-for-height)
      b. Excessive weight gain (>7 lb/mo)
    2. Underweight
      a. Low pregravid weight (>10% below weight-for-height)
      b. Inadequate weight gain (<2 lb/mo after first trimester)
      c. Excessive vomiting (with weight loss, ketonuria, or both)
II. Diet-related anemias
  A. Iron-deficiency anemia
  B. Pica
  C. Vegetarian
III. Medical problems
  A. Gestational diabetes
  B. Lactose intolerance
  C. Alcoholism
  D. Drug Use

Source: Medicine of the Fetus and Mother, p. 942 (1999).

positive affirmations from people who maintain a nonjudgmental approach and who have the time and ability to recognize each teen's unique problems while pointing out her individual strengths. Gutierrez (65) found that the most powerful factors contributing to good food practices during pregnancy was the mother's concern about the health and well-being of her baby, family support, and assumption of the maternal role.

VI. SUMMARY

Adolescent or teen pregnancy, while decreasing over the past decade, still accounts for nearly one in four pregnancies in the United States. The teenaged gravida presents a set of unique challenges for adequate nutrition during pregnancy. These are impacted by the fact that many, if not most, pregnant patients in this age group are continuing to experience somatic growth and have nutritional requirements that differ considerably from their adult counterparts. Other major challenges to attaining adequate nutrition for adolescents during pregnancy have to do with lifestyles and approaches to education that cannot be addressed with interventions that are designed for older populations. The majority of teen pregnancies are unintended and, as such, would not benefit from preconceptional planning. Consequently, principles of healthy nutrition and lifestyle need to be embedded in education programs provided by the schools that are attended by these young women. Strategies to encourage adequate nutrition cannot succeed without a basic knowledge of the specific dietary requirements that distinguish adolescents from adults. Encouragement of appropriate weight gain, based on age and prepregnancy weight, requires good coordination of the entire team involved in providing prenatal care and should not be considered the sole province of nutritionist and dieticians. It is hoped that this chapter provides a useful basis for health care professional who have taken up the challenge of caring for this special group of young patients.

REFERENCES

1. U.S. Department of Health and Human Services, National Center for Health Statistics: Division of Data Services, Hyattsville, MD, 2002.
2. Trissler RJ. The child within: a guide to nutrition counseling for pregnant teens. J Am Diet Assoc 1999; 99(8):916–917.
3. Trussell J. Teenage pregnancy in the United States. Fam Plann Perspect 1988; 20:252–256.
4. U.S. Department of Health and Human Services. New guide to help local communities establish teen pregnancy prevention programs. Hyattsville, MD, 2002.
5. U.S. Department of Health and Human Services. Preventing teenage pregnancy. Hyattsville, MD, 2002.
6. Treffers PE, Olukoya AA, Ferguson BJ, Liljestand J. Special communication from the World Health Organization: care for adolescent pregnancy and childbirth. Int J Gynecol Obstet 2001; 75:111–121.
7. Guttmacher Institute. Into a New World: Young Women's Sexual and Reproductive Lives. New York: The Instituter, 1998.
8. Grunbaum J, Kann L, Kinchen S, Ross J, Gowda V, Collins J, Kolbe L. Youth risk behavior surveillance national alternative high school youth risk behavior survey, United states, 1998. J Sch Healt 2000; 70(1):5–17.
9. U.S. Department of Health and Human Services. Live Births by Age of Mother and Race: United States, 1933-1998, Hyattsville, MD, 2002.
10. Story M. Promoting healthy eating and promoting adequate weight gain in pregnant adolescents: issues and strategies. Ann NY Acad Sci 1997; 817:321–333.
11. Mohomed K, Ismail A, Masona D. The young pregnant teenager—why the poor outcome? Cent Afr J Med 1989; 35:403–406.
12. Koje JC, Palmer A, Watson A, Hay DM, Imrie A. Early teenager pregnancies in hull. Br J Obstet Gynecol 1992; 99:969–973.

13. Olausson PO, Cnattingius S, Haglund B. Teenage pregnancies and risk of late fetal death and infant mortality. Brit J Obstet Gynecol 1999; 106:116–121.

14. National Center for Health Statistics, NHANES: Immunizations. Hyattsville, MD, 2002.

15. National Vital Statistics Report. Revised birth and fertility rates for the United States, 2000 and 2001; 51(6) 1–6, 2003.

16. Chromitz VR, Cheung WY, Lieberman E. The role of lifestyle in preventing low birth weight. The Future of Children: Low Birth Weight 1995; 5:121–138.

17. Randall B, Boast L. Study of WIC Participants and Program Characteristics. Alexandria, VA: USDA Food and Nutrition Service, 1992.

18. Skinner JD, Carruth BR, Pope J, Varner L, Goldberg D. Food and nutrient intake of white and black adolescents. J Am Diet Assoc 1992; 92:1127–1129.

19. Institute of Medicine. Prenatal Care: Reaching Mothers, Reaching Infants. Washington, DC: National Academy Press, 1988.

20. Singh S, Torres A, Forrest JD. The need for prenatal care in the United States: evidence from the 1980 National Natality Survey. Fam Plann Perspect 1985; 17:118–124.

21. Blankson ML, Cliver SP, Goldenberg RL, Hickey CA, Jin J, Dubard MB. Health behavior outcomes in sequential pregnancies of black and white adolescents. J Am Med Assoc 1993; 269:1401–1403.

22. Cornelius MD, Richardson GA, Day NL, Cornelius JR, Geva D, Taylor PM. A comparison of prenatal drinking in two recent samples of adolescent and adults. J Stud Alchol 1994; 55:412.

23. Story M, Alton I. Adolescent nutrition: current trends and critical issues. Top Clin Nutr 1996; 3:56–69.

24. Scholl ML, Hediger IG, Ances IG. Weight gain in pregnancy in adolescence: predictive ability of early weight gain. Obstet Gynecol 1990; 75:948–957.

25. Institute of Medicine. Committee on Nutritional States During Pregnancy and Lactation. Washington, DC: National Academy Press, 1990.

26. Rees J. Overview: nutrition for pregnant childbearing adolescents. Ann NY Acad Sci 1997; 817:241–245.

27. National Health and Nutrition Examination Survey. Overweight among U.S. children and adolescents. Hyattsville, MD 2002:1–2.

28. Lind T, Billewicz WJ, Brown G. A serial study of changes occurring in the oral glucose tolerance test in pregnancy. Brit J Obstet Bynecol 1973; 86:1033–1039.

29. Knopp R. Hormone-mediated changes in nutrient metabolism in pregnancy: a physiological basis for normal fetal development. Ann NY Acad Sci 1997; 817:251–271.

30. Miodovnik M, Mimouni F, Siddiqi TA. Preconceptual metabolic states and risk of spontaneous abortion in insulin-dependent diabetic pregnancies. Am J Perinatal 1988; 5:368.

31. Wahl R. Nutrition in the adolescent. Ped Annals 1999; 28:107–111.

32. Giddens JB, Krug SK, Tsang RC, Guo S, Miodovnik M, Prada JA. Pregnant adolescents and adult women have similarly low intakes of selected nutrients. J Am Diet Assoc 2000; 100(11):1334–1340.

33. Lenders C, Hediger M, Scholl T, Chor-San K, Slap G, Stallings V. Effects of high sugar intake by low-income pregnant adolescents on birth weight. J Adol Health 1994; 15:596–602.

34. Lenders C, McElrath T, Scholl T. Nutrition in adolescent pregnancy. Pediatrics 2000; 12:291–296.

35. Loris P, Dewey KG, Poirier-Brode K. Weight gain and dietary intake of pregnant teenagers. J Am Diet Assoc 1985; 85:1296–1305.

36. Lynch S. The potential impact of iron supplementation during adolescence on iron status in pregnancy. Am Soc Nutr Sci 2000; 130:448–451.

37. Bruner AB, Joffe E, Duggan AK, Casella JF, Brandt J. Randomized study of cognitive effects of iron supplementation in nonanemic iron-deficient adolescent girls. Lancet 1996; 348:992–996.

38. Preziosi P, Prual A, Pilar G, Daouda H, Boureima H, Hercberg S. Effects of iron supplementation on the iron status of pregnant women: consequences for the newborn. Am J Clin Nutr 1997; 66:1178–1182.

39. Neinstein LS, Schack LE. Nutrition:Adolescent Health Care: A Practical Guide. 3rd ed. Baltimore, MD: Williams & Wilkins, 1996:139–149.

40. Miller CA, Fine A, Adams-Taylor S. Monitoring Children's Health: Key Indicators. Washington, DC: American Public Health Association, 1989:1–164.

41. Edwards G, Stanisstreet M, Boyes E. Adolescents' ideas about the health of the fetus. Midwifery 1997; 13:17–23.

42. Parker T, Edwards G, Stanisstreet E, Boyes E. Vitamins and pregnancy: teenagers' belief. Pract Midwife 1998; 3:23–24.

43. Hosking D. Calcium homeostasis in pregnancy. Clin Endocrin 1996; 54:11.

44. Haran K, Thordarsh H, Dewig T. Calcium homeostasis in pregnancy and lactation. Acta Obstet Gynecol Scand 1993; 72:509.

45. Kohlmer L, Marcus R. Calcium disorders of pregnancy. Endocrinol Metab Clin N Amer 1995; 24:15–18.

46. Okah F, Tsang R, Sierra R, Brady K, Specker B. Bone turnover and mineral metabolism in the last trimester of pregnancy: effects of multiple gestation. Obstet Gynecol 1996; 88:168–171.

47. Petkin R, Reynolds W, Williams W, Haejs G. Calcium metabolism in normal pregnancy: a longitudinal study. Am J Obstet Gynecol 1979; 133:781–790.

48. Dubois S, Coulombe C, Pencharz P, Pinsonneault O, Duquette M. Ability of the Higgins Nutrition Intervention Program to improve adolescent pregnancy outcome. J Am Diet Assoc 1997; 97:871–878.

49. Hediger M, Scholl T, Schall J. Implications of the Camden study of adolescent pregnancy: interaction among maternal growth, nutritional status, and body composition. Ann NY Acad Sci 1997; 817:281–291.

50. Stevens-Simon C, McAnarney E. Determinants of weight gain in pregnant adolescents. J Am Diet Assoc 1992; 92:1348–1351.

51. Hunt D, Stoecker B, Hermann J, Kopel B, Williams G, Claypool P. Effects of nutrition education programs on anthropometric measurements and pregnancy outcomes of adolescents. J Am Diet Assoc 2002; 102(suppl):100–102.

52. Gutierrez Y, King J. Nutrition during teenage pregnancy. Pediatr Ann 1993; 22:99–108.

53. Lederman S. The effects of pregnancy weight gain on later obesity. Obstet Gynecol 1993; 82:148–155.

54. Scholl T, Hediger M, Schall J. Excessive gestational weight gain and chronic disease risk. Am J Hum Bio 1996; 8:735–741.

55. Rees J. Overview: nutrition for pregnant and childbearing adolescents. Ann NY Acad Sci 1997; 817:241–245.

56. Reece E, Hobbins J. Medicine of the Fetus and Mother. 2d ed. Philadelphia: Lippencott-Raven, 1999:943.

57. Rees J, Lederman S, Kiely J. Birth weight associated with lowest neonatal mortality: infants of adolescent and adult mothers. Pediatrics 1996; 98:1161–1166.

58. Roche A, Davila G. Late adolescent growth in stature. Pediatrics 1972; 66:247–261.

59. Wallace J, Bourke D, Da Silva P, Aitken R. Nutrient partitioning during adolescent pregnancy. Reproduction 2001; 122:347–357.

60. Wallace J, Aitken R, Cheyne M. Nutrient partitioning and fetal growth in rapidly growing adolescent ewes. J Repro Fertil 1996; 107:183–190.

61. Wallace J. Nutrient partitioning during pregnancy: adverse gestational outcome in overnourished adolescent dams. Nutrition Soc 2000; 59:107–117.

62. Wallace J, Bourke D, Aitken R. Nutrition and fetal growth: paradoxical effects in the overnourished adolescent sheep. J Repro Fertil 1996b; 52(suppl):385–399.

63. Janas B, Hymans J. New Jersey school nurses' perceptions of school-based prenatal nutrition education. J Sch Health 1997; 67:62–67.

64. Long V, Moe R, Martin T, Janson-Sand C. The Great Beginnings Program: impact of a nutrition curriculum on nutrition knowledge, diet quality, and birth outcomes in pregnant and parenting teens. J Am Diet Assoc 2002; 102(suppl): s86–s89.

65. Guierrez Y. Cultural factors affecting diet and pregnancy outcome of Mexican American adolescents. J Adol Health 1999; 25:227–237.

14

Artificial Hydration and Nutrition in the Neonate
Ethical Issues

Steven R. Leuthner
Medical College of Wisconsin, Milwaukee, Wisconsin, U.S.A.

Brian S. Carter
Vanderbilt Children's Hospital and Vanderbilt University Medical Center, Nashville, Tennessee, U.S.A.

I. INTRODUCTION

A. Perinatal Period

A unique relationship exists between the obstetrician, the pregnant woman, the fetus, and the pediatric specialist during the perinatal period. This unique maternal–fetal relationship leads to ethical issues when considering maternal or fetal therapies. Potential conflicts might arise in how the woman views her health and self-integrity versus how she or the obstetrician views the fetal best interests.

From a nutritional standpoint these issues might center on the adolescent pregnancy, the vegetarian or fad diet in pregnancy, obesity or diabetes in pregnancy, and how maternal nutrition effects fetal growth and development. There is a wealth of writing on the ethical and legal issues involved in maternal substance use, including smoking, alcohol, and illicit drug use and nutrient delivery. A pregnant woman may have a new diagnosis of cancer requiring radiation and/or chemotherapy, or she may be terminally ill and possibly need maternal hyperalimentation. Fetal conditions may raise ethical issues in perinatal nutrition, including the intrauterine growth-restricted (IUGR) fetus or the fetus with a congenital anomaly.

While these scenarios may lead to interesting ethical issues, they are outside the scope of this chapter except to acknowledge that the unique relationship exists. These issues all center on the main question of whether the fetus is a patient and whether the woman has a moral obligation to undergo treatment directed toward fetal well-being. It has been argued by some that the obstetrician has two patients, where access to one (fetus) is only through the other (pregnant woman). This requires the complex balancing of fetal best interests and a pregnant woman's health and integrity. In choosing to carry her pregnancy to term, she accepts some moral responsibility to make reasonable efforts toward preserving fetal health. We recommend in considering nutritional therapies in the perinatal period that they be strongly advocated for if the therapy meets the criteria put forth by Chervenak and McCullough for fetal therapies (1). They suggest that fetal interventions be used if the therapy is judged to have:

1. A high probability of being life-saving or preventing serious and irreversible disease, injury, or disability for the fetus and future child
2. Low mortality risk and manageable risk of injury to the fetus
3. Mortality risk and risk of injury or disability to the pregnant woman that is low or manageable

B. Neonatal Period

In neonatology, the provision of intravenous and medically administered fluids and nutrition is fundamental as part of both basic care and critical care for premature and ill infants. The goals of such interventions may be to:

1. Match in utero fetal growth rates in the premature newborn and ensure normal development
2. Provide energy substrate to meet basic metabolic needs and any increased needs attendant to acute or chronic illness
3. Ensure the nutrient balance necessary to support proper immune function and wound healing

As with other treatments, the provision of artificially administered hydration and nutrition should be conducted in such a manner as to be consistent with the body of clinical and research evidence. It should be done in a manner that will achieve its stated goals safely, benefit the patient, and be consistent with the overall plan of care for the infant.

II. WITHDRAWAL OF TECHNOLOGICAL NUTRITION AND HYDRATION: WHAT WE CAN LEARN FROM THE ADULT MODEL

The consideration of hydration and nutrition from an ethical perspective first gained wide attention in clinical medicine and ethics at the close of the 1970s and in the early 1980s. In the adult literature, there was an "emerging stream" of thought that fluids and nutrition could be withheld. The argument for withdrawal rests on two propositions:

1. Nutritional and hydration support is a medical intervention.
2. Judgment about withholding/withdrawing medical interventions is based on a calculus of benefits and burdens (proportionality).

Seigler and Weisbard (2) argued against this emerging stream, stating that while these two propositions are true, they found it "troublesome" that physicians or families could possibly conclude that the "burdens of withdrawal" might outweigh the "benefits" of treatment (e.g., a sustained life).

Such thinking may well be flawed. It certainly appears to be against how clinicians commonly approach such weighty decisions. When deciding to continue or withdraw a ventilator, for example, clinicians do not balance the benefits of the treatment against the burdens of treatment withdrawal. Instead, what is considered are the benefits and burdens of the treatment itself, should it be started, continued, or withdrawn. It is important to understand the consequences of not providing the treatment, which also have their benefits and burdens. But to report the treatment as beneficial and the withdrawal as burdensome immediately shows a value bias, not a rational weighing of proportionality.

Later in the 1980s, Mark Yarborough (3) proposed that physicians may be mislead by the symbolism that is often attached to artificial feeding—especially tube feeding for terminally ill adults. The perception voiced by many physicians was that these measures were essential—even when other medical interventions were being withdrawn. The argument made by clinicians generally held that the withdrawal of artificial hydration and nutrition would be the equivalent to "starving a patient to death" or allowing the patient to "die of thirst." Yarborough probed the issue further by asking clinicians to consider the provision of medically administered hydration and nutrition not as an essential good but, rather, as "force feeding." He stated that

1. The burden of proof should rest with those who insist on tube feeding to demonstrate benefit rather than on those who would forego it to explain [potential] harms.

2. The emotional attachment that clinicians have to artificial hydration and nutrition interferes with more reasoned ethical decisions—highlighting the need for facts about the risks and benefits of such measures in the terminally ill patient.

3. Research into the potential that forced artificial hydration and nutrition might even be considered a form of torture rather than a means of providing comfort for a supposed state of suffering.

Indeed, many physician professional societies (and ethicists) see no difference in artificially administered hydration and nutrition and any other medical intervention that might become inappropriate in a given patient's condition and thereby be considered for withdrawal (4–6).

In 2000, Stephen Winter reviewed the benefits and burdens of nutritional support and of withholding/withdrawing (WH/WD) it in regards to survival, response to therapy, and comfort or correction of metabolic abnormalities in adults (7). He reported that studies have consistently failed to demonstrate a meaningful clinical benefit of nutritional support at or near the end of life. Importantly, he reviewed studies demonstrating that parenteral hydration and nutrition has a general complication rate of at least 15% (infection, thrombosis, etc.). In reviewing artificially administered enteral feedings, which are often thought to be less invasive, he found that only 24% of patients did not have some major or minor complication.

Winter also reviewed the benefits and burdens of not providing these interventions (7). Benefits reported in not providing artificially administered hydration and nutrition included a reduction in the metabolic rate, urea load, respiratory secretions, coughing, nausea, vomiting, diarrhea, urine output—all of which make the clinical or custodial care of the patient easier. Fasting also was reported to lead to psychological or behavioral changes—including induced endogenous endorphins, which may lead to an analgesia effect, with a rise in pain threshold or euphoria even amid the preservation of mental function. Ketones produced with fasting are also known to reduce hunger.

III. WITHDRAWAL OF TECHNOLOGICAL NUTRITION AND HYDRATION: PEDIATRICS

While in the adult literature there is support that artificial means of hydration and nutrition near the end of life do not prolong life, this might not be true in pediatrics. There are pediatric populations for whom gastrostomy tube feedings or parenteral nutrition will prolong the life of the child even though the child will eventually die from the underlying disease. An example may be the premature child with an extremely short gut or a child with severe hypoxic–ischemic encephalopathy (HIE). Of course it may be because these lives can be prolonged that one ought to engage the family in the dialogue about what constitutes a valued life or, alternatively, what may be considered as prolonging death. Families need information and the opportunity to have time for reflection as well as room to contribute to a most difficult decision. What may first be considered as absolutely essential care for every infant may need to be viewed in light of the underlying diagnosis, prognosis, and limits of what medicine has to offer. As Ronald Cranford has stated, "Anyone who believes that eating and drinking in normal children are remotely similar to providing a feeding tube for severely brain damaged children has never been present at the bedside of these patients and has no good sense of the medical reality" (8).

A. Decision Making

In considering the decision-making process for the WH/WD of artificially administered hydration and nutrition, many issues must be examined. While the focus needs to remain on the infant and his/her perceived best interests, all pertinent decision makers need to be identified, facts obtained and values contemplated, and external concerns such as legal precedents weighed.

B. Decision Makers

The prerogative of parents as principal decision makers for their children is well established. Their role in the neonatal intensive care unit (NICU), however, has been variably considered in the last 40 years (9–11). Myths concerning the parent(s)' capabilities need to be dismissed, barring evidence of their being incapacitated, acting with harmful intent, or being absent or uninvolved (12). These may include such myths as parents being unable to hear and understand facts, being overwhelmed by emotions, or speaking out of concern for their own interest rather than the infant's interests. Health care professionals obviously have an interest in the well-being and long-term outcome of their patients. In the NICU, where outcomes may be uncertain, the inclination to treat or intervene seems rational when growth, development, healing, and some measure of health can be attained. However, there are tragic situations in which cure-oriented care needs to recede and give way to comfort measures, in view of terminal prognoses (see Table 1). The state also may hold an interest in preserving an infant's life if it is clear that the life will be meaningful in a human relational sense. Similarly, if perceived suffering can be reduced and parents do not allow for such, the state's interests may prevail and parental rights be limited or terminated through court actions.

Table 1 Diagnoses in which Withdrawal or Withholding of Hydration and Nutrition are Likely to be Considered

Anencephaly
Trisomy 13/18
Potter's syndrome
Lethal dwarfism
Congenital heart disease (inoperable)
Hypoxic–ischemic encephalopathy
NEC and total bowel necrosis
Total bowel Hirschprung's/neuronal dysplasia
Werdnig Hoffman
Severe short gut syndrome (e.g., from necrotizing enterocolitis or midgut volvulus)

C. Factual Considerations

The facts that need to be considered in making decisions to WH/WD artificially administered hydration or nutrition fall into two categories. First, the medical facts that pertain to the underlying diagnosis, its response to any previously given treatments, its likely response to appropriate treatments or interventions not yet offered, and the ultimate prognosis for the infant's condition need to be determined and discussed. Is there any of the following?

1. An underlying lethal condition (e.g., Trisomy 18)
2. A refractory chronic and debilitating condition (severe broncho-pulmonary dysplasia with respiratory failure on assisted ventilation at >3 months of age)
3. A circumstance of multiple organ–system failure (perhaps overwhelming sepsis)
4. An irreparable loss of vital tissue or organ function (e.g., severe short gut)

Or is the condition one that can be overcome with time or for which there exists nutritional, medical, or surgical options (even organ transplantation) given time, relative health, and access to such measures at home or in the hospital?

The second category of factual considerations is human value in nature. What is it that the parents anticipate, expect, or desire for this infant—even amid an unexpected or complicated course in the NICU? What values, principles, or other constructs motivate their likelihood to consider risk, weigh options, and proceed with decision making? And also, what values are upheld or pursued by the involved health care team? These facts often are not explicitly discussed on rounds. They may require formats such as patient/

family care conferences, ethics consultation, or other more deliberately planned sessions to uncover values that are important in shaping choices. The American Academy of Pediatrics has given guidance about decision making for critically ill newborns and infants, which speaks to the need for these human-value facts to be as clearly elaborated as medical facts in order to pursue an informed, shared decision-making process (13–15). Leuthner has further elaborated on the negotiated best-interest standard as an essential and most beneficial means by which to accomplish a mutually recognized good for the infant by parents and health care professionals alike (16). Thus, human-value facts must be discovered and discussed.

D. Legal Issues

Finally, the external considerations that may shape decisions for WH/WD of artificially administered hydration and nutrition must be examined as real people within society and institutions make choices that may lead to precedents for others. There have been a total of eight judicial decisions regarding the withdrawal of technological hydration and nutrition: Four addressed patients in a persistent vegetative state (PVS) and four addressed never-competent persons (17). Many appellate court decisions regarding nasogastric or gastrostomy tube feedings, as well as parenteral nutrition, hold these measures to be equivalent to life-sustaining technologies such as mechanical ventilation. In a recent issue of the Journal of the American Medical Association, seven legal barriers to end-of-life care were addressed as myths, realities, or having grains of truth (18). The authors describe the myth that WH/WD of artificial fluids and nutrition from terminally ill or permanently unconscious patients is illegal. They state the reality is that like any other medical treatment, these can be withheld/withdrawn if the patient refuses or, in the case of an incapacitated patient, the appropriate surrogate decides. In those situations that require a surrogate, however, the "grains of truth" are different among the states, many having different levels of legal standards. Some states, including Wisconsin, may not allow the option to WH/WD artificially administered hydration and nutrition at the request of a surrogate decision maker unless the patient is terminal or in a persistent vegetative state or there is some explicit refusal of this treatment prior to the respective patient's losing decision-making capacity. But the value of human dignity extends to both competent and incompetent individuals. Cognitive or developmental incompetency should not result in a denial of the right of being free from medical interventions.

Where does this leave children? The incompetent child has a right to refuse medical treatment, and that decision properly belongs to the parents.

The assumption that life-sustaining treatment should continue until death is imminent, if the patient has not previously indicated otherwise, makes the infant or child a passive object of medical technology (17). It would seem necessary, again, to place the burden of proof on the medical staff to demonstrate that a parent/guardian is not acting in the best interests of the infant before usurping this authority from them.

State interests in the infant's life for any particular case may be pertinent, however, if the infant's condition is not terminal or irreversible. The so called Baby Doe rules (Child Abuse Amendments) may pertain should physicians, parents, or others question the consideration of artificially administered hydration and nutrition as "medically indicated" treatment or construe it as clinically "appropriate" in all cases.

The 1984 Federal Child Abuse Prevention and Treatment Act states,

> The term ["withholding of medically indicated treatment"] does not include the failure to provide treatment (other than *appropriate* nutrition, hydration, or medication) to an infant when, in the treating physician's... *reasonable* medical judgment ...
>
> a. the infant is *chronically and irreversibly* comatose,
> b. the provision of such treatment would
>
>   (i)   merely prolong dying,
>   (ii) not be effective in *ameliorating* or correcting all of the infant's life-threatening conditions, or
>   (iii) otherwise be *futile* in terms of the survival of the infant; or,
>
> c. the provision of such treatment would be *virtually futile* in terms of the survival of the infant and the treatment itself under such circumstances would be *inhumane* (italics added for emphasis).

Such language (see italics) is subject to varied interpretations:

1. Every infant provided with medical means of nutrition all the time, or
2. Every infant should receive nutrition appropriate for his/her medical situation.

Realistically, this law does not apply directly to physicians, nurses, or parents. Nor does it create federally mandated standards of care (20). It does not authorize any civil or criminal penalties. What it addresses is the receipt of federal dollars for patient care and the potential that such money may be curtailed if an institution is reported, investigated, and found to be in breach of the Child Abuse and Neglect Amendments by withholding care against the standards stated earlier. Given the broad interpretation of *appropriate* nutrition, hydration, or medication, the purview of reasonable clinical judgment, there should not be a restrictive interpretation of these rules to prohibit the withdrawal of nutrition.

E. Emotional Considerations

There are strong psychological forces that lead many people, both parents and professionals alike, to think of nutrition and hydration as different from medical treatments. Pediatric professionals demonstrate this when they make a distinction between artificial breathing and feeding and their practice patterns of treatment withdrawal. The Pediatric Section of the Society for Critical Care Medicine demonstrated that 98% of physicians were apt to withhold cardiopulmonary resuscitation (CPR), 86% to withdraw ventilators, and only 42% to withdraw tube feedings (21). A pediatric house-staff survey (3rd-year residents) revealed a practice that 100% would withhold CPR and vasoactive drugs, 97% would withdraw ventilator support, but only 45% would withdraw fluids and nutrition (22). A 1991 Child Neurology Society survey demonstrated that 75% of pediatric neurologist never withheld nutrition and hydration, even in cases of persistent vegetative state in children (23). And in a 2003 inpatient review of the care provided to terminally ill infants and children, while CPR or assisted ventilation was withheld or withdrawn in 55% and 64%, respectively, of dying infants and children, only 23% had their nutritional support removed prior to their death (24).

Those who argue against withdrawing artificially administered hydration and nutrition generally hold that there is something basic about eating or being fed. This intuitive desire to help provide food to infants and children seems to have even more symbolic importance to parents than to other family members who might be asked to consider it in an adult relative, because of the nature of parenting and the very biological and social roles that parents fulfill. Parents nurture their infants by doing many things, including feed them. Yet, while it would indeed be wrong to withhold hydration and nutrition from otherwise-healthy infants, some infants are not—or may never be—healthy at all (see Table 1) (25). Hence, the moral or ethical confusion of any obligatory provision of hydration and nutrition to all infants and children should be avoided (17).

In a 2000 article by Johnson and Mitchell, the issue of WH/WD artificial means of hydration and nutrition is addressed (26). They agree there is no moral distinction between an endotracheal breathing tube (ETT) and a feeding tube of any sort—plastic tubes that enter a body orifice for the purpose of providing necessary elements for survival, be they sugar, protein, fat, or oxygen, have no moral distinction. Additionally, they and others address a few of the psychological issues pertinent to this issue (17,26). Such considerations as the societal beliefs that children are not supposed to die, that medicine may have a "cure" for any given condition "just around the corner," and that clinicians therefore should not "give up" on any infant or child all must be recognized. Perhaps the most pertinent real concern, both factually and emotionally, is the potential uncertainty of outcomes for a given condition in a young infant. This may be true for neurologic and metabolic diagnoses and even for some other chronic conditions.

Many of the psychological stumbling blocks may revolve around the concept of *starving* and the issue of *time*. If a clinician withdraws a ventilator from an infant, the infant typically does some breathing on his/her own. It may be only one agonal breath in a critically ill infant, but continued respiratory function may continue for some time in others—for some infants it may be days. Typically, if an infant does some intermittent breathing, allowing it to live for a few hours or days, it is not argued that clinicians should reinstate the ETT because the infant is taking in only half the oxygen she or he needs. Instead, the standard of care is to apply palliative care through giving oxygen and medication for comfort.

Yet this is the conclusion that many arrive at in cases concerning artificially administered feedings. It is argued that if the infant may take in half of the feeding required to survive, there is justification in providing the other half through artificial means (26). The course of reasoning for this is that without feedings, the infant's dying (and alleged suffering) will be protracted—therefore, a slow "starving" of the infant should be avoided. This rationale may well be the first of a few psychological traps into which any caregiver may fall. The exploration of what is meant when people say the word *starving* seems necessary.

Typically when *starving* is used, there are two parts to the word that come to mind. The first of these is the lack of nutrition. This includes the lack of calories, proteins, fats, and sugars. It may well be true that taking in only half of the necessary feedings necessary to sustain life, accomplish growth, or heal disease may lead to a slow death through lack of nutrition. But the question must be asked: Is this really any different than the infant who takes intermittent breaths of oxygen—not enough to survive, but enough to prolong things a little? Why would the response to these two scenarios be different?

The second part to be considered when using the word *starving* is that there is a connotation of suffering that accompanies the lack of nutrition. It is this meaning of the word that people rely upon for an emotional response. Suffering is a well-recognized thing to be avoided. The goals of medicine include the reduction or elimination of suffering. Such a consideration, then, has moral weight. But the moral weight is no different than that for the infant for whom the ventilator is withdrawn. In this latter case it is argued to give morphine to take away the suffering attributed to air hunger. Is this any different than providing morphine or some other medication to take away food hunger? If the infant will be suffering, clinicians do not want to cause a long-suffering death. Ronald Cranford states, "Patients do not show any of the terrible signs of starvation described by pro-life supporters" (8).

The difference that may exist between the withdrawal of these two interventions really seems to be in the length of time from withdrawal of the intervention until death. Should it be asked if there is any moral significance in the "time" from WH/WD to death? This consideration of time may represent a second psychological stumbling block for caregivers. If, indeed, time is the issue, it probably underscores why most clinicians have so easily come to grips with stopping ventilation—the infant usually dies rather quickly. Without much time on their hands to fret over whether this is the "right decision," it may be more readily accepted. Comfort care is provided for a relatively short time, and it is generally considered that the right thing was done for the infant. On the other hand, when all hydration and nutrition is discontinued, it can take up to 2–3 weeks for an infant to die. This gives us plenty of "time" to question the moral stance of involved parties, the infant included. If the infant takes in half the necessary volume of feedings orally, this time may be even more prolonged, in the range of months. But if this time is spent without suffering, is it wrong? Is it really different than if it only was a few hours or days?

In the end, if the infant has a condition she or he will eventually die from, there is no real moral weight to "time" other than the importance that it be spent free of suffering, with optimal human contact, and in comfort. Such a consideration, then, may equally support the removal of all artificially administered hydration and nutrition and the provision of active comfort measures (27). It could be argued not to provide artificial tubes but instead to turn hopes toward providing the best care and comfort for the baby in the remaining time that he/she has with family.

Should an infant be provided some volume of feedings as a first measure of comfort, it will likely satisfy his/her hunger—so there will not be hunger "pains." In such a setting, there is likely not any second component to the definition of starving—no suffering. The fact is, however, that artificial feedings can issue more discomfort than benefit for the dying child. Risks attendant to the administration of hydration and nutrition are noteworthy (see Table 2). And, as in the case with adults, that such measures are truly beneficial to the infant remains to be demonstrated beyond the simple fact of prolonging the infant's biologic life—perhaps without any potential for perceiving benefit or interacting in a human relational sense (28).

Table 2 Risks Associated with the Administration of Artificial Hydration and Nutrition

Intravenous delivery	Enteral delivery
Difficult access	Agitation
Pain	Epistaxis
Complications of central line placement:	Airway obstruction
Pneumothorax	Sinusitis
Chylothorax	Aspiration pneumonia
Sepsis	Intestinal obstruction
Catheter-site infection	Abdominal distention
Venous thrombosis	Emesis
	Diarrhea

Both
Metabolic aberrations: Hyperglycemia, hypophosphatemia, hypomagnesemia, hypercalcemia
Hyperosmolar state
Cholestasis

Source: Adapted from Ref. 3.

IV. PRACTICAL STRATEGIES IN THE NICU

Given the necessity, at times, of considering to WH/WD artificially administered hydration and nutrition in the NICU, what guidance can be given in developing a plan of care (see Table 3)?

Of foremost consideration is the necessity to maintain communication between the parents, the extended family, and the health care staff. All involved should be aware of the infant's signs and symptoms that may develop with the withdrawal or artificial hydration and nutrition—and the time frame over which these will likely appear following withdrawal until death. Any staff member that is uncomfortable with a decision to WH/WD hydration and nutrition should be allowed to step down from the care of the infant, just as with withdrawal of any other therapy.

If there is going to be a withdrawing of other support, such as a ventilator or vasoactive support, and death is expected in minutes to hours, then intravenous access may be important for comfort medicine and need not be removed until after death. It is reasonable to cap the intravenous line. While some feel more comfortable removing these other modalities first and then addressing the withdrawal of hydration later, this is an unnecessary step and may lead to more psychological distress than removing all therapies at

Table 3 Plan of Care for the Infant Under Palliative Care Treatment Plans and Having a "Do Not Resuscitate" Status

- Change philosophical focus to caring, not curing. Identify the goals of care.
- Appropriately address pain and symptom management.
- Identify infant and family needs and the resources to meet them.
  Spiritual
  Psychosocial
  Child life resources
  Cultural
  Grief counseling and bereavement support
  "How to Parent" the terminally ill infant—roles of care
  What can be expected? How long?
  Home/hospice care
- Support health care theme issues.
  Education
  Communication
      Open forum to discuss possible disagreements
      Care conferences
      Consultation with Ethics Committee or Palliative Care Team
      Care plan and timetable, changes to be expected
  Decision-making strategies
  Emotional support

once. It is also important to withdraw nutrition and hydration together, because withdrawal of nutrition only prolongs the death without the biological advantages of dehydration on relieving other symptoms.

Assuming the infant has survived the withdrawal of other therapies, it is important to understand the potential time frame of death from withdrawing/withholding artificially administered hydration and nutrition. This is dependent somewhat on the disease process and the size of the infant. For example, the preterm infant who had NEC and has severe short gut syndrome will likely die within a week or so from stopping. The full-term infant with gastroschesis and short gut from infarction of the intestine, on the other hand, may survive up to 3 weeks. While it will be impossible to predict when a child might die at the outset, it is important that the staff and family be prepared that this might take a while. If the infant can take in some oral feedings and acts hungry, they should be provided. In this setting, it is important to remain focused on the overall goals of comfort care, for this infant might live weeks to months. Encouraging a shift of focus from wondering and sadly wishing for the death to be quick toward one of enjoying each extra day as a gift goes a long way in coping and avoiding second-guessing.

Another issue to address is where the family wishes the death to take place. Some may want to stay in the NICU because of the support they feel from the staff. Others might choose to go home with hospice care. Still others may wish to move to a more private room in the hospital. The "environment" of the death includes both space and personal support, both of which require individualized attention with each family. The family should be counseled that they can determine what additional personnel are to be considered family supports and who needs to know about the issues. Respecting family privacy and confidentiality is always important, but in this scenario it may be even more of an issue because those not immediately involved may only prove a disservice by holding out unrealistic or inconsistent ideas, such as expecting this infant to be a "miracle baby." The ease with which a family chooses where their infant will die will likely depend on their comfort in understanding and being supported psychologically, spiritually, and in symptom management.

Pertinent symptom management for infants receiving palliative care is listed in Table 4. Generally, infants who die from the WD/WH of hydration and nutrition do so comfortably. While there will likely be significant

Table 4 Goals of Feeding and Palliative Care Symptom Management

Typical medical goals
Growth and maturation = 120 kcal/kg/day

Palliative care goals
Comfort... the infant should be symptom free.

Parental goals
Fulfill parenting instincts. Know that the infant is not starving. Recognize signs
  and symptoms of hunger:
    Continual whining or whimpering without other cause
    Agitation/irritability/inability to settle without other cause

Symptom management
Hunger: allow oral feeds for comfort (eye dropper, finger feeding, suckling)
Mouth care: daily mouth exam for thrush; toothettes, mucous membrane care
  swabs every 4 hours
Skin care: Vaseline or nonperfumed lotion to skin; hygiene to diaper area, but no
  need for full bath
Eye care: Artificial tears every 8 hours
Sedation: hydroxyzine or lorazepam IV or sublingual prn; chloral hydrate per
  rectum prn.
Pain control: temperature control; repositioning and swaddling; morphine
  sublingual, per eye dropper PO, or IV

electrolyte disturbances, seizures are extremely rare and usually occur only in infants who have an underlying seizure disorder or neurological condition. If a child is going home with a family, lorazepan should be available for any sign of agitation, and it can be given IV, IM, PO, or subcutaneously for a seizure. Morphine should also be available for any signs of discomfort. Both of these medicines can be given sublingually or by dropper. Good skin and mucous membrane care is important in helping prevent any potential symptom of thirst or discomfort. It is also an outward sign that the infant is well cared for by the family.

When the infant stops making urine, death can soon be anticipated. It usually will be only a number of days from the point of anuria. Typically, the infant will have more and more sleep periods, eventually not ever consciously waking. Death is usually described as happening comfortably in the infant's sleep.

REFERENCES

1. Chervenak FA, McCullough LB. Ethical issues in recommending and offering fetal therapy. West J Med 1993; 159:396–399.
2. Seigler M, Weisbard AJ. Against the emerging stream. Should fluids and nutritional support be discontinued? Arch Intern Med 1985; 145:129–131.
3. Yarborough M. Why physicians must not give food and water to every patient. J Fam Pract 1989; 29:683–684.
4. Council on Scientific Affairs and Council on Ethical and Judicial Affairs. Persistent vegetative state and the decision to withdraw or withhold life support. JAMA 1990; 263:426–430.
5. Hastings Center. Guidelines on the Termination of Life-Sustaining Treatment and Care of the Dying. Briarcliff Manor, NY: Hastings Center, 1987.
6. Society of Critical Care Medicine Ethics Committee. Attitudes of critical care medicine professionals concerning forgoing life-sustaining treatments. Crit Care Med 1992; 20(3):320–326.
7. Winter S. Terminal nutrition: framing the debate for the withdrawal of nutritional support in terminally ill patients. Am J Med 2000; 109:723–726.
8. Cranford RE. Withdrawing artificial feeding from children with brain damage: is not the same as assisted suicide or euthanasia. Br Med J 1995; 311:464–465.
9. Harrison H. The principles for family-centered neonatal care. Pediatrics 1993; 92:643–650.
10. Anderson B, Hall B. Parents' perspectives of decision making for children. J Law, Med Ethics 1995; 23:15–19.
11. Carter BS, Leuthner SR. Decision making in the NICU—strategies, statistics, and "satisficing." Bioethics Forum 2003; 18(3/4):7–15.
12. President's Commission for the Study of Ethical Problems in Medicine and Biomedical and Behavioral Research. Deciding to Forego Life-Sustaining

Treatment: A Report on the Ethical, Medical, and Legal Issues in Treatment Decisions. Washington, DC: U.S. Government Printing Office, 1983:171–192.

13. American Academy of Pediatrics, Committee on Fetus and Newborn. The initiation or withdrawal of treatment for high-risk newborns. Pediatrics 1995; 96:362–363.

14. American Academy of Pediatrics, Committee on Fetus and Newborn and American College of Obstetricians and Gynecologists, Committee on Obstetric Practice. Perinatal care at the threshold of viability. Pediatrics 1995; 95:974–976.

15. American Academy of Pediatrics, Committee on Bioethics. Ethics and the care of critically ill infants and children. Pediatrics 1996; 98:149–152.

16. Leuthner SR. Decisions regarding resuscitation of the extremely premature infant and models of best interest. J Perinatol 2001; 21:1–6.

17. Nelson LJ, Rushton CH, Cranford RE, Nelson RM, Glover JJ, Truog RD. Forgoing medically provided nutrition and hydration in pediatric patients. J Law Med Ethics 1995; 23:33–46.

18. Maisel A, Snyder L, Quill T. Seven legal barriers to end-of-life care: myths, realities, and grains of truth. JAMA 2000; 284(19):2495–2501.

19. U.S. Child Abuse Protection and Treatment Amendments of 1984. Pub L No. 98-457.

20. Barnett TJ. Baby Doe: nothing to fear but fear itself. J Perinatol 1990; 10:307–311.

21. Task Force on Ethics of the Society of Critical Care Medicine. Consensus report on the ethics of foregoing life-sustaining treatments in the critically ill. Crit Care Med 1990; 18(12):1435–1439.

22. Rubenstein JS, Unti SM, Winter RJ. Pediatric resident attitudes about technologic support of vegetative patients and the effects of parental input—a longitudinal study. Pediatrics 1994; 94(1):8–12.

23. Ashwal S, Bale JF, Coulter DL, et al. Child Neurology Society Ethics Committee. The persistent vegetative state in children: results of the questionnaire sent to members of the Child Neurology Society [abstr]. Ann Neurol 1991; 30(3):472–473.

24. Howenstein M, Carter BS, Gilmer MJ, et al. Circumstances surrounding pediatric death in hospital [abstr]. J Invest Med, 2003, 51.

25. Carter BS, Sandling J. Decision making in the NICU: the question of medical futility. J Clin Ethics 1992; 3:142–143.

26. Johnson J, Mitchell C. Responding to parental requests to forego pediatric nutrition and hydration. J Clin Ethics 2000; 11(2):128–135.

27. Catlin AJ, Carter BS. Creation of a neonatal end-of-life palliative care protocol. J Perinatal 2002; 22:184–195.

28. Morris EB, Carter BS. Decision making for severely brain-injured newborns. Pharos; Spring, 2001, 4–9.

Index

Set up meeting

Week of June 9th

ideal Thurs 6/12
12th

Post — Adrienne & Leslie
Conference
invite all members

Health Fair Post A
Action mee
1-2 pm
11:30 pm